Geriatric Dentistry Through Case Studies

Geriatric Dentistry Through Case Studies

Editor: Abel Foster

AMERICAN
MEDICAL PUBLISHERS
www.americanmedicalpublishers.com

AMERICAN
MEDICAL PUBLISHERS
www.americanmedicalpublishers.com

American Medical Publishers,
41 Flatbush Avenue,
1st Floor, New York,
NY 11217, USA

Geriatric Dentistry Through Case Studies
Edited by Abel Foster

ISBN 979-8-88740-639-8 (Hardback)

Contents

Preface

Every book is initially just a concept; it takes months of research and hard work to give it the final shape in which the readers receive it. In its early stages, this book also went through rigorous reviewing. The notable contributions made by experts from across the globe were first molded into patterned chapters and then arranged in a sensibly sequential manner to bring out the best results.

Geriatric dentistry, also known as geriodontics or geriatric oral health, is a specialized field of dentistry that focuses on providing dental care to older adults. It focuses on addressing the unique oral health challenges and dental conditions which affect people as they grow older. Some important aspects of geriatric dentistry are oral health assessment, denture care and treatment of dental diseases. Oral health assessment involves the examination of the teeth, gums, oral tissues, and evaluation of the overall oral hygiene. Dentures refer to prosthetic devices which are used to replace missing teeth. They are used by a large number of older adults and their care encompasses fitting, adjustments, repairs, and maintenance to ensure optimal fit and function. This book unfolds the innovative aspects of geriatric dentistry which will be crucial for the progress of this field in the future. For all those who are interested in this field, it can prove to be an essential guide.

It has been my immense pleasure to be a part of this project and to contribute my years of learning in such a meaningful form. I would like to take this opportunity to thank all the people who have been associated with the completion of this book at any step.

Editor

A Case of Myxoma Arising in the Buccal Mucosa

Masahiko Okubo,[1,2] Yoshie Sano,[1] Yosuke Fukushima,[1] Taketo Tomoda,[1] Shoichiro Kokabu ,[3] and Tsuyoshi Sato[1]

[1]*Department of Oral and Maxillofacial Surgery, Faculty of Medicine, Saitama Medical University, 38 Morohongo, Moroyama-machi, Iruma-gun, Saitama 350-0495, Japan*
[2]*Kamimura Dental and Orthodontic Clinic, 3-246-1, Sagami-chou, Koshigaya-shi, Saitama 343-0823, Japan*
[3]*Division of Molecular Signaling and Biochemistry, Department of Health Improvement, Kyushu Dental University, 2-6-1 Manazuru, Kokurakita-ku, Kitakyusyu-shi, 803-8580, Japan*

Correspondence should be addressed to Shoichiro Kokabu; r14kokabu@fa.kyu-dent.ac.jp

Academic Editor: Rui Amaral Mendes

Myxomas arising in the oral and maxillofacial areas are extremely rare. This study reports a case of myxoma arising in the soft tissue beneath the buccal mucosa of an 86-year-old man.

1. Introduction

Myxomas are benign tumors that usually arise in the heart, skin, bone, or muscle. Cases of the maxillofacial region, in which the main site of occurrence is the maxilla or mandibular bone, are relatively rare [1]. Here, we report a case of myxoma arising in the soft tissue beneath the buccal mucosa.

2. Case Report

An 86-year-old male was referred to Saitama Medical University Hospital (Moroyama, Saitama, Japan) from a local dentist in July 2015 due to the presence of an intraoral mass. The patient had not noticed the mass until the dentist brought it to his attention. His previous history included transitional cell cancer of the bladder, but his family history was unremarkable. The round mass, measuring 12 mm in diameter, was located in the left buccal mucosa (Figure 1). The mass was soft, nontender, and nonadherent to the surrounding tissue, and the surface exhibited normal mucosa. Magnetic resonance imaging (MRI) of the left buccal region showed a mass with intensity lower than that of skeletal muscle tissue on T1-weighted imaging (Figure 2(a)) and with intensity higher than that of adipose tissue on T2-weighted imaging (Figure 2(b)). This was diagnosed as a benign buccal tumor and was subsequently resected under local anesthesia. The tumor was easily dissected from the surrounding tissue and appeared to be covered with a thin fibrotic capsule. The resected specimen measured 2 cm at its largest diameter (Figure 3(a)) and was filled with glossy, mucoid, and milky white materials (Figure 3(b)). Microscopically, the tumor cells in the sparse mucoid matrix (Figure 4) exhibited a spindle or stellate shape without nuclear atypia (data not shown). The tumor matrix had abundant collagen fibers and was strongly stained with alcian blue, indicating the presence of acidic polysaccharides (data not shown). On immunohistochemistry, the tumor cells were negative for S-100 protein, ASMA, and CD3 (data not shown). The final histopathological diagnosis was a myxoma. The tumor was completely resected, and five years later, the patient exhibited no recurrence or distant metastasis.

3. Discussion

Myxoma is a relatively rare benign tumor derived from soft tissue and was first described by Virchow as a tumor histologically resembling the mucinous substance of the umbilical cord. Myxoma was defined as a neoplasm without

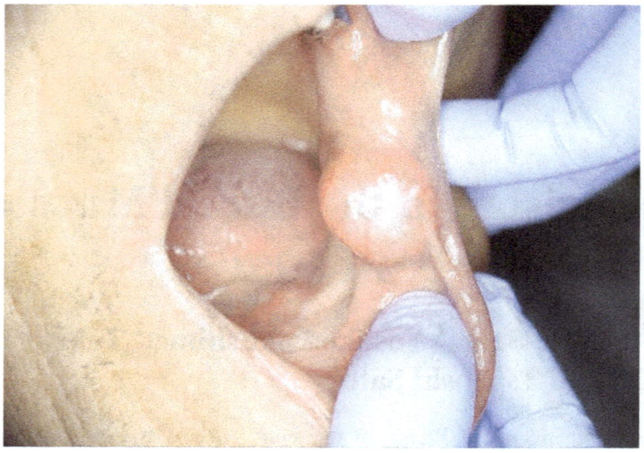

Figure 1: Intraoral clinical findings. The mass was round and located in the left buccal mucosa. The surface showed normal mucosa.

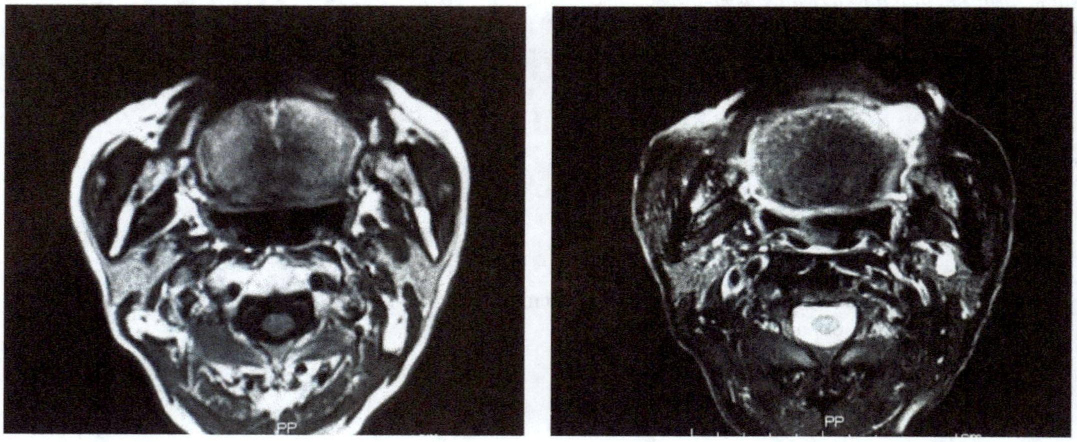

(a) (b)

Figure 2: Magnetic resonance imaging of the tumor. (a) T1-weighted MRI showed a mass with low intensity in comparison with skeletal muscle tissue (yellow dot) while (b) T2-weighted MRI revealed a lesion with high intensity in comparison with adipose tissue (yellow dot).

mesenchymal cells, such as chondrocytes, myoblasts, or adipocytes, and without metastatic capacity [1].

Myxomas most frequently occur in the myocardium, followed by the subcutaneous and intramuscular regions of the lower leg or shoulder. Myxomas arising in the oral and maxillofacial areas are extremely rare. Moreover, most of these cases occur in the maxillary or mandibular bones as odontogenic myxoma derived from odontogenic cells. Thus, only a few reports on soft tissue myxomas are available in the literature [1].

Patients usually recognize a slowly growing indolent mass for myxomas occurring in the soft tissue of the oral and maxillofacial regions. Following gradual enlargement, functional disorders such as difficulty in chewing and/or swallowing may develop, depending on the location [2]. In our case, the patient was asymptomatic and did not recognize the mass until it was noticed by his dentist.

Myxoma usually appears as a mass with smooth margins, with low intensity on T1-weighted MRI and with high intensity on T2-weighted MRI. However, these are not features specific to myxomas and are relatively common in benign soft tissue tumors. The same findings were present in our patient, leading us to a clinical diagnosis of a benign tumor in the soft tissue.

In this case, cytoscreening was not performed. Generally, cytology by fine needle aspiration cannot be used to diagnose myxomas since the tumor has few cellular components. Histopathological analysis revealed spindle-shaped tumor cells with pyknotic nuclei and elongated protrusions, sparsely arranged in a matrix containing mucoid substances. Immunohistochemistry showed that the myxoma cells were positive for vimentin, an intermediate filament specific to mesenchymal cells, and were negative for desmin and S-100 protein [3]. In addition, immunohistochemistry of other proteins may have some utility in investigating differential diagnoses of adipoma, chondroma, fibroneuroma, or myxoid liposarcoma [4]. The treatment of myxoma is essentially surgical resection. Many cases of myxoma do not have thick capsules, resulting in a tendency to expand and invade the surrounding tissue. Therefore, myxomas should be resected with normal surrounding tissue to prevent recurrence [5].

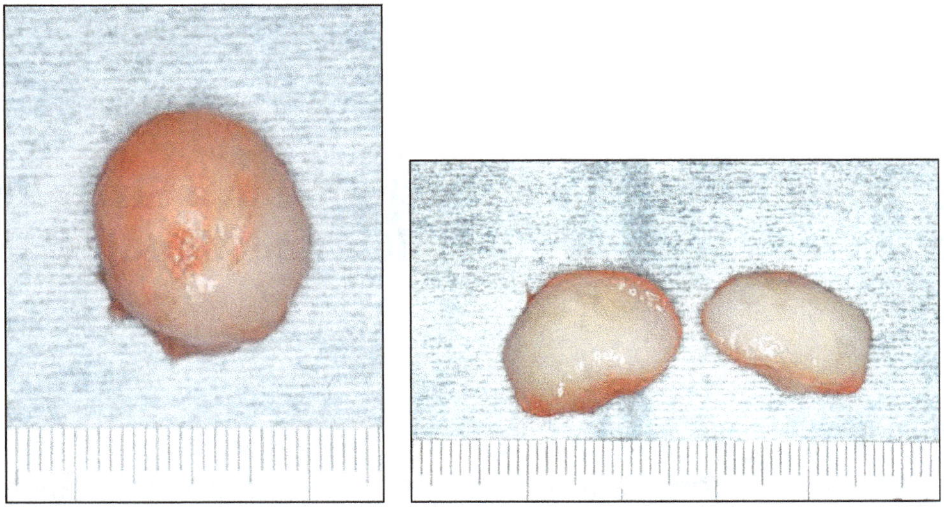

(a) (b)

Figure 3: Gross appearance of the resected specimen (a). The surgical specimen measured 2 cm at its largest diameter and was filled with glossy, mucoid, and milky white secretions (b).

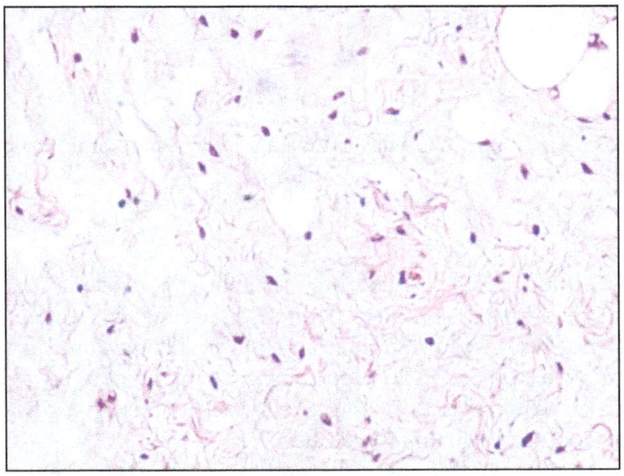

Figure 4: Histopathological findings. On hematoxylin and eosin staining, tumor cells were present in the sparse mucoid matrix. The original magnifications were ×200.

4. Conclusion

We encountered a case of myxoma arising in the buccal mucosa. Myxomas have no metastatic capacity but may occasionally recur. Thus, careful long-term follow-up is needed.

Consent

Consent to publish the case report was not obtained. The report does not contain any personal information that could lead to identifying the patient.

References

[1] M. Nisi, R. Izzetti, M. Gabriele, and A. Pucci, "Oral intramuscular myxoma: case report and brief review of the literature," *Oral Surgery, Oral Medicine, Oral Pathology, Oral Radiology*, vol. 131, no. 2, pp. e52–e58, 2021.

[2] S. ITO, Y. KURACHI, M. MANABE et al., "A case of myxoma of the lower gingiva. In Japanese," *Japanese Journal of Oral & Maxillofacial Surgery*, vol. 29, no. 11, pp. 2090–2095, 1983.

[3] P. B. Deron, N. Nikolovski, J. C. den Hollander, H. A. Spoelstra, and P. P. Knegt, "Myxoma of the maxilla: a case with extremely aggressive biologic behavior," *Head & Neck*, vol. 18, no. 5, pp. 459–464, 1996.

[4] L. E. Landa, M. H. Hedrick, M. C. Nepomuceno-Perez, and G. C. Sotereanos, "Recurrent myxoma of the zygoma: A case report," *Journal of Oral and Maxillofacial Surgery*, vol. 60, no. 6, pp. 704–708, 2002.

[5] T. Andrews, K. Stilianos E, and A. A. Maillard, "Myxomas of the head and neck," *American Journal of Otolaryngology*, vol. 21, no. 3, pp. 184–189, 2000.

2

Achieving Lingualized Balanced Occlusion in a Fixed-Removable Rehabilitation for a Maxillary Complete and Mandibular Kennedy Class II Case

Ibrahim Tulunoglu and Samuel Cohen

Case Western Reserve University School of Dental Medicine, Department of Comprehensive Care, 2124 Cornell Rd, Cleveland, 44106 OH, USA

Correspondence should be addressed to Ibrahim Tulunoglu; ixt45@case.edu

Academic Editor: Hüsamettin Oktay

In this case report, a method to achieve an adequate compensating curve and bilateral balanced lingualized occlusion in a case requiring maxillary complete denture and mandibular Kennedy Class II removable partial and fixed prosthodontic rehabilitation is described.

1. Introduction

With the aging population in the advent of the baby boomers, tooth replacement is becoming more of a frequent procedure, especially with the increasing demands on patients' quality of life. Postponed or lack of replacement of missing teeth is an impending detriment to the remaining dentition. The mesial, distal, and coronal migration of unopposed teeth can be mitigated by the prosthetic restoration of edentulous spaces.

Occlusion plays a critical role in influencing the retention, stability, and the overall masticatory performance of removable prostheses. There is ample literature on lingualized, bilateral balanced, and neutrocentric occlusion [1–5], although there is no clinical evidence pertaining to the superiority of a certain tooth form or arrangement over others [6]. On the other hand, lingualized occlusion, based on a merging of esthetic and food penetration advantages of anatomic form teeth and the mechanical freedom of the nonanatomic form [3], has become more widely accepted in recent years [2].

Using a system that incorporates the tools and the artificial teeth for a lingualized tooth arrangement is useful in providing ease and consistency of the initial tooth set-up, as well as in achieving a balanced occlusion in excursive movements.

Although the methodology for fabrication of maxillary and mandibular complete dentures is well documented, it has not been well established in cases involving a maxillary complete denture (CD), opposing a mandibular removable partial denture (RPD) and fixed restorations to provide harmonious lingualized occlusion.

This paper defines a method to achieve an adequate compensating curve and bilateral balanced lingualized occlusion in a case requiring fixed and removable prosthodontic rehabilitation.

2. Case Report

2.1. Examination. A 64-year-old female presented to the DMD admitting clinic at the School of Dental Medicine with an ill-fitting maxillary acrylic-based removable partial denture. The patient's chief complaint was to get "a new set of teeth," seeking an improvement in her esthetics and masticatory function. The patient had no major related medical conditions aside from suffering from depression and anxiety. Oral hygiene was fair and there was no periodontal disease present.

Clinical and radiographic examination revealed edentulous spaces in both arches, extensive presence of nonrestorable teeth, and active caries. The patient's plane of

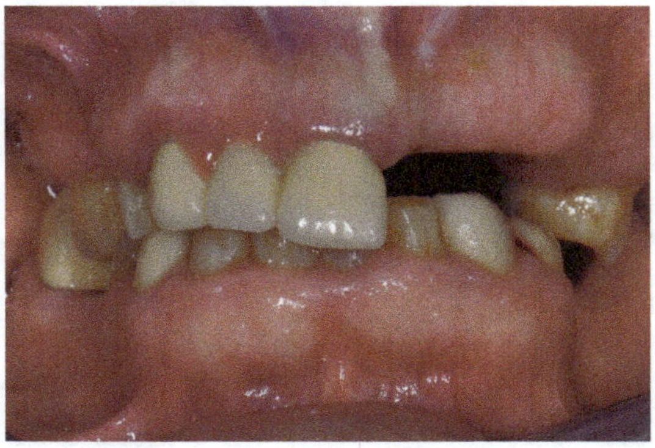

FIGURE 1: Fontal view of teeth in occlusion before treatment.

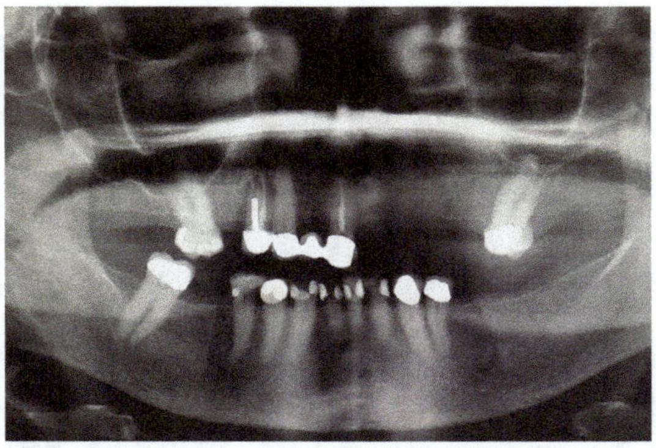

FIGURE 2: Panoramic radiograph before treatment.

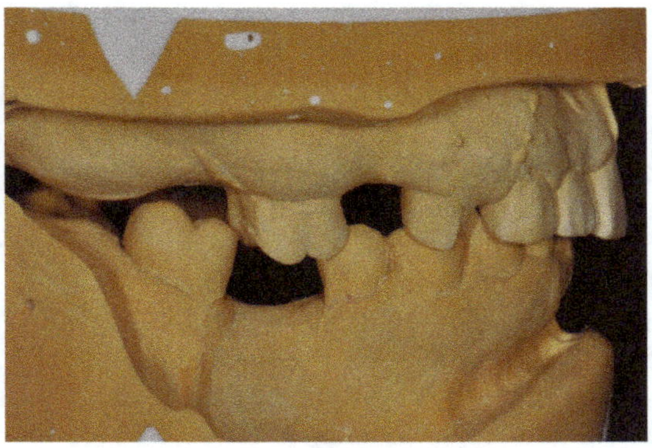

FIGURE 3: A view of mounted diagnostic casts.

occlusion was not harmonious, and the lack of a stable posterior occlusion led to moderate wear of her remaining anterior teeth and a collapse in her vertical dimension of occlusion which were not addressed with the previous fixed partial restorations on teeth #14, 13, and 11 (Figures 1–3). The difference between the vertical dimension of rest (VDR) and vertical dimension of occlusion (VDO) of the patient was found to be 9 mm.

After removal of the restorations, teeth #14, 13, and 11 revealed deep carious lesions, and #5 vertical root fracture. Teeth 17 and 27 showed furcation defects on the distal aspects. The patient was given various treatment plans, including full arch-supported fixed prosthodontic rehabilitation with periodontal treatment on furcation defects and crown lengthening for teeth #13, 11, 32, 31, 41, and 42 and

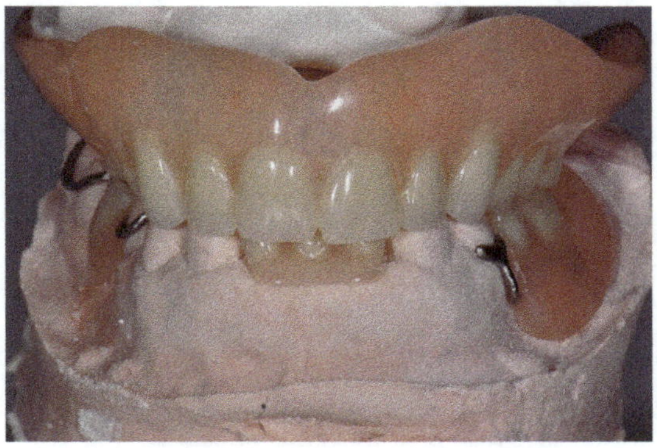

FIGURE 4: Clinical remount of interim prostheses.

placement of implants to support the fixed partial denture restorations replacing the tooth loss at the edentulous spans, and opted for the treatment plan involving crowning of teeth #35, 34, 43, 45, and 47 and the fabrication of a maxillary complete and mandibular removable partial denture because of the patient's avoidance from surgical placement of implants and the cost of an implant-supported rehabilitation.

2.2. Treatment. After thorough oral hygiene instructions, the patient's active disease was stabilized with surgical, operative, and prosthodontic intervention. An interim maxillary complete denture and mandibular partial denture was delivered immediately after the extraction of the remaining maxillary teeth and mandibular incisors (Figure 4). In this provisional phase, the patient was rehabilitated at a 2 mm increased VDO that allowed her to be monitored in terms of any possible adverse reactions or changes in the stomatognathic system. After 6 months of osseous healing and observation period, the definitive phase of prosthetic treatment began as no adverse effect was observed in the stomatognathic system.

The maxillary wax occlusal rim was adjusted intraorally to provide the correct location and position of the occlusal plane relative to the VDO lip line and smile line of the patient. Using a semiadjustable articulator (Stratos 100, Ivoclar Vivadent, Schaan, Liechtenstein), the maxillary master cast was mounted using the maxillary wax occlusal rim and the Maxillary Mounting Table (Stratos 100, Ivoclar Vivadent, Schaan, Liechtenstein) of the system. The mandibular arch was mounted in centric relation (CR). Maxillary anterior teeth (Vivadent DCL, Ivoclar Vivadent, Schaan, Liechtenstein) were set using the Mounting Table that represents the defined occlusal plane location, and the mandibular teeth were set as to obtain 1 mm of overbite and 1.5 mm of overjet. Then, the maxillary cast was removed from the upper member of the articulator, and the guide plane jig for compensating curve (2.5D Setup Template, Ivoclar Vivadent, Schaan, Liechtenstein) was inserted. The simulation of tooth preparations was made on the mandibular cast to ideal dimensions before the wax-up was made (Figure 5). An artificial tooth set-up for the maxillary posterior teeth was made to fabricate the fixed restorations accordingly.

After preparations for abutment teeth for PFM crowns #35, 34, 43, 45, and 47, the final impression was made in PVS impression material (3M Imprint 3 Heavy Body and

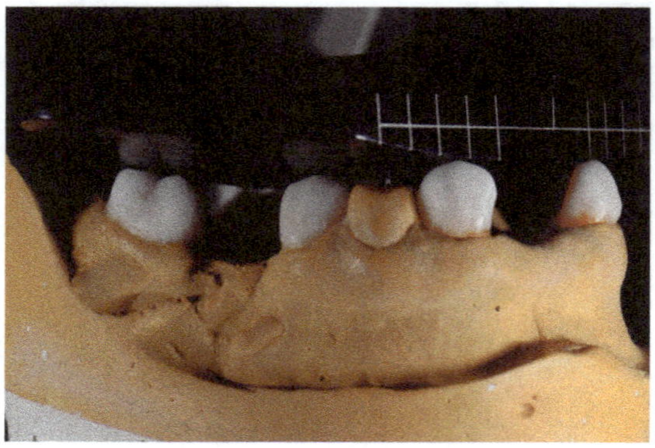

Figure 5: Wax-up for PFM crowns on teeth #21, 22, 27, 29, and 31.

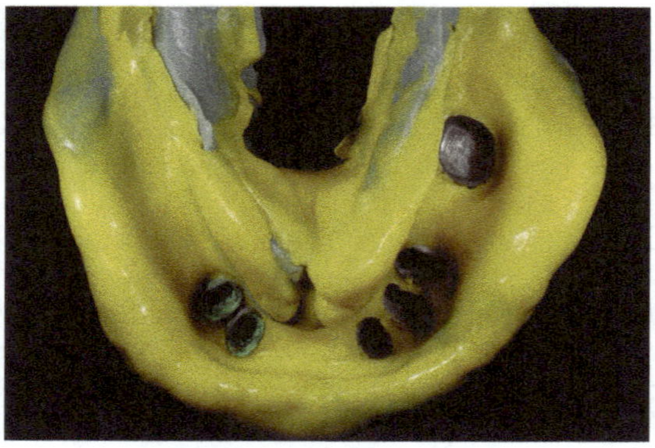

Figure 6: Pick-up impression of metal copings made.

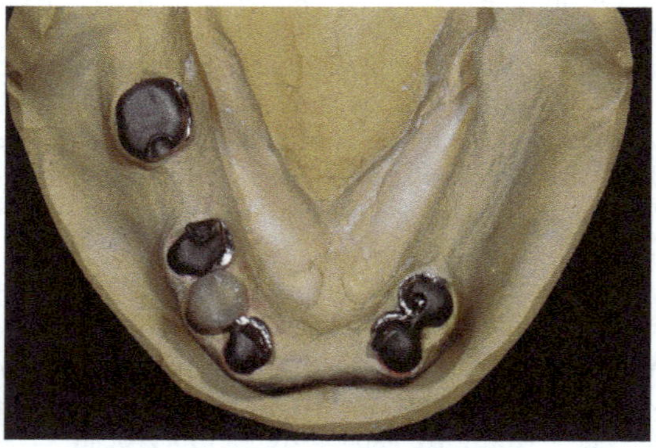

Figure 7: Metal copings with their exact spatial relations obtained on the master cast.

3M Imprint 3 Light Body). A jig for proper VDO was made on the articulator against the maxillary tooth arrangement. This jig is used as a vertical stopper for the intermaxillary relationship record to replicate the VDO. Surveyed crown restorations with guide planes parallel to the defined path of insertion and ledges were made, to improve retention, stability, and support of the RPD and tried intraorally. A coping pick-up impression was made with the PVS impression material (Figure 6) and poured with stone (Microstone, Whip Mix Corp.) (Figure 7). The guide planes and gingival ledges were refined and milled once more, including the dovetail-shaped rests between the splinted copings on 21 and 22. Then, porcelain was built on the copings following

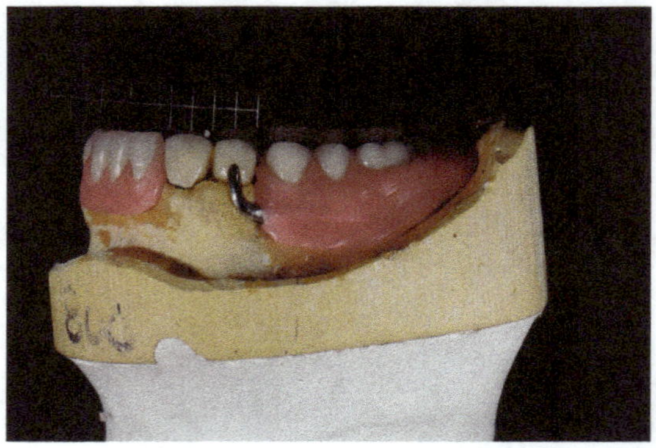

Figure 8: Final mandibular tooth arrangement made using the 2.5D guide plane.

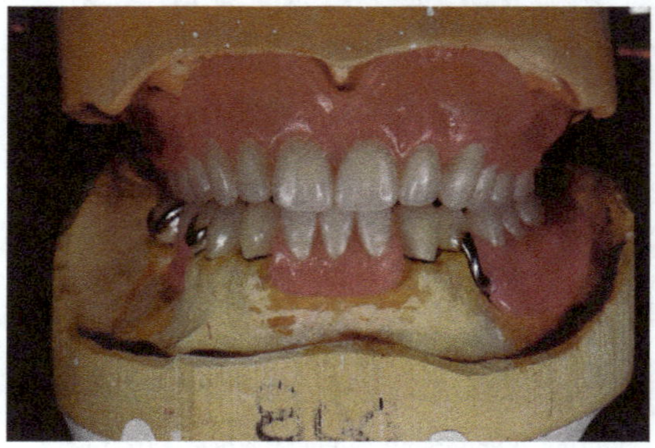

Figure 9: View of final tooth arrangement made.

the 2.5D template and the maxillary tooth arrangement was also made according to the same template (Figure 8). After the crowns were made, the RPD metal framework was fabricated for the Kennedy Class II mod II mandibular arch. The metal framework and the crowns were tried in together, and the final tooth arrangement was made with the same template (Figure 9). Final try-in of the maxillary CD, mandibular RPD, and fixed prostheses allowed for minor adjustments in the tooth set-up. The final tooth arrangement in wax shows the harmonious occlusion between the fixed and removable elements of the prostheses. At delivery, minimal occlusal adjustments were done intraorally to achieve lingualized occlusion with balanced centric and eccentric contacts (Figure 10).

3. Discussion

With such a dilapidated dentition and loss of vertical dimension, it was of utmost importance to restore the patient's occlusal plane so that proper function could be obtained. Not only is having proper centric contacts on all teeth essential for function, but having those contacts orientated in the correct occlusal plane and compensating curve was imperative. Extractions, surveyed metal-ceramic restorations with parallel guide planes, a mandibular removable partial denture (RPD), and maxillary complete denture (CD) were treatment avenues used to rehabilitate this patient. An approach utilizing the Stratos 100 Articulator and 2.5D guide plane

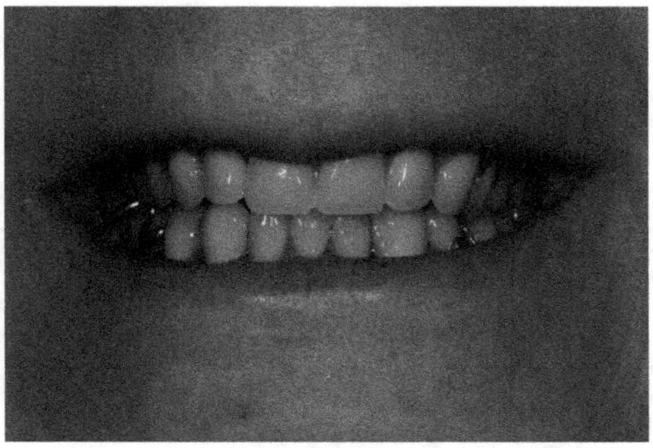

FIGURE 10: View of patient's smile at delivery.

was sought to harmonize the occlusion between the fixed and removable elements of the mandibular prostheses.

A concern that will inherently come with any system that does not include a face bow transfer may be whether this would cause a big discrepancy between a patient stomatognathic system and articulator. Kumar et al. compared two methods, one with and one without face bow transfer and concluded that balanced occlusion can be achieved successfully with a system that does not require face bow transfer [7]. In this clinical case, we did not observe a difference between the interarch relationship in the patient's mouth and the articulator. The system allowed to establish the desired occlusal plane location and position as well as the contact patterns that are designed as part of the standards established with the Stratos system. This included establishing the occlusal configurations as well as the positions and locations of both fixed restorations and artificial teeth on removable dentures with minimal adjustment at delivery. Instead of maxillary and mandibular posterior teeth with steep cuspal angles, using artificial teeth fabricated purposely for lingualized occlusion also contributed to the fact that fewer adjustments overall necessitated.

The *Glossary of Prosthodontic Terms* defines the compensating curve as "the anteroposterior curving (in the median plane) and the mediolateral curving (in the frontal plane) within the alignment of the occluding surfaces and incisal edges of artificial teeth that is used to develop balanced occlusion" [8]. A balanced occlusion is desirable for all removable complete denture rehabilitations. In other words, this is one of the five major determinants of balanced occlusion expressed in Hanau's Quint and Thielemann's formula [2, 3]. The compensating curve is provided by the 2.5D template, and the cusp heights are also provided by the artificial teeth set produced specifically for lingualized occlusion.

4. Conclusion

Using the principles of lingualized occlusion in complete dentures, it is possible to achieve lingualized balanced occlusion in a maxillary edentulous and mandibular Kennedy Class II fixed-removable rehabilitation case.

References

[1] T. E. Jacobson and A. J. Krol, "A contemporary review of the factors involved in complete denture retention, stability, and support. Part I: retention," *The Journal of Prosthetic Dentistry*, vol. 49, no. 1, pp. 5–15, 1983.

[2] V. Rangarajan, B. Gajapathi, P. B. Yogesh, M. M. Ibrahim, R. G. Kumar, and P. Karthik, "Concepts of occlusion in prosthodontics: A literature review, part I," *The Journal of Indian Prosthodontic Society*, vol. 15, no. 3, pp. 200–205, 2015.

[3] V. Rangarajan, B. Gajapathi, P. B. Yogesh et al., "Concepts of occlusion in prosthodontics: a literature review, part II," *The Journal of Indian Prosthodontic Society*, vol. 16, no. 1, pp. 8–14, 2015.

[4] R. L. Engelmeier and R. D. Phoenix, "The development of lingualized occlusion," *Journal of Prosthodontics*, vol. 28, no. 1, pp. e118–e131, 2019.

[5] C. M. Becker, C. C. Swoope, and A. D. Guckes, "Lingualized occlusion for removable prosthodontics," *The Journal of Prosthetic Dentistry*, vol. 38, no. 6, pp. 601–608, 1977.

[6] A. Farias-Neto, "Complete denture occlusion: an evidence-based approach," *Journal of Prosthodontics*, vol. 22, no. 2, pp. 94–97, 2013.

[7] M. Kumar and D. S. J. D'Souza, "Comparative evaluation of two techniques in achieving balanced occlusion in complete dentures," *Medical Journal Armed Forces India*, vol. 66, pp. 362–366, 2010.

[8] K. J. Ferro, "The Glossary of Prosthodontic Terms: Ninth Edition," *The Journal Prosthetic Dentistry*, vol. 117, no. 5S, 2017.

3

Pink Tooth of Mummery in the Maxillary Left Canine after Fixed Partial Denture (FPD) Preparation

Eger V. Korolevsky,[1] Takashi Komabayashi,[1,2] and Denise Foran[1]

[1]*Department of Veterans Affairs, New York Harbor Healthcare System, New York City, NY, USA*
[2]*University of New England College of Dental Medicine, Portland, ME, USA*

Correspondence should be addressed to Takashi Komabayashi; tkomabayashi@une.edu

Academic Editor: Giuseppe Alessandro Scardina

Pink tooth of Mummery is typically found after trauma. However, this case report describes an unusual occurrence of pink tooth in a 67-year-old Caucasian male after fixed partial denture (FPD) tooth preparation. Pink tooth in this case may be due to one or more factors: tooth reduction and heat generation during tooth preparation; heat generation during polymerization of provisional material; and hyperocclusion of a provisional FPD. This case highlights the importance of choosing the appropriate materials and techniques to avoid pulpal complications after dental prosthesis work.

1. Introduction

A tooth with a pinkish hue is classically described as the pink tooth of Mummery, named after the 19th century anatomist James Howard Mummery. It is speculated that a pink tooth is due to the loss of internal dentin; this loss creates a large pulp space and allows more blood vessels to fill the area, which results in a pinkish hue. A pulpal hemorrhage is defined as the escape of blood from a ruptured vessel, and blood is trapped inside of the pulp chamber, giving off a pink hue. Thus, the pink tooth is usually associated with internal resorption in the coronal area of a tooth [1]. While pink tooth often emerges after a dental trauma or following orthodontic treatment [2], few reports refer to the appearance of pink tooth after a fixed partial denture (FPD), also known as bridge, tooth preparation.

The aim of this case report is to describe an unusual case of a pink tooth of Mummery occurring during fixed partial denture (FPD) tooth preparation and to identify possible causes.

2. Case Report

2.1. Previous Treatment and Diagnosis. A 67-year-old Caucasian male presented to the Veterans Affairs New York Harbor Medical Center's Manhattan Endodontics Department for evaluation of dental pain on maxillary left canine, tooth #11. Six weeks prior to this evaluation appointment, maxillary teeth had been prepared by a dentist for a fixed partial denture (FPD) spanning from tooth #6 (maxillary right canine) to tooth #11 (maxillary left canine). Teeth #6 and #11 are abutment teeth. Teeth #7 (maxillary right lateral incisor), #8 (maxillary right central incisor), #9 (maxillary left central incisor), and #10 (maxillary left lateral incisor) are pontics of the FPD. The patient's chief complaint four weeks after the initial preparation of teeth #6 and #11 was the lingering sensitivity to cold in the maxillary left quadrant. When the patient presented to the endodontic department six weeks after the teeth were prepared for the FPD, his sensitivity had subsided.

His medical history was significant for sciatica, osteoarthritis with herniated disc, anxiety, and depression. He was taking gabapentin 300 mg tab twice a day for back pain, methocarbamol 750 mg tab three times a day for muscle relaxation, venlafaxine 75 mg tab once a day for depression, sertraline 200 mg tab once a day for anxiety, quetiapine fumarate 400 mg tab twice a day for depression, and diazepam 5 mg tab once a day for anxiety. He had drug allergies to haloperidol and risperidone. His dental history included

Table 1: Summary of diagnostic tests.

Tooth	#6 (maxillary right canine)	#11 (maxillary left canine)
Percussion pain	No	Yes
Palpation pain	No	No
Cold test response	Yes	Yes
Mobility	No	No
Swelling	No	No
Probing	<4 mm	<4 mm
Discoloration	No	Yes

a full mouth rehabilitation with low caries risk and acceptable oral hygiene.

The extraoral exam and perioral soft tissue exams were within normal limits. His temporomandibular joint function was normal without any deviation upon opening or discomfort upon palpation, and the intraoral hard examination revealed no evident abnormalities; the soft tissues had no signs or symptoms of pathology. Clinically, teeth #6-11 were temporized with Luxatemp LC (DMG America, Englewood, NJ, USA) provisional cemented with Durelon (3M, Two Harbors, MN, USA). There was discomfort upon percussion and no tenderness upon palpation (Table 1). His chief complaint was not reproducible with Endo Ice (Coltène Whaledent, Cuyahoga Falls, OH, USA) when tested with the FPD in place. Teeth #6 and #11 responded to cold without lingering sensitivity. The FPD was removed without local anesthesia to further evaluate the teeth. Tooth #11 appeared to have a bright red hemorrhage-like hue whereas tooth #6 appeared normal (Figures 1(a) and 1(b)). A radiographic examination revealed an intact periodontal ligament (PDL) space around tooth #11 with no obvious periapical pathology (Figures 1(c) and 1(d)). Pulpal diagnosis was asymptomatic irreversible pulpitis, and apical diagnosis was symptomatic apical periodontitis. Treatment options were discussed with patient, including no treatment, nonsurgical root canal treatment (NSRCT), or extraction. Considering risks and benefits of all treatment options, an agreement was made to proceed with NSRCT and informed consent was obtained.

2.2. Endodontic Treatment. The endodontic treatment for this tooth was initiated the day of the evaluation. Patient was anesthetized via maxillary infiltration with 1.8 ml of 2% lidocaine with 0.036 mg of epinephrine. Tooth isolation was achieved with a ligated endodontic clamp and a latex rubber dam (Figure 2(a)). With the use of a dental operating microscope, hemorrhagic vital pulp tissue was found inside the pulp chamber upon access (Figure 2(b)). Although the pulp tissue was still vital, the tissue did not have a healthy appearance (Figure 2(c)). Pulp extirpation was accomplished using hand instrumentation with K-type and Hedstrom files (Dentsply Sirona, Tulsa, OK, USA) and rotary instrumentation using HyFlex EDM files (Coltene, Cuyahoga Falls, OH, USA). Working lengths were determined with the use of an electronic apex locator (Root ZX II, J. Morita, Kyoto, Japan), and measurement radiographs were taken with a size 30K file. Copious irrigation of 6% sodium hypochlorite solution was used during the cleaning and shaping process, followed by a final rinse of 17% ethylenediaminetetraacetic acid (EDTA) to remove the smear layer (Figure 2(d)). Gutta percha 0.04 taper size 25 (Henry Schein, Melville, NY, USA) was selected to obtain an appropriate apical fit and tug back. After taking a master cone radiograph, the canal was dried with medium size paper points (DiaDent, Seoul, Korea) and obturated using a warm vertical condensation technique with a BL-alpha II heating plugger (B&L Biotech USA Inc, Fairfax, VA, USA) in conjunction with Sealapex root canal sealer (SybronEndo, Glendora, CA, USA). The backfill was accomplished with Continuous Wave Obturation system (Kerr Dental, Orange, CA, USA) to achieve a three-dimensional fill and to eliminate possible voids (Figure 3(a)). After obturation was completed, the tooth access was temporized with a cotton pellet and Cavit (3M, Two Harbors, MN, USA). The provisional FPD was recemented with Durelon (Figure 3(b)).

2.3. Postoperative Follow-Up. The patient was referred to his prosthodontist for permanent restoration and continuation of care. The patient was recalled for a 6-month follow-up to treatment, and the outcome was excellent. The patient has remained asymptomatic since the completion of NSRCT, and radiographic exam remained free of periapical pathosis.

3. Discussion

To identify possible causes of this unusual pink tooth case [1], tooth reduction during tooth preparation [2], heat generation during tooth preparation [3], heat generation during polymerization of the provisional material intraorally [4], and hyperocclusion of provisional FPD were carefully reviewed in the order of treatment sequence.

Tooth reduction during tooth preparation maybe a possible cause, according to other case reports. In short term, Goodacre and Spolnik described that the incidence of endodontic treatment required after tooth preparation ranged from 3% to 23%. FPDs have had higher incidence rates than single crowns. It has been assumed that the higher rates are a result of the greater tooth reduction sometimes required to align multiple teeth [3]. Davis et al.'s research has suggested that 2 mm or more of remaining dentine is critical in protecting the pulp following tooth preparation [4]. In long term, Cheung et al. reported that the pulp survival rate in vital teeth restored with a single-unit ceramic metal crown (CMC) was 84.4% after 10 years. Pulp survival rate of teeth used as abutments for FPD's was 70.8% after 10 years. In addition, maxillary anterior teeth serving as FPD abutments developed pulpal necrosis more frequently than any other tooth type [5]. Figures 1(c) and 1(d) show both teeth #6 and #11 look similar with respect to tooth reduction, and estimated 1.5mm remaining dentin after tooth preparation.

Another possible cause is heat generation during tooth preparation. Historically, Langeland K and Langeland LK

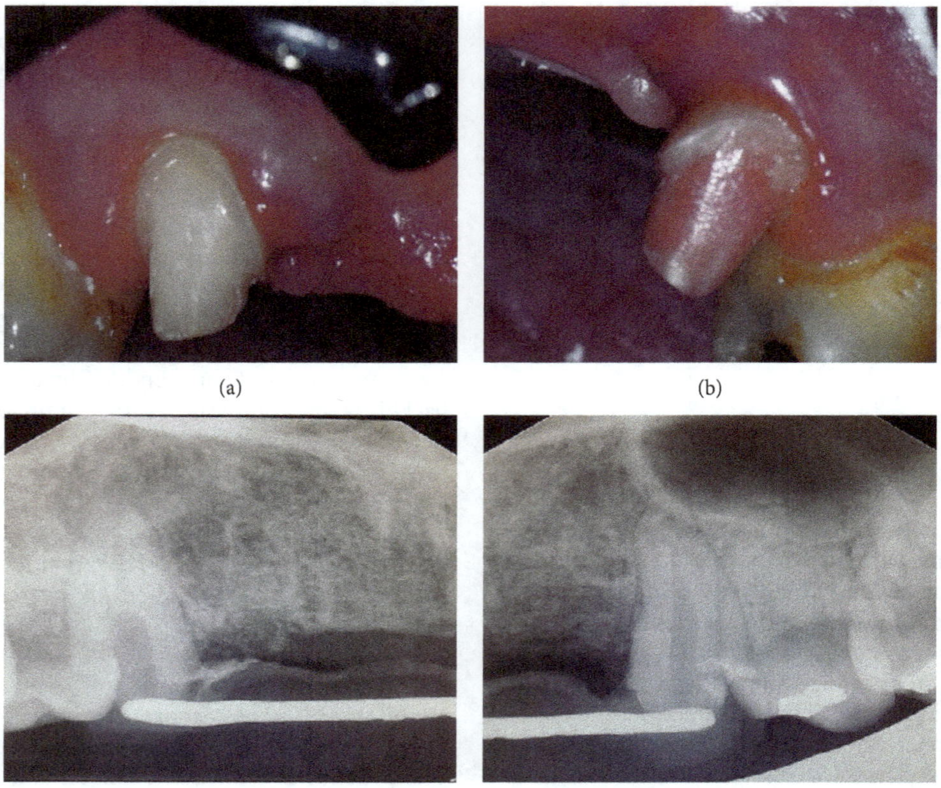

Figure 1: (a) Clinical photograph of tooth #6 after the removal of provisional FPD, normal clinical appearance. (b) Clinical photograph of tooth #11 after the removal of provisional FPD, red hue appearance. (c) Radiograph of tooth #6 before the removal of provisional FPD. (d) Radiograph of tooth #11 before the removal of provisional FPD.

obtained histological evidence that crown preparation in human teeth produced no initial pulpal reaction as long as it was carried out with adequate water spray. However, if the water spray was insufficient, the dentine showed evidence of burning, and odontoblast cell bodies were displaced into the ends of the cut dentinal tubules [6]. A temperature rise of 5.6°C can lead to a 15% loss of vitality in the pulp, and an 11°C temperature rise will lead to a vitality loss of approximately 60%. In addition, a 16.6°C temperature rise may cause 100% necrosis of the pulp [7]. In our unique pink tooth case, the dentist who prepared teeth #6 and #11 reported using the same well-maintained handpiece with water throughout the procedure.

Heat generation during fabrication of a provisional FPD using a direct technique could be another factor. Direct and indirect methods are used for the fabrication of a provisional FPD. Driscoll et al. found that the temperature increase produced by the polymerization of dental materials ranged from 14.8 to 27.3°C. A disadvantage of the direct technique is the generation of heat during polymerization of the provisional material intraorally [8]. Due to its accuracy and pulpal protection from polymerization heat, the indirect method is preferred over the direct method; however, time limitation and inadequate laboratory support may require the clinician to use the direct technique [9]. Even though the temporary FPD for this pink tooth case was lab fabricated, it was then relined intraorally with acrylic material, which is a direct technique. It can be speculated that a higher volume of acrylic was used to reline the retainer of tooth #11 than for tooth #6.

It is generally believed that the pink tooth of Mummery is caused by granulation tissue undermining a necrotic area of the coronal pulp. This may be found in asymptomatic teeth with internal root resorption or external cervical resorption [1]. However, in our case, the coronal pulp was vital and there was no clinical evidence of granulation tissue (Figures 2(a)–2(c)). In addition, there was no radiographic evidence of resoptive lesions.

Finally, hyperocclusion of a provisional FPD could be another factor causing pink tooth in this case. It is reported that pink tooth often emerges after a dental trauma or following orthodontic treatment [2]. The patient had sensitivity with percussion pain on tooth #11 (Table 1). Radiographic examination of tooth #11 (Figure 1(d)) was unremarkable. Hyperocclusion may have resulted been a local force exerted on tooth #11. Radiographs of anterior maxilla reveal teeth #6 and #11 and a six unit provisional FPD (Figures 1(c) and 1(d)). Since only two abutment teeth (#6 and #11) were supporting all forces exerted on the six unit provisional FPD (#6, #7, #8, #9, #10, and #11), it is possible that local force was concentrated more on tooth #11 than tooth #6.

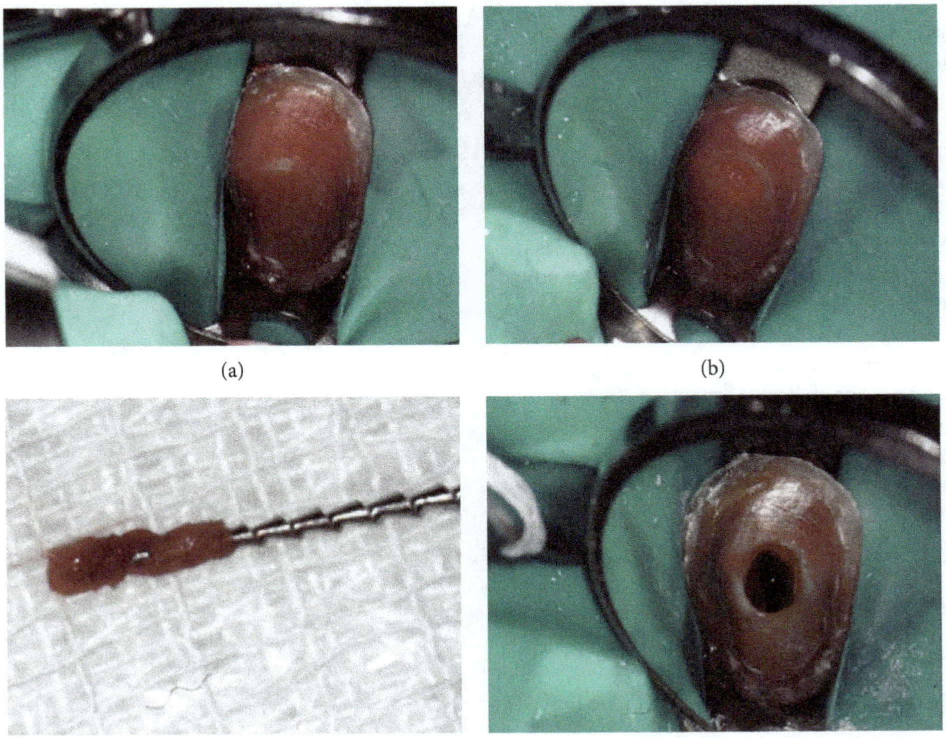

(a) (b) (c) (d)

FIGURE 2: (a) Rubber dam isolation of tooth #11. (b) Initial access preparation showing hemorrhagic pulpal tissue. (c) Extirpated pulpal tissue on hedstrom file. (d) Irrigation with 6% sodium hypochlorite solution in a pulp chamber. Tooth immediately changed color due to oxidation of hemoglobin.

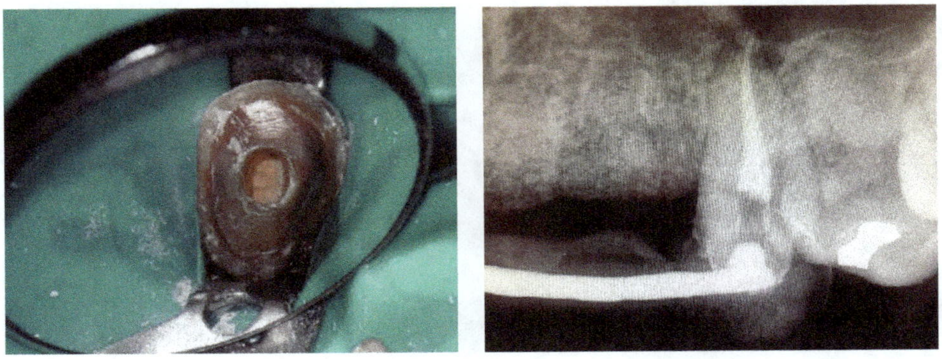

(a) (b)

FIGURE 3: (a) Clinical photograph of the obturated tooth #11 prior to placing a temporary filling and the provisional FPD. (b) Postoperative radiograph of the obturated tooth #11 with the provisional FPD cemented.

In conclusion, the pink tooth of Mummery may occur after a routine tooth preparation in addition to the more traditionally accepted etiology. The tooth discoloration described in this case report may have resulted from tooth preparation [1], heat generation during tooth preparation [2], heat generation during polymerization of the provisional material [3], and/or hyperocclusion of the provisional FPD [4]. By better understanding the multiple etiologies of the pink tooth of Mummery, clinicians may be better able to predict and prevent adverse outcomes of tooth prepration and provisionalization.

Acknowledgments

The authors thank Elizabeth Dyer for reference support and Lori Rand for writing consultation and editing.

References

[1] S. Patel, D. Ricucci, C. Durak, and F. Tay, "Internal root resorption: a review," *Journal of Endodontia*, vol. 36, no. 7, pp. 1107–1121, 2010.

[2] F. F. Silveira, E. Nunes, J. A. Soares, C. L. Ferreira, and I. Rotstein, "Double 'pink tooth' associated with extensive internal root resorption after orthodontic treatment: a case report," *Dental Traumatology*, vol. 25, no. 3, pp. e43–e47, 2009.

[3] C. J. Goodacre and K. J. Spolnik, "The prosthodontic management of endodontically treated teeth: a literature review. Part I. success and failure data, treatment concepts," *Journal of Prosthodontics*, vol. 3, no. 4, pp. 243–250, 1994.

[4] G. R. Davis, R. A. Tayeb, K. G. Seymour, and G. P. Cherukara, "Quantification of residual dentine thickness following crown preparation," *Journal of Dentistry*, vol. 40, no. 7, pp. 571–576, 2012.

[5] G. S. Cheung, S. C. Lai, and R. P. Ng, "Fate of vital pulps beneath a metal-ceramic crown or a bridge retainer," *International Endodontic Journal*, vol. 38, no. 8, pp. 521–530, 2005.

[6] K. Langeland and L. K. Langeland, "Pulp reactions to crown preparation, impression, temporary crown fixation, and permanent cementation," *The Journal of Prosthetic Dentistry*, vol. 15, no. 1, pp. 129–143, 1965.

[7] L. Zach and G. Cohen, "Pulp response to externally applied heat," *Oral Surgery, Oral Medicine, and Oral Pathology*, vol. 19, no. 4, pp. 515–530, 1965.

[8] C. F. Driscoll, G. Woolsey, and W. M. Ferguson, "Comparison of exothermic release during polymerization of four materials used to fabricate interim restorations," *The Journal of Prosthetic Dentistry*, vol. 65, no. 4, pp. 504–506, 1991.

[9] T. Akova, A. Ozkomur, C. Dundar, and N. Aytutuldu, "Intrapulpal heat generation during provisionalization: effect of desensitizer and matrix type," *Journal of Prosthodontics*, vol. 17, no. 2, pp. 108–113, 2008.

4

A 37 mm Spindle Cell Lipoma on the Floor of the Mouth

Eve Malthiery,[1] Valérie Costes-Martineau,[2] Marie-Alix Fauroux,[1] and Jacques-Henri Torres[1]

[1]*Service d'Odontologie, Centre Hospitalier Universitaire, 34295 Montpellier Cedex 5, France*
[2]*Laboratoire d'Anatomie et de Cytologie Pathologiques, Centre Hospitalier Universitaire, 34295 Montpellier Cedex 5, France*

Correspondence should be addressed to Jacques-Henri Torres; j-torres@chu-montpellier.fr

Academic Editor: Eugenio Maiorano

Spindle cell lipoma (SCL) is a rare variety of lipoma that mostly arises in male patients and rarely affects the oral cavity. The floor of the mouth is an uncommon site for SCL, and very few cases have been reported in this location. A case of SCL is reported in a 70-year-old woman who had noticed a swelling of the floor of the mouth without any functional consequence. Both ultrasonography and RMI suggested a diagnosis of ranula, whereas clinical palpation showed a nonfluctuant mass. The lesion was excised under local anesthesia. A 37×32 mm encapsulated yellow mass was removed. Histological features (mature adipocytes and CD34+ spindle cells) led to a diagnosis of SCL. Medical imaging assessment of this lesion could have been influenced by the high frequency of the ranulas in the floor of the mouth. This case appears to be quite infrequent because of its location (floor of the mouth), its size (over 3.5 cm), and the patient's gender (female).

1. Introduction

Lipomas are not frequent in the oral cavity. They only represent 0.1 to 5% of oral tumors [1]. They usually appear as soft yellowish nodular swellings covered by normal mucosa. Lipomas seldom affect the floor of the mouth (2 among the 46 lipomas reported by Fregnani et al., while 10 were in the buccal mucosa) [1].

Several histopathological types of lipomas have been described: fibrolipoma, sialolipoma, myelolipoma, osteolipoma, chondrolipoma, chondroid lipoma, angiolipoma, angiomyolipoma, myolipoma, intramuscular lipoma, pleomorphic lipoma, and spindle cell lipoma (SCL) [2]. Enzinger and Harvey first described SCL in 1975 [3]. These tumors typically arise in the subcutaneous tissue of the upper back, posterior neck, and shoulders of males aged 40–70 and scarcely involve the oral cavity [4].

In 2003, Fregnani et al. reported 46 cases of lipomas of the oral cavity [1]. Five of them were in the floor of the mouth, none of which were SCL. Although SCL was predominant in the lip in the Furlong et al. 2004 report of 95 lipomas of the oral region, only 1 SCL was detected among the 5 cases reported in the floor of the mouth [5]. In 2006, Billings et al. found 16 published SCL cases of the oral cavity in the literature [4]. They reported 7 new cases of SCL, of which only 1 was located in the floor of the mouth. In their 2010 series of 41 cases of lipomas, Juliasse et al. reported 1 SCL among 3 cases of lipomas in the floor of the mouth [2]. In 2013, Manor et al. found 33 reported cases of SCL of the oral cavity and added 2 personal cases [6]. The average size of these lesions was 20.87 mm; male predilection was 2 : 1. Among these 35 cases, only 5 affected the floor of the mouth.

We are reporting a new case of SCL in the floor of the mouth in a 70-year-old woman.

2. Observation

A 70-year-old Caucasian woman was referred to the hospital by her dentist for a swelling noticed 3 weeks before in the floor of the mouth. It had no functional consequence on her speech or mastication and neither on tongue mobility. An echography was performed, which lead to the conclusion of a ranula. The patient's medical conditions of osteoporosis, hypothyroidism, and mild depression were treated

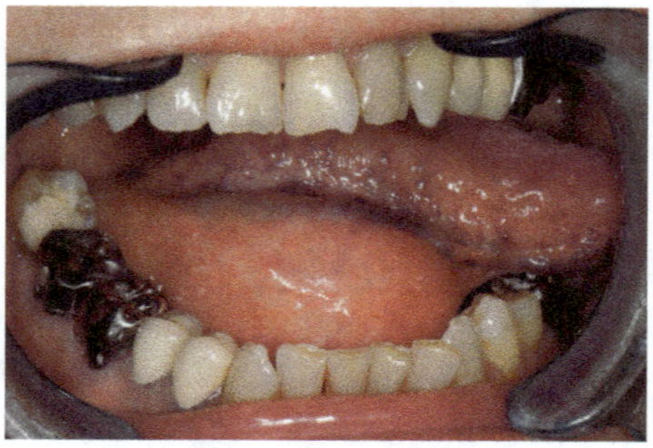

Figure 1: Clinical aspect of the mass located in the right sublingual region (tip of the tongue turned to the left side). The superior limit is above the occlusal surface of the molars.

by alendronic acid, levothyroxine, and fluoxetine. Physical examination revealed a tender mass, in the right sublingual region, though its posterior limit could not be clearly defined (Figure 1).

The swelling was not attached to the mandible bone or to other surrounding tissues. The mucosa covering the mass had a normal appearance and color. No inflammation, erosion, or ulceration were noted. Salivary flow from the right submandibular gland was not affected by the swelling. Palpation revealed a nonfluctuant mass without cervical lymphadenopathy.

An MRI scan was prescribed, which showed a 37 mm well-defined lesion with both T1 and T2 hypersignals (Figure 2); the conclusion was that the sublingual mass could be a ranula. The patient was proposed an excision, and the procedure was performed under local anesthesia.

An encapsulated yellow mass was removed (Figure 3).

Histopathological examination established a diagnosis of spindle cell lipoma (Figure 4).

A proliferation of adipocytes in a myxoid background was seen, associated to small bland spindle cells with small chromatic nuclei without mitosis or atypia, low cellular density, and without wavy collagen fibers. Adipocytes size was regular, without significant anisocytosis unlike the recently described anisometric cell lipoma [7]. Immunohistochemical examination was HMGA2 and MDM2 negative. Spindle cells were immunoreactive for CD34 and negative for PS100 (Figures 5 and 6).

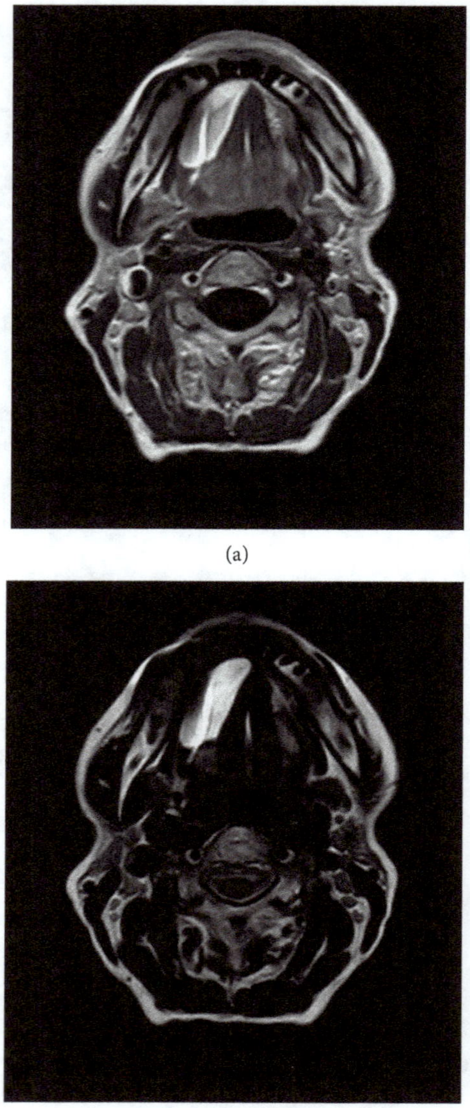

(a)

(b)

Figure 2: RMI features of the lesion: both T1- (a) and T2- (b) weighed images show hypersignal.

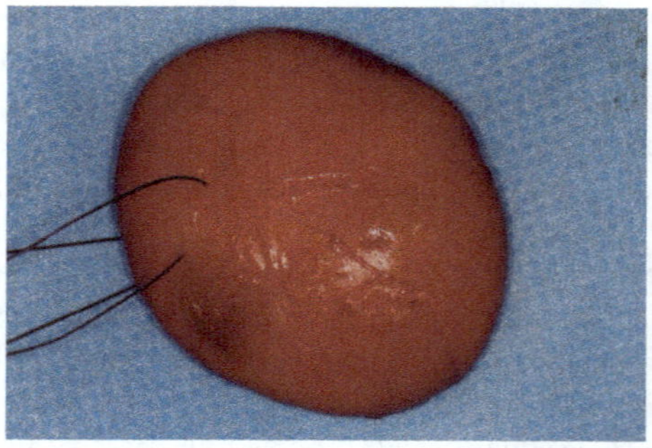

Figure 3: Resection specimen: 37 × 32 mm encapsulated yellow mass.

3. Discussion

Like in the case reported here, oral lipomas are usually asymptomatic. However, large lipomas have been reported to cause functional impairment: a lipoma measuring 5 cm disturbed lower denture stability [8]. An 8.5 cm sublingual lipoma has been reported to cause submandibular salivary gland swelling [9].

In the case series reported by Manor et al. [6], only one SCL in the floor of the mouth was larger (45 mm) than the one reported here (37 mm). Despite the size of the lesion, local anesthesia was chosen for surgery in this case because of patient's cooperation and preference to avoid general anesthesia.

In this case, ultrasonography could not eliminate a diagnosis of the ranula. Yet, a ranula typically appears as an anechoic or hypoechoic cystic component, whereas a

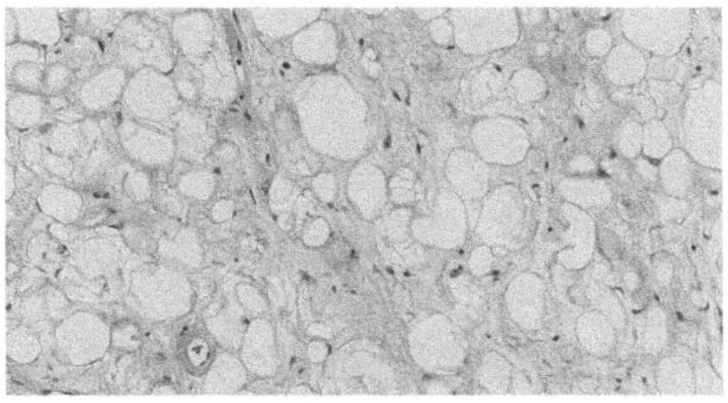

FIGURE 4: Histology showing mature adipocytes, uniform spindle cells, and short bundles of collagen in a myxoid matrix (HE staining, × 20).

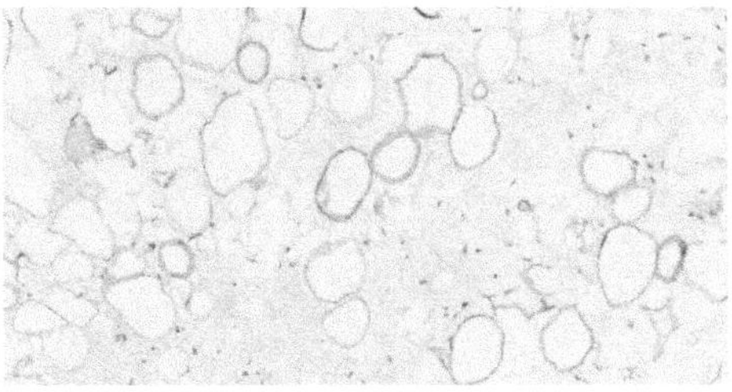

FIGURE 5: Immunohistochemical anti-PS100 staining (× 20): adipocytes are PS100 positive.

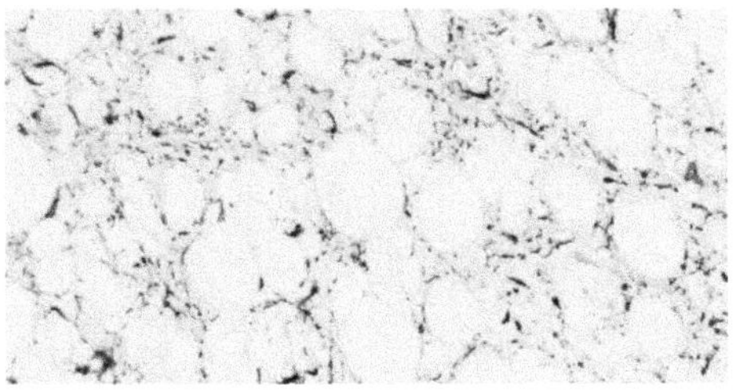

FIGURE 6: Immunohistochemical anti-CD34 staining (× 20): adipocytes are CD34 negative and spindle cells are CD34 positive.

lipoma has an isoechoic appearance with multiple internal fine echogenic lines [10]. Clinical palpation was more efficient, showing that the mass was not liquid. At this stage, the most likely clinical diagnosis was a sublingual gland pleomorphic adenoma. On RMI, imaging features of such lesions are typically T1 low signal and T2 marked hyperintensity [11]. The RMI exam, which has not been performed in the hospital, showed T1 and T2 hypersignals. However, the RMI report proposed a diagnosis of ranula. It may also be supposed that the location of the mass influenced the assessment; a ranula is indeed much more frequent than an adenoma or a lipoma of the floor of the mouth. Both lipoma and ranula are supposed to give homogenous internal structure, but lipoma T1-T2 images are expected to be high/high whereas ranula T1-T2 images are supposed to be low/markedly high [12]. In the present case, the RMI appearance was in favor of a lipoma.

From a histologic point of view, SCLs are made up of mature adipocytes and CD34+ spindle cells in a myxoid matrix with bands of birefringent collagen. Their histological differential diagnosis includes benign lesions such as classic lipoma, schwannoma, neurofibroma, leiomyoma, solitary fibrous tumor (whose prognosis is regarded as uncertain) and truly malignant ones such as atypical lipomatous tumors (well-differentiated liposarcoma), and dermatofibrosarcoma protuberans [13]. In particular, secondary degenerative modifications and atrophy observed in SCL must not be mistaken with the malignant histologic features seen in liposarcomas [14].

4. Conclusion

This case appears to be very infrequent because of its location (floor of the mouth), its size (over 3.5 cm), and the patient's gender (female). It also reminds the clinicians to prudently consider data from imaging interpretation of tumors.

References

[1] E. R. Fregnani, F. R. Pires, R. Falzoni, M. A. Lopes, and P. A. Vargas, "Lipomas of the oral cavity: clinical findings, histological classification and proliferative activity of 46 cases," *International Journal of Oral and Maxillofacial Surgery*, vol. 32, no. 1, pp. 49–53, 2003.

[2] L. E. R. Juliasse, C. F. W. Nonaka, L. P. Pinto, R. A. Freitas, and M. C. C. Miguel, "Lipomas of the oral cavity: clinical and histopathologic study of 41 cases in a Brazilian population," *European Archives of Oto-Rhino-Laryngology*, vol. 267, no. 3, pp. 459–465, 2010.

[3] F. M. Enzinger and D. A. Harvey, "Spindle cell lipoma," *Cancer*, vol. 36, no. 5, pp. 1852–1859, 1975.

[4] S. D. Billings, J. D. Henley, D.-J. Summerlin, S. Vakili, and C. E. Tomich, "Spindle cell lipoma of the oral cavity," *The American Journal of Dermatopathology*, vol. 28, no. 1, pp. 28–31, 2006.

[5] M. A. Furlong, J. C. Fanburg-Smith, and E. L. B. Childers, "Lipoma of the oral and maxillofacial region: site and subclassification of 125 cases," *Oral Surgery, Oral Medicine, Oral Pathology, Oral Radiology, and Endodontology*, vol. 98, no. 4, pp. 441–450, 2004.

[6] E. Manor, N. Sion-Vardy, P. A. Brennan, and L. Bodner, "Spindle cell lipoma of the oral cavity: a clinico-pathologic analysis of 35 reported cases," *Surgical Science*, vol. 4, no. 03, pp. 196–201, 2013.

[7] H. L. Evans, "Anisometric cell lipoma: a predominantly subcutaneous fatty tumor with notable variation in fat cell size but not more than slight nuclear enlargement and atypia," *AJSP: Reviews & Reports*, vol. 21, pp. 195–199, 2019.

[8] Y. Anavi, M. Gross, and S. Calderon, "Disturbed lower denture stability due to lipoma in the floor of the mouth," *Journal of Oral Rehabilitation*, vol. 22, no. 1, pp. 83–85, 1995.

[9] A. R. Gray and G. R. Barker, "Sublingual lipoma: report of an unusually large lesion," *Journal of Oral and Maxillofacial Surgery*, vol. 49, no. 7, pp. 747–750, 1991.

[10] L. Zhong, S. Zhao, G. Chen, and F. Ping, "Ultrasonographic appearance of lipoma in the oral and maxillofacial region," *Oral Surgery, Oral Medicine, Oral Pathology, Oral Radiology, and Endodontology*, vol. 98, no. 6, pp. 738–740, 2004.

[11] E. Matsusue, Y. Fujihara, E. Matsuda et al., "Differentiating parotid tumors by quantitative signal intensity evaluation on MR imaging," *Clinical Imaging*, vol. 46, pp. 37–43, 2017.

[12] T. Kurabayashi, M. Ida, M. Yasumoto et al., "MRI of ranulas," *Neuroradiology*, vol. 42, no. 12, pp. 917–922, 2000.

[13] N. V. M. Milhan, A. S. R. Cavalcante, Y. M. F. S. Marques, Y. R. Carvalho, and A. L. Anbinder, "Spindle cell lipoma occurring in the buccal mucosa: an unusual location of this benign lipomatous neoplasm," *Case Reports in Pathology*, vol. 2015, Article ID 805730, 5 pages, 2015.

[14] E. Manor, N. Sion-Vardy, B. Z. Joshua, and L. Bodner, "Oral lipoma: analysis of 58 new cases and review of the literature," *Annals of Diagnostic Pathology*, vol. 15, no. 4, pp. 257–261, 2011.

5

An Unusual Presentation of Multiple Superficial Mucoceles Occurring with Oral Lichen Planus

Dulyapong Rungraungrayabkul,[1] Puangwan Lapthanasupkul,[2] Naruemon Panpradit,[1] and Nis Okuma[1]

[1]*Department of Oral Medicine and Periodontology, Faculty of Dentistry, Mahidol University, 6 Yothi Rd. Rajthewee, Bangkok, Thailand 10400*
[2]*Department of Oral and Maxillofacial Pathology, Faculty of Dentistry, Mahidol University, 6 Yothi Rd. Rajthewee, Bangkok, Thailand 10400*

Correspondence should be addressed to Dulyapong Rungraungrayabkul; dulyapong.run@mahidol.ac.th

Academic Editor: Noam Yarom

Superficial mucoceles, a rare variant of the mucocele occurring simultaneously with oral lichen planus, are uncommon. This report introduces a case of multiple superficial mucoceles developing with oral lichen planus in a 76-year-old Thai female and provides information to avoid misdiagnosis and over-management of this lesion. Pathogenesis and clinicopathological characteristics of this phenomenon are also discussed.

1. Introduction

Superficial mucoceles are an unusual variant of mucocele in the oral cavity that were firstly described by Eveson in 1988 [1]. These lesions are a result of a mucous extravasating phenomenon that particularly originated from minor salivary glands. Superficial mucoceles present as small translucent tense subepithelial vesicles on the oral mucosa and may present as either isolated or multiple lesions. The lesions are frequently located at the labial mucosa, soft palate, retromolar trigone, and buccal mucosa. Unlike usual mucoceles, superficial mucoceles can resolve spontaneously and do not always require treatment except when recurrence is present. Due to the limited number of reports on the characteristics of superficial mucoceles, this disease was often misdiagnosed as other serious oral vesiculobullous diseases such as bullous lichen planus (BLP) and mucous membrane pemphigoid [2].

Previous reports revealed that superficial mucoceles are associated with several events such as trauma, allergy, radiation [3, 4], and various oral diseases such as oral lichen planus (OLP), oral lichenoid lesion from chronic graft-versus-host disease (GVHD), and mycoplasma-induced mucositis [1, 5, 6]. Among these oral diseases, superficial mucoceles are most commonly found with OLP. The latest case series reported by Lv et al. [2] described nine cases of superficial mucoceles developing concomitantly with OLP. All of the patient's superficial mucoceles were refractory to anti-inflammatory treatment [2]. Nowadays, pathogenesis of this phenomenon still remains unknown.

In this report, a 76-year-old female patient presenting with superficial mucoceles and concomitant oral lichen planus was described. The pathogenesis of this phenomenon and treatment are discussed.

2. Case Presentation

A 76-year-old woman was referred by an otorhinolaryngologist to the Faculty of Dentistry, Mahidol University. The patient reported burning sensation in the oral cavity for 6 months, and that was then followed by abundant small vesicles for 3 months. Upon examination, multiple tense and fluid-filled vesicles 1-4 mm in diameter were observed on the upper and lower labial mucosa, buccal mucosa, ventral surface of the tongue, left retromolar trigone, and soft

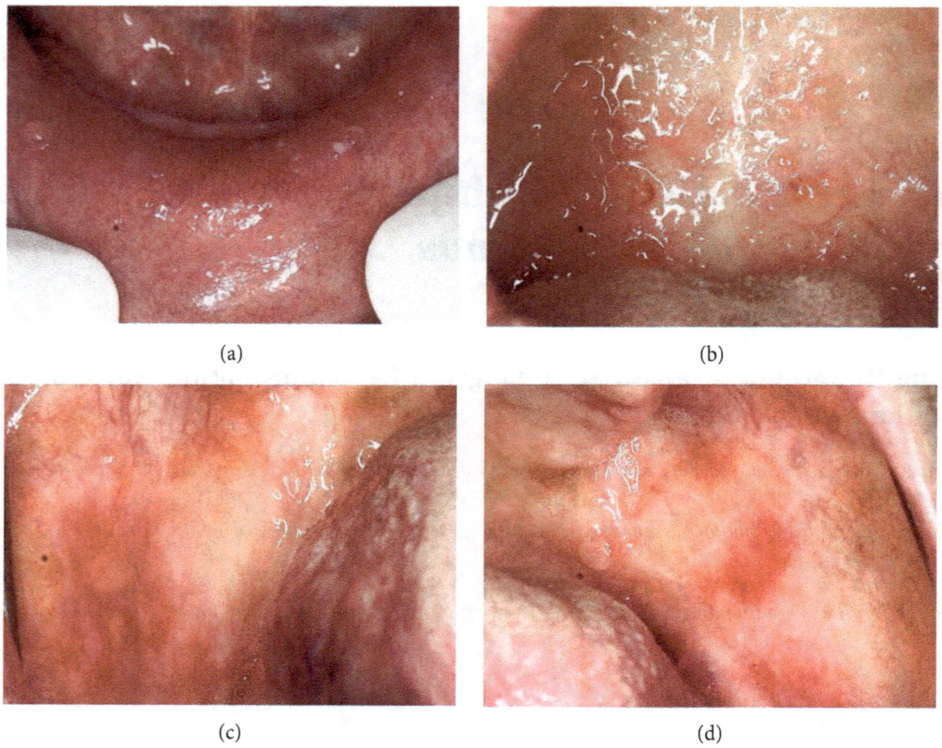

FIGURE 1: Multiple superficial mucoceles at the lower labial mucosa (a) and at the soft palate with no OLP lesion (b). White striation, erythema, and ulcerated areas at the bilateral buccal mucosa with superficial mucoceles in the adjacent area (c, d).

palate (Figures 1(a) and 1(b)). White striation, erythema, and ulcers were found on the edentulous ridge's mucosa and the bilateral buccal mucosa (Figures 1(c) and 1(d)). The laterodorsal area of the tongue showed a depapillated surface. Most of the vesicles were not associated with erythema and white striation. Extraoral examination revealed polygonal and purple papules with white striation on the extensor surface of both legs and the dorsal surface of both feet (Figure 2(a)). Both of her toenails also showed dystrophy (Figures 2(b) and 2(c)). Her past medical history included hypertension, dyslipidemia, and scoliosis. Her medications included losartan, atorvastatin, glucosamine sulfate, calcium carbonate, folic acid, and vitamins B1-6-12.

According to the patient's history and clinical findings, the diagnosis of superficial mucoceles concomitant with OLP was suggested. Incisional biopsies were performed from two sites. The first specimen was taken from the lower labial mucosa, and histopathological examination of superficial mucocele was confirmed. Histopathologically, the specimen showed intraepithelial vesicles containing a mucin pool with scattered lymphocytes (Figure 3(a)). The second specimen representing a red and white lesion was taken from the buccal mucosa. The tissue was bisected and sent for histopathological examination and direct immunofluorescence (DIF). The histological features showed a subepithelial infiltration of lymphocytes and macrophages as well as basal cell degeneration with civatte bodies, confirming the diagnosis of OLP (Figure 3(b)). The DIF finding showed fibrinogen positivity at the basement membrane with a shaggy pattern. Regarding the gold standard of OLP diagnosis [7] and the pathological diagnosis of superficial mucoceles, the definitive diagnosis of superficial mucoceles concomitant with OLP was therefore established.

According to the diagnosis, the high-potency topical steroids including mouth rinse formulated by 0.5 mg dexamethasone dissolved in 10 ml water and 0.1% fluocinolone acetonide in Orabase were prescribed for use three times a day. Additionally, nystatin oral suspension (1 : 100,000 units) was ordered twice a day in conjunction with the topical steroid for prophylaxis of fungal infection. After one month, OLP lesions were remitted, and the superficial mucoceles were decreased in number but remained only at the soft palate and the labial mucosa. The affected areas were temporally relieved as the lesions still developed every meal time, causing patient's discomfort. However, after an 8-month-treatment period, the superficial mucoceles showed complete resolution, and the patient was satisfied with this outcome (Figures 4(a)–4(d)).

3. Discussion

Superficial mucoceles arising with OLP are unusual. The vesiculobullous characteristics of superficial mucoceles often lead to a misdiagnosis of BLP. BLP is a rare distinct subtype of OLP caused by epithelial separation. The vesicles of BLP are usually larger, more fragile, and opaque, in comparison to superficial mucoceles [2]. Another remark is that oral BLP is often superimposed with or adjacent to the white striation [8]. In contrast, superficial mucoceles typically develop at the areas of minor salivary glands and can be either within or distant from the OLP lesion [1].

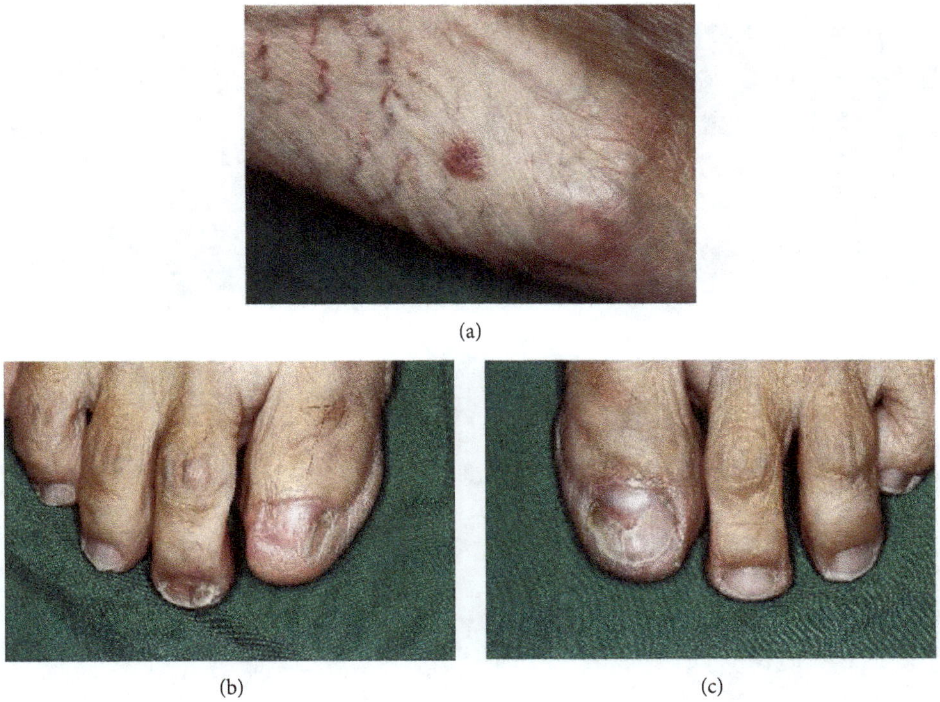

FIGURE 2: Extraoral examination revealed a polygonal purple papule with white striation on the dorsal surface of the foot (a) and dystrophic toenails (b, c).

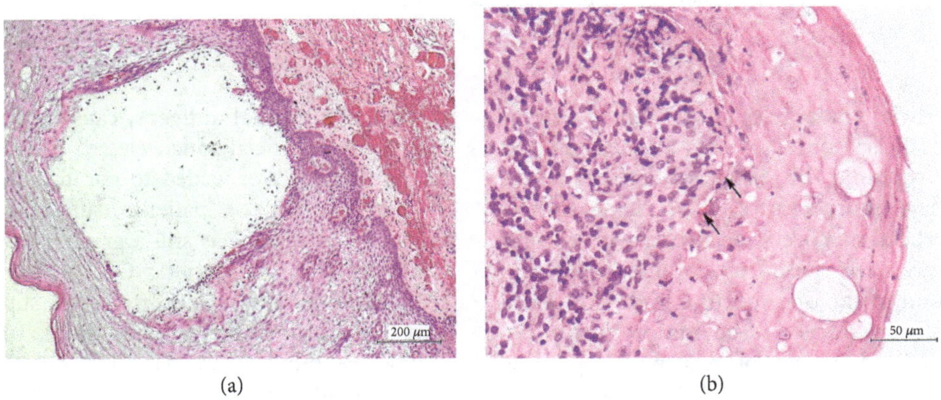

FIGURE 3: Histopathologic features of superficial mucoceles illustrated an intraepithelial vesicle containing mucin pool with scattered lymphocytes (original magnification, 100x) (a). Histopathologic features of OLP showed basal cell degeneration with subjacent inflammatory cell infiltrate. The arrows indicate civatte bodies (original magnification, 400x) (b).

Previous studies reported that multiple superficial mucoceles show a predilection for females and are more frequently found at the age of 30 years and older; that is consistent with our case [1, 9]. However, the most recent case series from Lv et al. did not find any sex predilection [2]. The dermatologic lesion of lichen planus presented in our case resembles that reported by Bermejo et al. [9], whereas other reports did not find any dermatologic condition in the cases of multiple superficial mucoceles occurring with OLP [1, 2, 9]. However, our case showed a difference in location involvement. The superficial mucoceles in our case developed in multiple areas including the labial mucosa, buccal mucosa, ventral surface of the tongue, retromolar trigone, and soft palate. None of the cases from previous reports showed multiple locations [1, 2]. This phenomenon raises a significant disturbance in our patient and confirmed that superficial mucoceles can develop in various oral mucosal sites containing minor salivary glands. In the present case, the soft palate and the ventral surface of the tongue were devoid of OLP lesions. Nevertheless, the most common location of superficial mucocele occurring with OLP reported from previous studies was the soft palate, followed by the buccal mucosa and labial mucosa [2, 9].

It has been proposed that increased intraductal pressure in salivary ducts could lead to ductal obstruction or rupture,

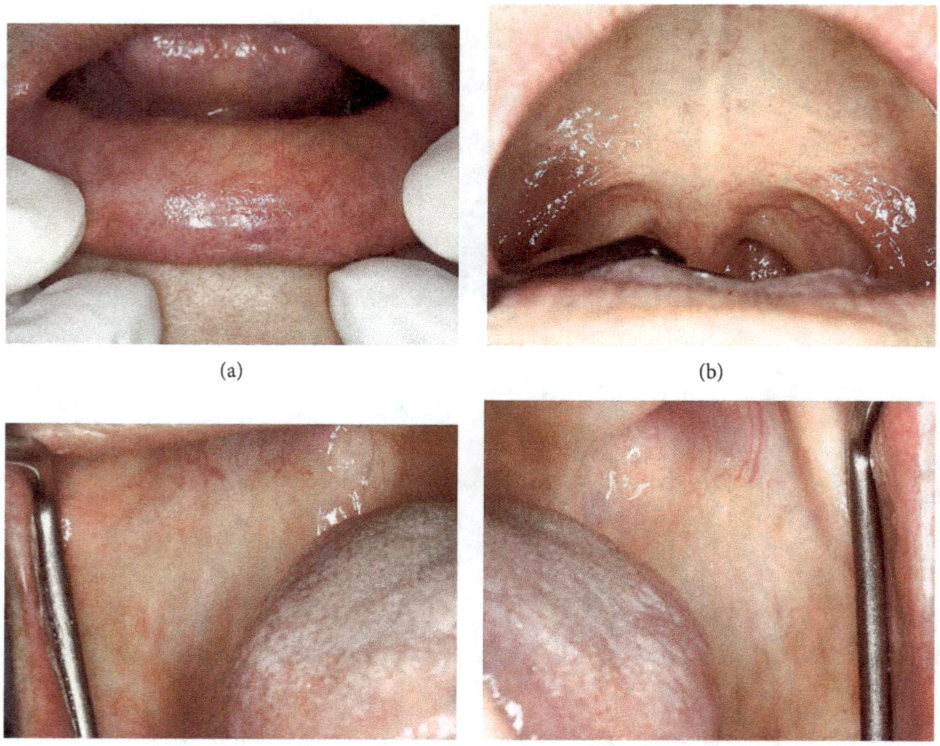

(a) (b) (c) (d)

FIGURE 4: Clinical illustration after 8-month treatment period; complete resolution of superficial mucoceles at the lower labial mucosa (a) and the soft palate (b). Remission of OLP lesions at the bilateral buccal mucosa (c, d).

resulting in superficial mucoceles [5]. Many authors believed that the salivary ducts of the affected mucosa were blocked or ruptured by lichenoid inflammation, resulting in superficial mucoceles [2, 5, 9]. Some authors proposed that superficial mucoceles occurring with chronic erosive lichen planus were caused by continuous erosion and reepithelialization of the oral mucosa, leading to damage of adjacent salivary ducts of the minor glands [9]. Campana et al. reported a case of recurrent superficial mucoceles developing with cutaneous lichen planus with an absence of OLP [10]. Consistently, the case reported by Lv et al. showed recurrent superficial mucoceles on the soft palate without OLP [2]. They proposed that this occurrence may be related to immunologic disturbance [2]. However, this was unable to explain a cause of superficial mucoceles located far away from the OLP lesion. Lourenco et al. firstly described a term "lichen planus sialadenitis" as a lichenoid infiltration surrounding excretory ducts of affected salivary glands [11]. This report also described that this phenomenon closely resembled lichen planopilaris which is a variant of cutaneous lichen planus affecting hair follicles [11, 12]. In our opinion, the pathogenesis of superficial mucoceles occurring with OLP may be similar to that of lichen planopilaris and is possibly a result of lichen planus sialadenitis. The periductal inflammation of minor salivary glands may be not only related to lichenoid infiltration of the affected mucosal area but also an activation of T-lymphocytes specifically targeting the ductal epithelial antigens, causing ductal inflammation and then superficial mucoceles at distant areas. However, further studies are needed to confirm this notion.

Management of patients suffering from superficial mucoceles with OLP is still a great challenge. The first-line treatment for symptomatic OLP is topical corticosteroid [13]. Previous studies reported that superficial mucoceles were refractory to topical steroids [2, 10] except for betamethasone mouthwash [4]. In our patient, we simulated Motallebejad et al.'s treatment by swishing and spitting out with 0.5 mg dexamethasone dissolved in 10 ml water. The outcome of temporary relief was still a burden for the patient. However, the long-term use of topical steroid conjunction with 0.1% fluocinolone in Orabase and dexamethasone mouth rinse could provide a remission of superficial mucoceles in our case. There are many reports claiming that surgical excision can be used for management of superficial mucoceles [1, 2, 14]. However, the definite treatment for multiple lesions has not been established due to postoperative complications, such as scar and tissue deformation [2]. Jinbu et al. reported that laser vaporization for recurrent multiple superficial mucocele treatment showed no complications [15]. Besides, some authors prefer reassuring patients and periodic observation for asymptomatic condition [2, 10, 16].

In conclusion, superficial mucoceles occurring with OLP are uncommon. We emphasize on recognition of distinct features of this condition to avoid misdiagnosis of other serious oral vesiculobullous diseases. In our case, the long-term use of topical steroids could provide a remission for superficial mucoceles.

Consent

No written consent has been obtained from the patient as there is no patient identifiable data included.

References

[1] J. W. Eveson, "Superficial mucoceles: pitfall in clinical and microscopic diagnosis," *Oral Surgery, Oral Medicine, and Oral Pathology*, vol. 66, no. 3, pp. 318–322, 1988.

[2] K. Lv, J. Liu, W. Ye, G. Wang, and H. Yao, "Multiple superficial mucoceles concomitant with oral lichen planus: a case series," *Oral Surgery, Oral Medicine, Oral Pathology, Oral Radiology*, vol. 127, no. 4, pp. e95–e101, 2019.

[3] A. C. Prado-Ribeiro, A. R. Santos-Silva, K. M. Faria et al., "Radiation-related superficial oral mucoceles: an under-recognized acute toxicity in head and neck cancer patients," *Medicina Oral, Patología Oral y Cirugía Bucal*, vol. 23, no. 5, pp. e518–e523, 2018.

[4] M. Motallebnejad, A. Shirzad, T. Molania, and M. Seyedmajidi, "Multiple recurrent vesicles in oral mucosa suggestive of superficial mucocele: an unusual presentation of allergic stomatitis," *Caspian Journal of Internal Medicine*, vol. 4, no. 4, pp. 793–796, 2013.

[5] F. V. M. J. Garcia, M. Pascual-Lopez, M. Elices, E. Dauden, A. Garcia-Diez, and J. Fraga, "Superficial mucoceles and lichenoid graft versus host disease: report of three cases," *Acta Dermato-Venereologica*, vol. 82, no. 6, pp. 453–455, 2002.

[6] M. Morand and A. Hatami, "Multiple superficial oral mucoceles after mycoplasma-induced mucositis," *Pediatric Dermatology*, vol. 35, no. 4, pp. e210–e211, 2018.

[7] E. H. van der Meij and I. van der Waal, "Lack of clinicopathologic correlation in the diagnosis of oral lichen planus based on the presently available diagnostic criteria and suggestions for modifications," *Journal of Oral Pathology & Medicine*, vol. 32, no. 9, pp. 507–512, 2003.

[8] A. Babu, S. Chellaswamy, S. Muthukumar, B. Pandey, M. Jayaraj, and S. Francis, "Bullous lichen planus: case report and review," *Journal of Pharmacy & Bioallied Sciences*, vol. 11, Suppl 2, pp. S499–S506, 2019.

[9] A. Bermejo, J. M. Aguirre, P. Lopez, and M. R. Saez, "Superficial mucocele: report of 4 cases," *Oral Surgery, Oral Medicine, Oral Pathology, Oral Radiology, and Endodontics*, vol. 88, no. 4, pp. 469–472, 1999.

[10] F. Campana, V. Sibaud, A. Chauvel, J. M. Boiron, A. Taieb, and J. C. Fricain, "Recurrent superficial mucoceles associated with lichenoid disorders," *Journal of Oral and Maxillofacial Surgery*, vol. 64, no. 12, pp. 1830–1833, 2006.

[11] S. V. Lourenco, A. C. Resende, S. B. Bologna, and M. M. Nico, "Lichen planus sialadenitis: a mucosal analog of lichen planopilaris and lichen planoporitis," *Journal of Cutaneous Pathology*, vol. 37, no. 3, pp. 396–399, 2010.

[12] P. Assouly and P. Reygagne, "Lichen planopilaris: update on diagnosis and treatment," *Seminars in Cutaneous Medicine and Surgery*, vol. 28, no. 1, pp. 3–10, 2009.

[13] L. Oberti, L. Alberta, P. Massimo, C. Francesco, and L. Dorina, "Clinical management of oral lichen planus: a systematic review," *Mini Reviews in Medicinal Chemistry*, vol. 19, no. 13, pp. 1049–1059, 2019.

[14] J. Yague-Garcia, A. J. Espana-Tost, L. Berini-Aytes, and C. Gay-Escoda, "Treatment of oral mucocele-scalpel versus CO_2 laser," *Medicina Oral, Patología Oral y Cirugía Bucal*, vol. 14, no. 9, pp. e469–e474, 2009.

[15] Y. Jinbu, K. Tsukinoki, M. Kusama, and Y. Watanabe, "Recurrent multiple superficial mucocele on the palate: histopathology and laser vaporization," *Oral Surgery, Oral Medicine, Oral Pathology, Oral Radiology, and Endodontics*, vol. 95, no. 2, pp. 193–197, 2003.

[16] G. Z. Xu, C. Yang, C. Q. Yu, D. He, and S. Zhang, "Multiple superficial mucoceles on lower lip, soft palate, retromolar region, and floor of mouth," *Journal of Oral and Maxillofacial Surgery*, vol. 68, no. 10, pp. 2601–2603, 2010.

6

Osteosarcoma of the Mandible in an Elderly Patient

Isao Hoshi,[1] Ryosuke Abe,[2] Kei Onodera,[1] Yu Ohashi,[1] Tadashi Kawai,[1] Ikuya Miyamoto,[1] Toshimi Chiba,[3] Yasunori Takeda,[4] and Hiroyuki Yamada[1]

[1]*Division of Oral and Maxillofacial Surgery, Department of Reconstructive Oral and Maxillofacial Surgery, School of Dentistry, Iwate Medical University, Morioka 020-8505, Japan*
[2]*Department of Oral and Maxillofacial Surgery, Iwate Prefectural Central Hospital, Morioka 020-0066, Japan*
[3]*Division of Internal Medicine, Department of Oral Medicine, Iwate Medical University, Morioka 020-8505, Japan*
[4]*Division of Clinical Pathology, Department of Oral and Maxillofacial Reconstructive Surgery, School of Dentistry, Iwate Medical University, Morioka 020-8505, Japan*

Correspondence should be addressed to Hiroyuki Yamada; yamadah@iwate-med.ac.jp

Academic Editor: Darko Macan

Osteosarcoma is a malignant tumor in which the cancerous cells produce an osteoid matrix or mineralized bone. Jaw bones are affected in 6% of all osteosarcomas and are the fourth most common site of origin. Surgical treatment of osteosarcoma in elderly patients is rarely reported. Here, we report successful treatment of osteosarcoma arising in the mandible of a 90-year-old man. The patient was referred to our institution for diagnosis and treatment of an oral lesion. Intraoral examination revealed that a hard mass measuring 35×27 mm was located on the floor of the oral cavity, attached to the bone, and its growth displaced the tongue posteriorly. Therefore, he experienced difficulty in speech and swallowing. Biopsy of the mandibular mass was suspicious for chondrosarcoma. Preoperative examination did not detect critical risks for general anesthesia or surgery. Based on a clinical diagnosis of a malignant bone tumor of the mandible, segmental mandibular resection with reconstruction using a titanium plate was performed. Surgical site infection occurred on postoperative day 12, which was resolved by drainage, local irrigation, and administration of antibiotics. There was no delirium or cardiovascular or pulmonary complications. Surgery resolved the patient's difficulties in speech and swallowing. There was no evidence of tumor recurrence or metastasis 4 years after surgery. This case showed that it was not necessary to exclude surgical treatment merely because the patient was 90 years old. Indications for surgery should be determined individually to improve the patient's quality of life.

1. Introduction

Osteosarcoma is a malignant tumor in which the cancerous cells produce an osteoid matrix or mineralized bone [1]. Jaw bones are affected in 6% of all osteosarcomas and are the fourth most common site of origin, following the femur, tibia, and humerus [2]. Osteosarcoma of the jaw (OSJ) tends to occur in the mandible twice as often as in the maxilla [3, 4]. No gender difference for the incidence of OSJ has been reported [2]. OSJ develops in older age and shows good prognosis when compared with that of tumors in the long bones [2]. Therefore, OSJ is considered to be distinct from osteosarcoma arising in the long bones [4]. The standard treatment for osteosarcoma of the long bones is surgery with perioperative chemotherapy [5]; however, it is not similarly applicable for OSJ [2]. A review of the English language literature revealed 214 cases of OSJ diagnosed over 40 years in patients with a maximum age of 83 years [4]. In another retrospective cohort study of 541 cases of OSJ, the maximum age was 91 years [6]. The mean age of patients with OSJ is reported to be 39–42 years; therefore, surgical treatment of osteosarcoma in elderly patients is rarely reported [3, 4, 6]. Here, we report successful treatment of osteosarcoma arising in the mandible in a 90-year-old man.

2. Case Presentation

A 90-year-old man was referred to our institution in May 2017 for diagnosis and treatment of an oral lesion. He had first noticed the lesion approximately 1 year earlier. The lesion grew gradually and showed rapid enlargement in the

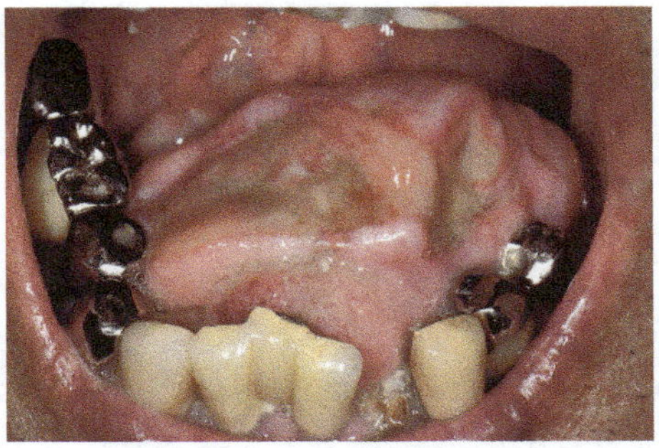

Figure 1: Intraoral photograph showing a large mass occupying the oral floor. The overlying oral mucosa is partially ulcerated.

last 6 months. The patient's medical history included atrial fibrillation treated with warfarin, hyperlipidemia, resected rectal cancer, and internal carotid artery stenosis treated by carotid endarterectomy. All of these conditions were followed up and controlled by the patient's physicians. He had smoked cigarettes from age 23 to 48 years, resulting in a Brinkman index of 3,000. His family history was unremarkable. Intraoral examination revealed that a hard mass measuring 35 × 27 mm was located on the floor of the oral cavity and attached to the bone. The overlying oral mucosa was partially ulcerated. The growth of the mass displaced the tongue posteriorly, resulting in a Mallampati score of IV (Figure 1); therefore, he experienced difficulty with speech and swallowing. There was no evidence of cranial nerve paralysis or cervical lymphadenopathy. Cone-beam computed tomography (CT) (3D Accuitomo F17; Morita, Kyoto, Japan) revealed that the mass was connected to the cortical bone of the mandible. The mass was inhomogeneous and spread to the left mandibular body (Figure 2). Magnetic resonance imaging was performed with a 3.0-Tesla system (MR750; General Electric Company, Boston, MA, USA). On T1- and T2-weighted axial images, the mass showed low signal intensity relative to muscle. Positron emission tomography (PET)/CT was performed with a Discovery PET/CT 600 scanner (General Electric Company). The image showed abnormal accumulation of fluorodeoxyglucose in the mandibular lesion (maximum standardized uptake value: 7.2) (Figure 3). There was no abnormal accumulation of fluorodeoxyglucose in any other organ. Biopsy of the mandibular mass was suspicious for chondrosarcoma. The American Society of Anesthesiologists (ASA) physical status was class 3. Echocardiography revealed an ejection fraction of 64% without ischemic or valvular heart disease. Spirography revealed that forced expiratory volume in 1 second was 64.8%, suggesting slight obstructive ventilation disorder. Magnetic resonance angiography of the internal carotid artery revealed no evidence of restenosis after carotid endarterectomy. Preoperative examination did not detect critical risks for general anesthesia and surgery, although their duration was reduced as much as possible. No method other than surgical treatment could have resolved his chief complaint. Heparin bridging was scheduled for atrial fibrillation treated with warfarin before surgery. Based on a clinical diagnosis of a malignant bone tumor of the mandible (cT1N0M0), segmental mandibular resection with reconstruction using a titanium plate was performed in June. Although the Mallampati score was IV, tracheal intubation was not difficult without trismus. During the operation, a surgical safety margin of about 10 mm was set in the

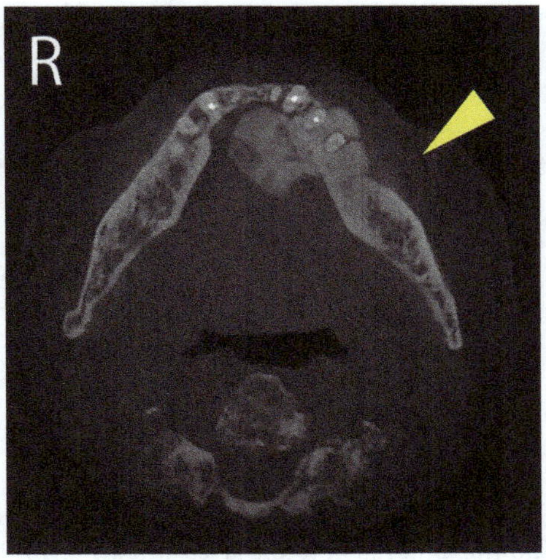

Figure 2: Cone-beam computed tomography showing the mass connected to the cortical bone of the mandible. The mass spread to the left mandibular body (arrowhead).

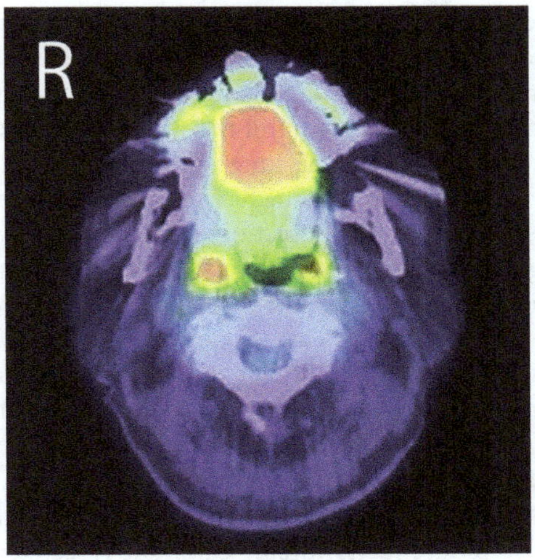

Figure 3: Positron emission tomography/computed tomography showing abnormal accumulation of fluorodeoxyglucose in the oral mass (maximum standardized uptake value 7.2).

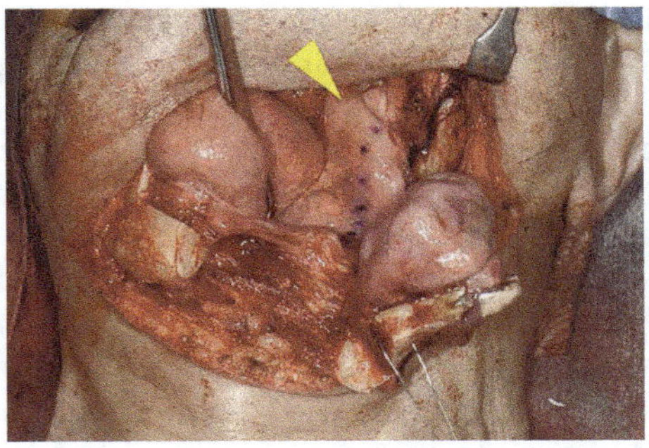

Figure 4: Intraoperative photomicrograph showing surgical safety margin of about 10 mm set in the normal-looking tissue (arrowhead).

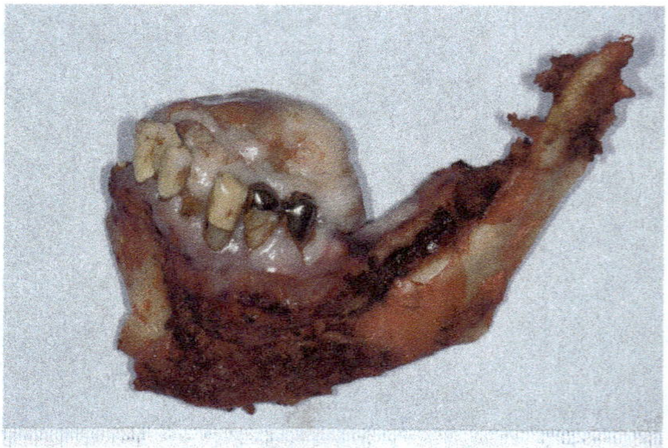

(a)

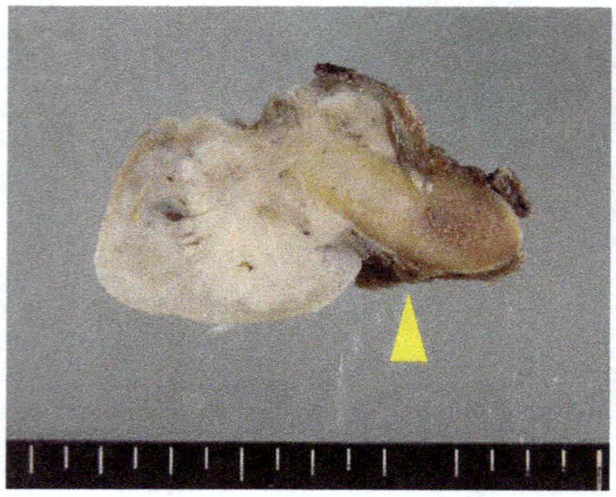

(b)

Figure 5: (a) Resected mandibular specimen revealing dominant exophilic proliferation. (b) Cut surface of the tumor after fixing with formalin showing infiltration to the alveolar bone (arrowhead).

normal-looking tissue. First, we reached the inferior border of the mandible through cervical incision. Next, we made an intraoral incision on the buccal gingiva. By resecting soft tissue around the tumor, we connected the oral wound to the cervical one. This procedure exposed the lateral surface of the tumor with surrounding soft tissue. The medial border was cut by the surgical saw, and the mandible was swung to the left side to visualize the inner surface of the tumor. By directly viewing the tumor attached to the bone, the oral floor was incised (Figure 4). Resection of the tumor with surrounding normal soft tissue was performed backward, and the inferior alveolar nerve and vascular bundles were ligated and cut. Finally, mandibular segmental resection was completed by cutting the mandibular ramus at the distal border. After removal of the tumor, the mandible was reconstructed using a titanium plate that was prepared preoperatively based on a 3D mandibular model. Operation time was 5 h, and the amount of bleeding was 389 g. After the operation, the patient received frequent nursing care. The resected mandibular specimen revealed dominant exophilic proliferation (Figure 5(a)), and the cut surface of the tumor after fixing with formalin showed infiltration to the alveolar bone (Figure 5(b)). Histopathological examination revealed that trabeculae with low calcification spread radially in the periphery of the tumor. Tumor cells with mild atypia were present densely with partial cartilage ossification (Figure 6). The surgically resected margins were negative for tumor. The final histopathological diagnosis was low-grade osteosarcoma (stage IA). Surgical site infection occurred on postoperative day 12, which was resolved by drainage, local irrigation, and administration of antibiotics. There was no delirium or cardiovascular or pulmonary complications. Surgery resolved the patient's speech and swallowing difficulties. He continued to come to our hospital alone on foot for regular clinical check-up. There was no evidence of tumor recurrence or metastasis 4 years after surgery by evaluation with panoramic radiography (Figure 7) and chest X-ray.

3. Discussion

Surgery in the oldest patients has various complications, including cardiovascular and pulmonary complications, surgical site infection, and delirium. The cardiovascular risk index is a newly proposed method for preoperative cardiovascular evaluation [7]. The index is based on 6 easily acquired data elements (age > 75 years, history of heart disease, symptoms of angina or dyspnea, hemoglobin < 12 mg/dl, vascular surgery, and emergency surgery) that can strongly predict the 30-day risk of postoperative cardiovascular events in patients undergoing noncardiac surgery. If the present case is evaluated using this index, age and history of heart disease are 2 positive elements, resulting in an intermediate risk retrospectively. Postoperative pulmonary complications are closely related to the surgical site. Their incidence is highest among patients who undergo cardiothoracic surgery (5.3%) and lowest in orthopedic and urological surgery (0.7%) [8]. Head and neck surgery carries an intermediate risk, and advanced age is an important independent predictor of postoperative pulmonary complications in noncardiothoracic surgery [9]. Cigarette smoking indicates a modest increase in complication risk [9]. At least 2 months of smoking cessation is recommended to reduce the risk of increased intraoperative sputum volume [10]. In the present case, a high Brinkman index was documented; however, smoking cessation had been continued for >40 years. Delirium is an acute fluctuating alteration of mental state,

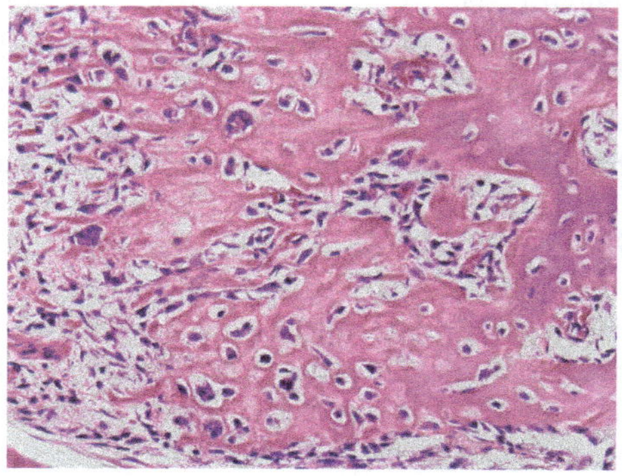

Figure 6: Photomicrograph showing trabeculae with low calcification spread radially in the periphery of the tumor. Tumor cells with mild atypia are present densely, with partial cartilage ossification (hematoxylin-eosin stain, ×400).

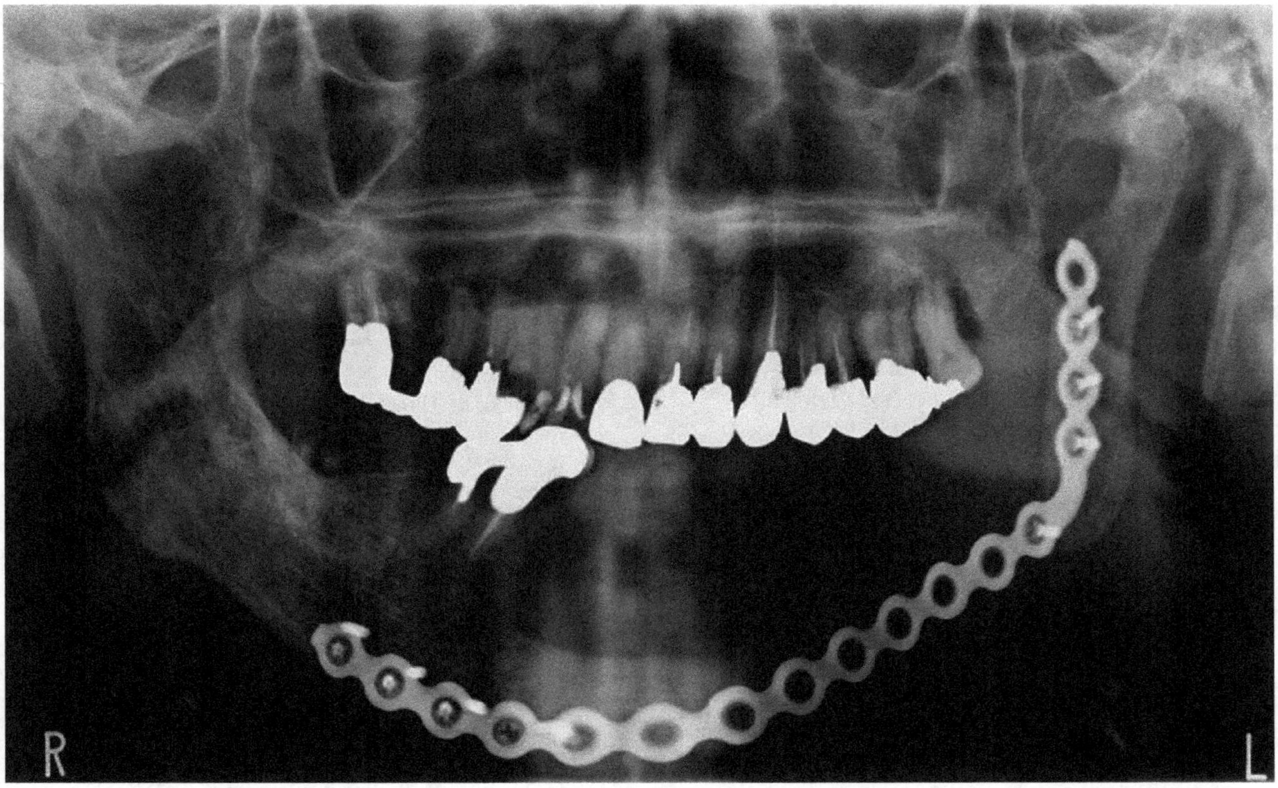

Figure 7: Postoperative panoramic X-ray showing the reconstructed mandible with a titanium plate.

reduced awareness, and disturbance of attention that may be triggered by acute medical illness, surgery, trauma, or drugs [11]. After head and neck surgery, the incidence of postoperative delirium is reported to be 19.26% [12]. The occurrence of postoperative delirium is significantly related to increased age, mental health status, ASA score, and drug dependence [13]. In the present case, good mental condition, absence of drug dependence, and frequent nursing care might have contributed to the absence of delirium. Consequently, major complications except for surgical site infection were avoided. The most equivocal differential diagnosis of low-grade osteosarcoma is benign fibro-osseous lesions. The presence of proliferative infiltration is the main histopathological finding to exclude fibro-osseous lesions. Moreover, immunohistochemically positive staining for murine double-minute type 2 and cyclin-dependent kinase 4 is useful to distinguish osteosarcoma from benign fibro-osseous lesions [14]. Although immunohistochemical analysis was not performed in the present case, the histopathological finding of infiltration of tumor cells to the alveolar bone, with cartilage ossification, was consistent with the diagnosis of osteosarcoma.

Osteosarcoma is also a common secondary malignancy following radiotherapy of a primary malignant tumor [15]. In the present case, irradiation to the head and neck was not performed previously. The surgically resected specimen did not clearly show the preexisting mandibular lesion. PET showed no abnormal accumulation of fluorodeoxyglucose in any other organ except for the mandible. Therefore, the present case was classified as primary rather than secondary osteosarcoma. The standard treatment for high-grade osteosarcoma is surgery with pre- and postoperative chemotherapy [5]. However, low-grade OSJ can typically be cured by complete resection [4]. In the present case, the result of preoperative biopsy was suspected chondrosarcoma. Because the standard treatment for chondrosarcoma is surgery [5], we selected surgery without preoperative chemotherapy. The final histopathological diagnosis of low-grade osteosarcoma, complete surgical removal of the tumor, and the patient's age of 90 years prompted us to select postoperative observation without chemotherapy. As a result, the patient survived for 4 years without tumor recurrence or metastasis. The vascularized fibula using a microsurgical technique is the most popular free flap for mandibular reconstruction [16] and should be selected if the patient is not elderly. However, this method requires a long operation time. In the present case, the duration of general anesthesia and surgery was reduced as much as possible. Therefore, minimally required operation was selected. Fortunately, soft tissue deficiency after segmental mandibular resection was small because of the exophilic nature of the tumor. The presence of mislocalized cytoplasmic p27 is reported to be associated with higher metastatic status and poorer survival of osteosarcoma [17]. As clinical factors, proximal location of osteosarcoma in the long bone of an extremity portends a worse clinical outcome than tumors located in the distal long bones [18]. The prognostic factors for OSJ have been reported in a few studies [4, 6]. The biomarker melanoma-associated antigen-A failed to predict the prognosis of OSJ [3]. The clinical factors of the lower tumor stage [6], surgery performed [6], clear surgical margin [4], and earlier age at diagnosis [6] show better prognosis. In the present case, although the patient was 90 years old, a safety margin of about 10 mm was set because of the exophilic nature of the tumor, resulting in histopathologically complete resection. In conclusion, we report a rare case of osteosarcoma arising in the mandible of a 90-year-old man. This case showed that it was not necessary to exclude surgical treatment merely because the patient was aged 90 years. Indications for surgery should be determined individually to improve the patient's quality of life.

Consent

The patient provided written informed consent for publication of this case report and any accompanying images. A copy of the written consent is available for review by the editor-in-chief of the journal.

Authors' Contributions

IH, TC, TK, IM, and HY reviewed the literature. HY, RA, KO, and YO performed the operation and analyzed and interpreted the patient's data. YT performed the histopathological analyses. RA, YO, KO, TC, and HY were clinically responsible for the patient's care. All authors have read and approved the final manuscript.

Acknowledgments

We thank Cathel Kerr, BSc, PhD, from Edanz (https://jp.edanz.com/ac) for editing a draft of this manuscript.

References

[1] A. Horvai, "Osteosarcoma," in *Robbins & Cotran Pathologic Basis of Disease*, V. Kumar, A. K. Abbas, and J. C. Aster, Eds., Elsevier, Philadelphia, 10th edition, 2021.

[2] D. Baumhoer, M. Lopes, and E. Raubenheimer, "Osteosarcoma," in *WHO Classification of Head and Neck Tumours*, A. K. El-Naggar, J. K. C. Chan, J. R. Grandis, T. Takata, and P. J. Slootweg, Eds., International agency for research on cancer, Lyon, 4th edition, 2017.

[3] C. Eder-Czembirek, D. Moser, S. Holawe et al., "Osteosarcoma of the jaw - experience at the Medical University Vienna and comparative study with international tumor registries," *Clinics (São Paulo, Brazil)*, vol. 74, article e701, 2019.

[4] D. Baumhoer, P. Brunner, S. Eppenberger-Castori, J. Smida, M. Nathrath, and G. Jundt, "Osteosarcomas of the jaws differ from their peripheral counterparts and require a distinct treatment approach. Experiences from the DOESAK registry," *Oral Oncology*, vol. 50, no. 2, pp. 147–153, 2014.

[5] P. G. Casali, S. Bielack, N. Abecassis et al., "Bone sarcomas: ESMO-PaedCan-EURACAN Clinical Practice Guidelines for diagnosis, treatment and follow-up," *Annals of Oncology*, vol. 29, Supplement 4, pp. iv79–iv95, 2018.

[6] R. J. Lee, A. Arshi, H. C. Schwartz, and R. E. Christensen, "Characteristics and prognostic factors of osteosarcoma of the jaws: a retrospective cohort study," *JAMA Otolaryngology. Head & Neck Surgery*, vol. 141, no. 5, pp. 470–477, 2015.

[7] H. A. Dakik, O. Chehab, M. Eldirani et al., "A new index for pre-operative cardiovascular evaluation," *Journal of the American College of Cardiology*, vol. 73, no. 24, pp. 3067–3078, 2019.

[8] M. Chughtai, C. U. Gwam, A. Khlopas et al., "The incidence of postoperative pneumonia in various surgical subspecialties: a dual database analysis," *Surgical Technology International*, vol. 30, pp. 45–51, 2017.

[9] G. W. Smetana, V. A. Lawrence, J. E. Cornell, and American College of Physicians, "Preoperative pulmonary risk stratification for noncardiothoracic surgery: systematic review for the American College of Physicians," *Annals of Internal Medicine*, vol. 144, no. 8, pp. 581–595, 2006.

[10] S. Yamashita, H. Yamaguchi, M. Sakaguchi et al., "Effect of smoking on intraoperative sputum and postoperative pulmonary complication in minor surgical patients," *Respiratory Medicine*, vol. 98, no. 8, pp. 760–766, 2004.

[11] P. Aceto, R. Antonelli Incalzi, G. Bettelli et al., "Perioperative Management of Elderly patients (PriME): recommendations from an Italian intersociety consensus," *Aging Clinical and Experimental Research*, vol. 32, no. 9, pp. 1647–1673, 2020.

[12] Y. Zhu, G. Wang, S. Liu et al., "Risk factors for postoperative delirium in patients undergoing major head and neck cancer surgery: a meta-analysis," *Japanese Journal of Clinical Oncology*, vol. 47, no. 6, pp. 505–511, 2017.

[13] D. A. Edwards, A. Medhavy, O. G. Hoffman, and G. R. Hoffman, "Postoperative delirium is associated with prolonged head and neck resection and reconstruction surgery: an institutional study," *Journal of Oral and Maxillofacial Surgery*, vol. 79, no. 1, pp. 249–258, 2021.

[14] F. Dujardin, M. B. Binh, C. Bouvier et al., "MDM2 and CDK4 immunohistochemistry is a valuable tool in the differential diagnosis of low-grade osteosarcomas and other primary fibro-osseous lesions of the bone," *Modern Pathology*, vol. 24, no. 5, pp. 624–637, 2011.

[15] W. Zhu, F. Hu, T. Zhao, C. Wang, and Q. Tao, "Clinical characteristics of radiation-induced sarcoma of the head and neck: review of 15 cases and 323 cases in the literature," *Journal of Oral and Maxillofacial Surgery*, vol. 74, no. 2, pp. 283–291, 2016.

[16] B. T. Goh, S. Lee, H. Tideman, and P. J. Stoelinga, "Mandibular reconstruction in adults: a review," *International Journal of Oral and Maxillofacial Surgery*, vol. 37, no. 7, pp. 597–605, 2008.

[17] X. Chen, J. M. M. Cates, Y. C. Du et al., "Mislocalized cytoplasmic p27 activates PAK1-mediated metastasis and is a prognostic factor in osteosarcoma," *Molecular Oncology*, vol. 14, no. 4, pp. 846–864, 2020.

[18] J. M. Cates and J. G. Schoenecker, "Proximal location in extremity long bones is a poor prognostic factor for osteosarcoma: a retrospective cohort study of 153 patients," *Acta Oncologica*, vol. 55, no. 8, pp. 1036–1039, 2016.

7

Plasma Cell Gingivitis Treated with Photobiomodulation, with No Recurrence for a Five-Year Follow-Up

Federica Pulicari,[1,2] Matteo Pellegrini ,[3] Maurizio Pascadopoli ,[4] Massimo Porrini,[1,2] Elisabetta Kuhn,[2,5] Andrea Scribante ,[4] and Francesco Spadari[1,2]

[1]*Maxillo-Facial and Odontostomatology Unit, Fondazione IRCCS Cà Granda Ospedale Maggiore Policlinico, Milan 20122, Italy*
[2]*Department of Biomedical, Surgical and Dental Sciences, University of Milan, Via della Commenda 10, Milan 20122, Italy*
[3]*Section of Dentistry, Department of Clinical, Surgical, Diagnostic and Pediatric Sciences, University of Pavia, Pavia 27100, Italy*
[4]*Unit of Orthodontics and Pediatric Dentistry, Section of Dentistry, Department of Clinical, Surgical, Diagnostic and Pediatric Sciences, University of Pavia, Pavia 27100, Italy*
[5]*Pathology Unit, Fondazione IRCCS Cà Granda Ospedale Maggiore Policlinico, Milan 20122, Italy*

Correspondence should be addressed to Andrea Scribante; andrea.scribante@unipv.it

Academic Editor: Paolo Giacomo Arduino

Introduction. Plasma cell gingivitis (PCG) is a chronic inflammatory disease usually affecting the vestibular portion of the gingival mucosa. Clinical presentation is marked by erythematous macules of intense red color, confluent, and delimited from the healthy neighboring mucosa. Generally asymptomatic, the gum lesions sometimes are accompanied by burning sensations and a sense of local tension. Recommended treatment is the use of topical steroids, but with apparent initial healing that is not stable over time. The present case report concerns a patient diagnosed with PCG in November 2017, with a five-year follow-up. This is the first patient with PCG successfully treated with non-surgical periodontal therapies associated with photobiomodulation (PBM). *Methods.* A 64-year-old male patient had intense erythema and edema on the vestibular side of the gingival mucosa area from 1.5 to 2.5. The patient's symptomatic subjectivity parameters were evaluated through dedicated questionnaires. Erythema and gingival bleeding were also evaluated. Periodontal charting was not pathological, but intense bleeding was noted. Multiple biopsies were performed, and microscopic findings confirmed the clinical hypothesis of PCG. *Results.* The treatment applied was PBM associated with periodontal therapy. The patient demonstrated a progressive improvement in clinical parameters considered and reported symptoms. During the five-year follow-up, no recurrence of the disease was observed. *Conclusions.* The combined PBM and periodontal therapies have proved to be sufficiently effective in the control of PCG, showing reduction of the intense inflammatory, erythematous component, and gingival bleeding, and are a valid treatment alternative to topical steroids.

1. Introduction

Plasma cell gingivitis (PCG) is a chronic inflammatory disease affecting the gingival mucous membranes. It is a rare occurrence with an etiopathogenetic matrix still uncertain [1–3]. Microscopically, it is characterized by a dense plasma cell infiltrate. Non-neoplastic plasma cell proliferation can involve different anatomical sites, including the upper aerodigestive tract, especially the gums, such as PCG. PCGs are broadly characterized by heterogeneous morphological features, high morbidity, and a lack of a shared therapeutic approach [1, 2]. The average age of onset is 45 years and there is a higher prevalence in males [2].

Although the etiology is still unclear, many hypotheses have been postulated regarding PCG onset, ranging from trauma to hypersensitive reactions to certain types of antigens (e.g., chewing gum components, toothpaste, khat, or specific foods) or physical somatization of psychological disorders [1, 2]. However, most of these lesions are currently considered idiopathic [1, 3].

PCG characteristically affects the vestibular portions of the adherent gingival mucous membranes and then extends up to the mucogingival junction. The palatal mucosa is rarely involved. The clinical-objective features are represented by erythematous mucous membranes with intense red color, velvety, edematous, and delimited by the surrounding mucosa. These lesions are accompanied by painful symptoms, burning, and frequent bleeding [1, 4–7].

PCG presents a histopathological feature characterized by lymphoplasmacellular infiltrate near the basal membrane, spongiosis, and marked exocytosis [1–3, 5]. It is known that chronic inflammatory modifications could lead to locoregional immunological dysregulation and induce plasma cell migration with pro-inflammatory cytokines that seem to have a key role in the immune-mediated mechanisms that trigger B-cell proliferation [2]. The diagnosis is fundamentally histopathological. In differential diagnosis, there are chronic gingivitis non-plaque dependent, atrophic erosive, bullous gingivitis, and possible plasma cell neoplastic infiltrates [3, 4, 6]. Furthermore, PCG could mimic a wide range of life-threatening entities, such as squamous cell carcinoma, autoimmune mucocutaneous bullous diseases, and lymphoproliferative disorders [1, 2, 4, 8, 9]. Plasma cell proliferation is also associated with some infectious diseases, such as syphilis [2], Castleman's disease [2, 10], primary infectious disease of the lymph node, and, recently, COVID-19 [2, 11].

The pharmacological treatment is usually symptom-related, based on local and systemic corticosteroids, immunomodulators, antibiotics, and plaque-control local mouthwashes that represent the most frequent choice as first-line therapy, to delete local irritants and to reduce immunological cell-mediated and cytokine-mediate response, preventing recurrence [1, 2, 12]. Gum improvements are always related to oral hygiene levels. However, relapses are common after stopping steroid therapy [4].

The purpose of this study is to describe a case of a patient, presented at operative unit, suffering from PCG, treated with a novel therapeutic approach based on photobiomodulation (PBM) using a laser therapy, as an alternative to pharmacological treatment, and followed up for over five years.

2. Case Report

2.1. Diagnosis and Etiology. A 64-year-old Italian male patient presented to observation at the Pathology and Oral Medicine Outpatient Clinic of Milan, in November 2017, complaining gingival bleeding.

During the collection of anamnestic data, the patient declared that he did not have allergies or voluptuous habits and that he was suffering from hypertension under treatment with nebivolol and diuretics. Following fillings of the teeth in 2016, he found erythematous hyperplastic gingivitis in the upper arch conditioning the feeding. He denied Raynaud's phenomenon, photosensitivity, lymph node swelling, weight loss, fever, xerostomia, and xerophthalmia. From the report of the specialist visit carried out by the rheumatologist, at blood tests he had isolated low anti-RNP antibody titers. Also, the patient reported no cases of psoriasis or rheumatic diseases in the family.

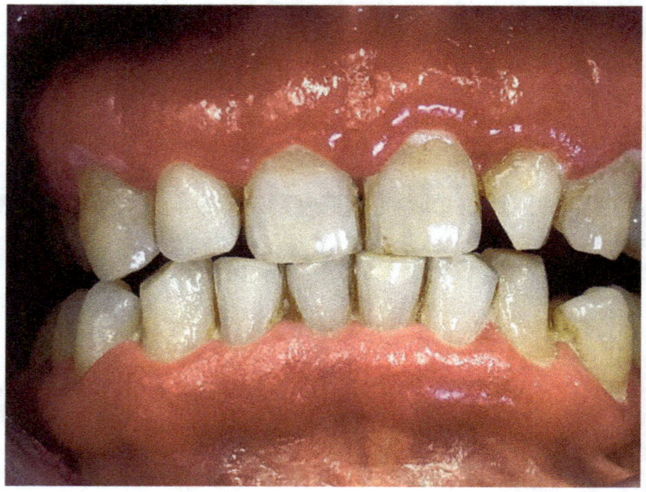

FIGURE 1: Intense edema and erythema localized to the adherent vestibular gingival mucosa, from elements 1.5 to 2.5.

The local objective clinical examination revealed intense edema and erythema localized to the adherent vestibular gingival mucosa, from elements 1.5 to 2.5 (Figure 1). The periodontal charting showed probing pocket depth <3 mm without loss of clinical attachment level, in the presence of intense bleeding. First and second level blood chemistry was prescribed and showed positivity for Proteinase 3 antibodies.

2.2. Treatment Objectives. The aim of this treatment is to find a therapeutic alternative for the treatment of PCG, which is effective and minimizes the risk of recurrence after the end of the treatment.

2.3. Treatment Alternatives. Many therapeutic treatments have been proposed over the years. Specifically, the use of topical or intralesional injection of steroids or systemic steroid therapies, contribute to the reduction of the size of the lesion, but to the suspension of the therapy do not guarantee a complete cure of the pathology [1, 2, 4]. Moreover, if the lesions are extended to the surrounding soft tissues, for example, there is the involvement of the larynx, a treatment based on chemotherapy and prednisone has been studied, favoring a temporary regression of the lesion, which recurs, however, when the therapy is suspended [1]. On the other hand, starting from the assumption that the cause of PCG is a *Candida albicans* infection, topical nystatin-based therapies have been proposed, but have been proved ineffective [1]. Another therapeutic approach indicated in the literature is low-dose radiation therapy and surgical excision. Low dose radiation caused a relative improvement in the treatment, but several studies confirm as gold standard the surgical excision by surgical blades, electrocoagulation, CO_2 laser, or cryotherapy even with the risk of recurrence [13–15]. Finally, a therapeutic approach discussed in the literature reports a non-surgical protocol found to be effective for the management of the disease, which consists of the

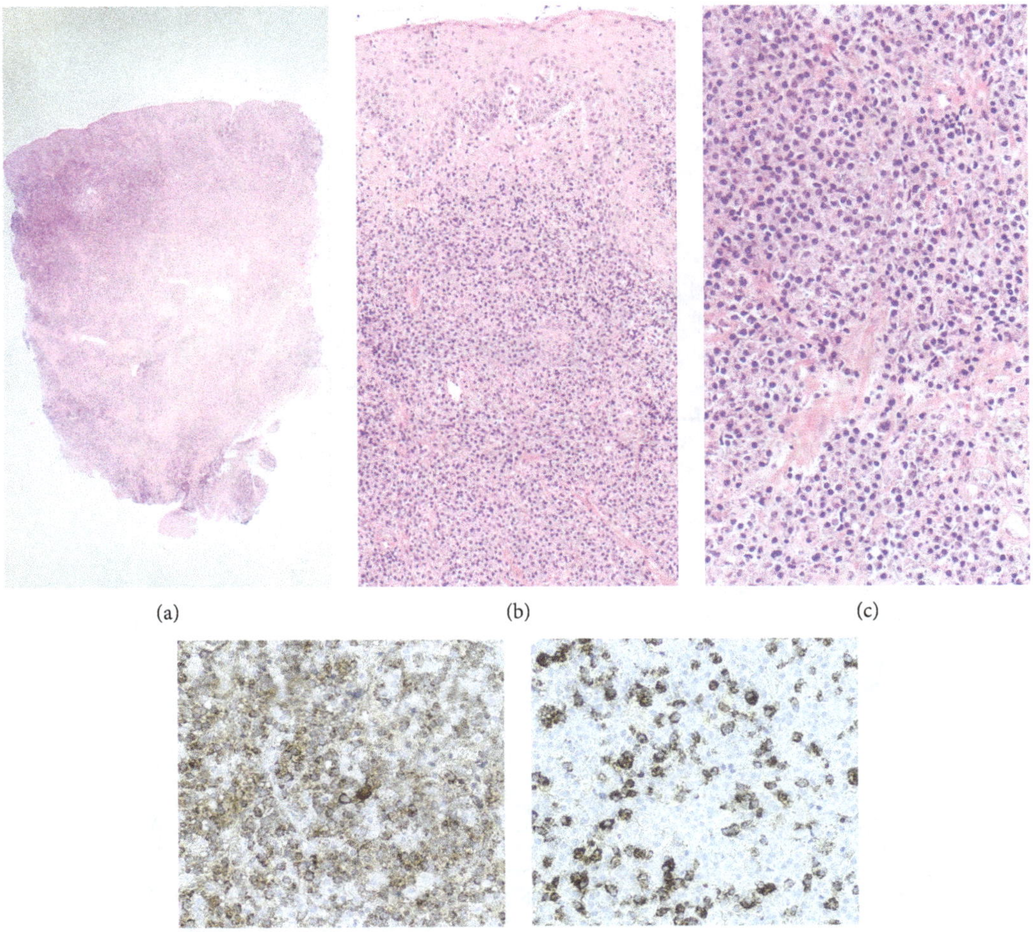

(a) (b) (c)

(d) (e)

FIGURE 2: (a) The panoramic histological picture shows an oral mucosa punch biopsy, with highly cellular stroma (hematoxylin–eosin 20×). (b) At higher magnification, the oral mucosa appears spongiotic with mononuclear cell exocytosis, associated with dense stromal inflammation (hematoxylin–eosin 100×). (c) The stroma displays an intense infiltration of normal-appearing plasma cells (hematoxylin–eosin 200×). (d) Plasma cells are polyclonal, expressing both kappa (kappa light chain immunostaining 200×). (e) Lambda light chains (lambda light chain immunostaining 200×).

administration of chlorhexidine twice a day for seven weeks, home oral hygiene instructions and patient motivation, supragingival scaling, and polish, and in separate sessions complete mouth scaling with the administration of tranexamic acid for the reduction of bleeding [16].

2.4. Treatment Progress. Two incisional biopsies were performed. The microscopic findings showed an intense inflamed infiltrate, predominantly plasmacellular, in the peripheral context of the lamina propria with edema and intra-epithelial spongiosis (Figures 2(a)–2(e)). Immunohistochemistry showed no immunoglobulin light chain restriction. The histopathological diagnosis confirmed the clinical hypothesis of PCG.

After informed consent signature, a PBM protocol associated with oral hygiene sessions and instructions for proper oral hygiene at home was planned. PBM treatments, which began in January 2018, were performed with a diode laser (SmartFile, Deka, Calenzano (FI), Italy) with a wavelength of 635 nm, 600-μm fiber, and a handpiece with a 1 cm diameter lens. A power of 300 mW was used, with continuous

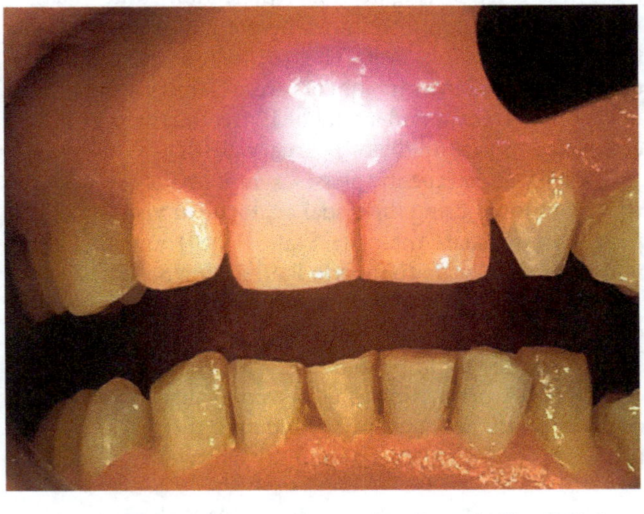

FIGURE 3: Intra-operative view, treatment performed with a diode laser, with a wavelength of 635 nm, 600-μm fiber, and a handpiece with 1 cm diameter lens. A power of 300 mW was used, with continuous emission mode and with application times not exceeding 1 minute/cm^2 (fluence 22 J/cm^2), carrying out grid-like scanning movements.

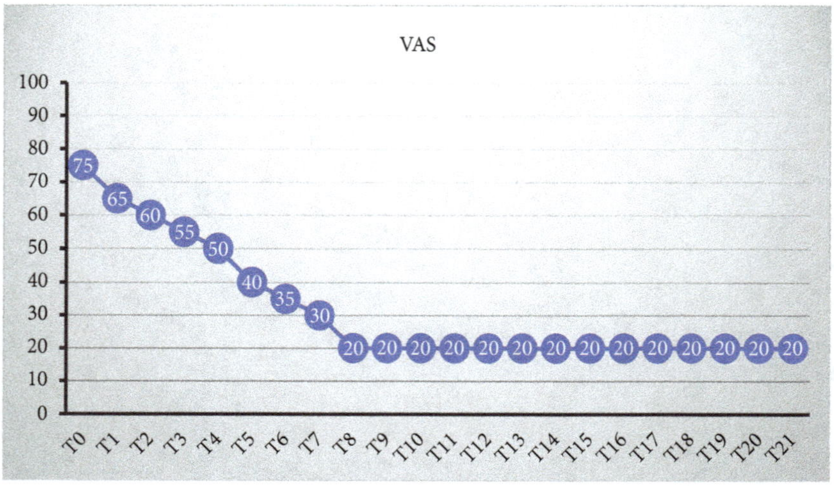

(a)

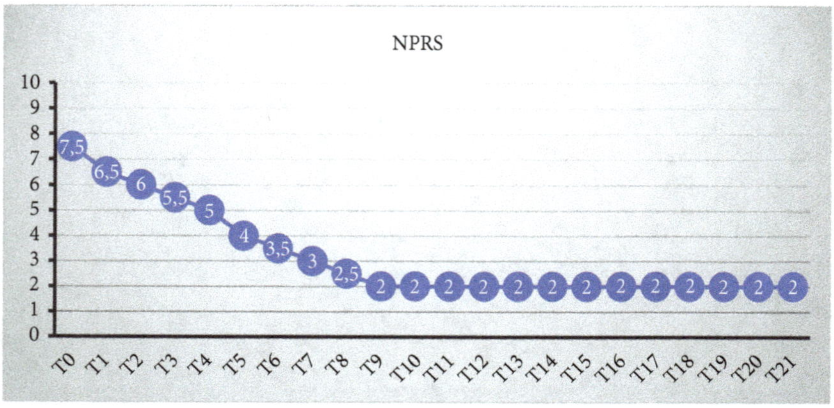

(b)

Figure 4: The trend of measured values over time-related to: (a) Visual Analogue Scale (VAS) and (b) Numeric Pain Rating Scale (NPRS) denotes a decrease in reported symptoms.

emission mode and with application times not exceeding 1 minute/cm^2 (fluence 22 J/cm^2), carrying out grid-like scanning movements (Figure 3). Application time was 12 minutes per session; 6 minutes before and 6 minutes after the hygiene session oral. The treated mucosal area was 6 cm^2. The combined treatments were 3 times a week, for a duration of 4 weeks and a total of 12 treatments, which were completed in the middle of February 2018.

During all therapeutic phases, symptomatic subjectivities were monitored using the visual analogue or visual analogue pain scale (Visual Analogue Scale [VAS]) and the verbal numerical pain scale (Numeric Pain Rating Scale [NPRS]).

Periodontal indices were also evaluated with the degrees of erythema and gingival bleeding. Clinical parameters considered showed an improvement in the four weeks of PBM constant and progressive. Furthermore, there were significant symptomatic reductions found after the first two therapeutic sessions (Figures 4(a) and 4(b)).

2.5. Treatment Results. Throughout 2018, the patient was visited monthly, without observing noteworthy relapses. A second biopsy and histopathological examination were performed about two months after the treatment ended. Histopathological examination showed a stable reduction in inflammation and plasma cell infiltrate. Then, the patient made a control visit every three months, and during the control visit in the year 2020, the blood tests were again requested, including chemistry as well as c-ANCA, p-ANCA, and IgG4 assay tests. The results of the blood chemistry tests indicated: S-Myeloperoxidase antibodies <1.0 (normal range <6.0 U/mL); Proteinase 3 antibodies: 21.8 (normally absent). Upon objective examination, the mucous membranes of the lining appear normo-chromic and normo-perfused in the absence of inflammation and symptoms (Figure 5). The patient was motivated to continue the indicated periodontal therapies and to follow scrupulous oral hygiene.

At the last check carried out in 2022, the patient's mucous membranes did not show signs of inflammation or recurrence of the original lesions (Figure 6).

3. Discussion

PCG is an extended form of plasma cell mucositis of unknown etiology. Only in some patients is it possible to recognize a specific irritant cause that could favor the disease, with consequent remission of the disease after removal [1, 2, 4, 6, 7].

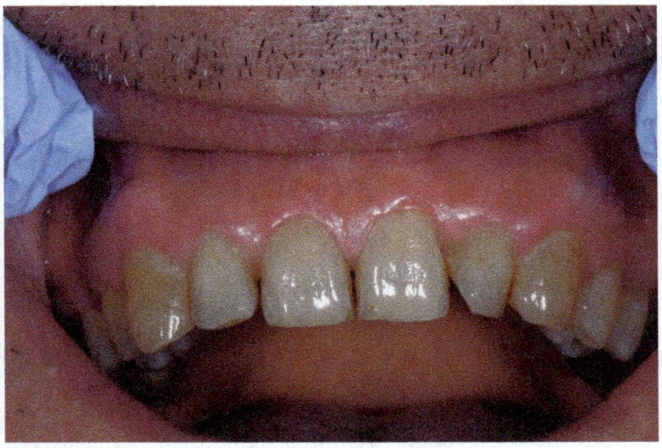

Figure 5: Six month after the end of treatment the mucous membranes of the lining appeared normo-chromic and normo-perfused in the absence of inflammation and symptoms.

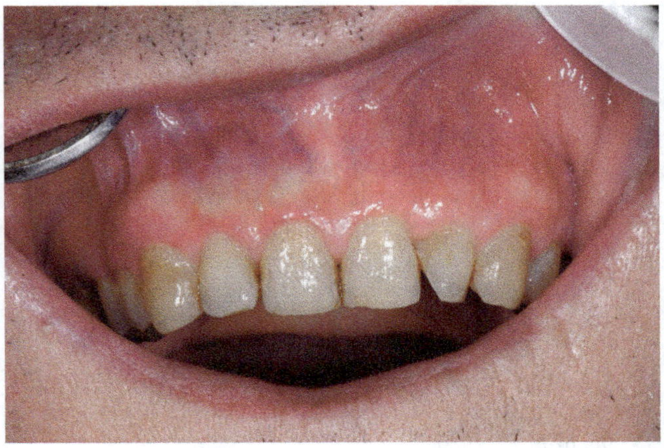

Figure 6: At the last check carried out in 2022, the patient's mucous membranes did not show signs of inflammation or recurrence of the original lesions.

The role that bacterial plaque plays in the etiology of the disease is not clear. Although the lesions often appear in anatomical areas compatible with plaque-induced gingivitis, patients generally do not have significant indices of periodontal inflammation, but a general condition of periodontitis is associated [1, 2, 4, 12].

PCG is histologically characterized by a prevalent plasma cell infiltrate near the basement membrane, associated with spongiosis, and marked exocytosis [4, 6, 7, 9, 15, 17–20]. The histopathological examination is fundamental because this pathology must be placed in a differential diagnosis with chronic non-plaque dependent gingivitis, atrophic-erosive gingivitis, bullous gingivitis, and possible plasma cell neoplastic infiltrates [4, 6, 7, 9, 15, 17–20].

In our clinical experience, we wanted to test the effectiveness of PBM on tissues affected by PCG, to find a valid and lasting therapeutic alternative in the treatment of this disease. In fact, in the literature it is highlighted that laser irradiation could induce a PBM effect on cells and tissues [21, 22], influencing modulation of cell behaviors, and enhancing the processes of tissue repair. PBM could also induce cell proliferation and stem cell differentiation. In addition, laser therapy has an analgesic and anti-inflammatory effect on the treated tissues [21, 22]. It could be interesting in the future to test PBM in combination with ozone therapy [23], probiotics [24], postbiotics [25], and other natural compounds [26] in order to understand if it would be possible to improve tissue repair.

In the illustrated case report, in the clinical evaluations, the parameters of symptomatic subjectivity of the patient were considered through the administration of the VAS and NRS scale, finding a progressive improvement of subjective symptoms. At histological examination, a substantial decrease in plasma cell inflammatory infiltrate in the peripheral context of the lamina propria was found after PBM treatment. To date, after five years of treatment, the patient presents healthy gingival tissue, without noteworthy recurrence of the lesion, with no need of topical steroid therapy.

4. Conclusion

Our case is the first to show the efficacy of PBM treatment with diode lasers in containing PCG, and, above all, the lack of side effects. The use of laser light, capable of inducing PBM effects, has proved to be a valid alternative to pharmacological treatments, which are not stable over time. Indeed, PBM treatment and supportive periodontal therapies have been found to be effective in reducing inflammatory components and gingival bleeding. Importantly, the therapeutic results obtained remained stable for a follow-up period of five-year, without any additional pharmacologic therapy.

Consent

A written informed consent was obtained from all patients before the commencement of the study.

Authors' Contributions

FP: writing—original draft. MPe: writing—original draft. MPa: editing. MPo: investigation, methodology, and writing—review and editing. EK: writing—review, editing, investigation, methodology, and supervision. AS: conceptualization, project administration, and supervision. FS: conceptualization, supervision, data curation, formal analysis, investigation, methodology, and project administration.

References

[1] H. A. Helmy, A. F. Fadel, K. M. Mansour et al., "Unusual presentation of maxillary plasma cell gingivitis mistakenly treated as aggressive periodontitis (a case report)," *International Journal of Surgery Case Reports*, vol. 93, article 106998, 2022.

[2] S. Leuci, N. Coppola, N. Adamo et al., "Clinico-pathological profile and outcomes of 45 cases of plasma cell gingivitis," *Journal of Clinical Medicine*, vol. 10, no. 4, p. 830, 2021.

[3] B. S. Negi, N. R. Kumar, P. S. Haris, J. A. Yogesh, C. Vijayalakshmi, and J. James, "Plasma-cell gingivitis a challenge to the oral physician," *Contemporary Clinical Dentistry*, vol. 10, no. 3, pp. 565–570, 2019.

[4] M. Porrini, M. Rossi, M. Bosotti, S. Marino, and F. Spadari, "Gengivite plasmacellulare, nuovo trattamento con fotobiomodulazione: 2 anni di follow-up," *Dental Cadmos*, vol. 88, no. 6, pp. 394–396, 2020.

[5] Y. Jadwat, R. Meyerov, J. Lemmer, E. J. Raubenheimer, and L. Feller, "Plasma cell gingivitis: does it exist? Report of a case and review of the literature," *SADJ*, vol. 63, no. 7, pp. 394-395, 2008.

[6] V. Vishnu, R. Ramesh, R. P. Radhakrishnan, and R. M. Sreelakshmi, "Plasma cell gingivitis mimicking granulomatous disease: a diagnostic dilemma," *Clinical Advances in Periodontics*, vol. 11, no. 4, pp. 220–224, 2021.

[7] S. Subhadarshani, J. Sarangi, and S. Yadav, "Plasma cell gingivitis," *Indian Dermatology Online Journal*, vol. 11, no. 5, pp. 874-875, 2020.

[8] L. Mahalingam, "The histological observation of laser biopsy versus scalpel biopsy on plasma cell gingivitis," *Journal of Indian Society of Periodontology*, vol. 26, no. 3, pp. 299–301, 2022.

[9] R. M. Lubow, R. L. Cooley, K. S. Hartman, and R. K. McDaniel, "Plasma-cell gingivitis: report of a case," *Journal of Periodontology*, vol. 55, no. 4, pp. 235–241, 1984.

[10] K. M. Schulte and N. Talat, "Castleman's disease—a two compartment model of HHV8 infection," *Nature Reviews. Clinical Oncology*, vol. 7, no. 9, pp. 533–543, 2010.

[11] G. Voiriot, A. Fajac, A. Gibelin, A. Parrot, and M. Fartoukh, "Alveolar lymphocytosis with plasmacytosis in severe COVID-19," *Respiratory Medicine and Research*, vol. 78, p. 100784, 2020.

[12] A. O. Parashis, E. Vardas, and K. Tosios, "Generalized aggressive periodontitis associated with a plasma cell gingivitis lesion: a case report and non-surgical treatment," *Clinical Advances in Periodontics*, vol. 5, no. 2, pp. 91–98, 2015.

[13] J. W. White, K. D. Olsen, and P. M. Banks, "Plasma cell orificial mucositis. Report of a case and review of the literature," *Archives of Dermatology*, vol. 122, no. 11, pp. 1321–1324, 1986.

[14] P. Marker and A. Krogdahl, "Plasma cell gingivitis apparently related to the use of khat: report of a case," *British Dental Journal*, vol. 192, no. 6, pp. 311–313, 2002.

[15] C. Joshi and P. Shukla, "Plasma cell gingivitis," *Journal of Indian Society of Periodontology*, vol. 19, no. 2, pp. 221–223, 2015.

[16] P. G. Arduino, F. D'Aiuto, C. Cavallito et al., "Professional oral hygiene as a therapeutic option for pediatric patients with plasma cell gingivitis: preliminary results of a prospective case series," *Journal of Periodontology*, vol. 82, no. 12, pp. 1670–1675, 2011.

[17] N. Lamdari and S. Pradhan, "Plasma cell gingivitis: a case report," *Journal of the Nepal Medical Association*, vol. 52, no. 186, pp. 85–87, 2012.

[18] H. O. Perry, "Idiopathic gingivostomatitis," *Dermatologic Clinics*, vol. 5, no. 4, pp. 719–722, 1987.

[19] J. S. Prasanna, D. A. Mutyap, V. R. Pantula, S. Akula, and B. Chinthapalli, "Plasma cell gingivitis - a conflict of diagnosis," *Journal of Clinical and Diagnostic Research*, vol. 10, no. 11, pp. ZD01–ZD03, 2016.

[20] G. N. Ketkar and G. Kaarthikeyan, "An atypical presentation of plasma cell gingivitis with generalized skin lesions," *Journal of Oral and Maxillofacial Pathology*, vol. 25, no. 4, pp. S54–S57, 2021.

[21] C. Dompe, L. Moncrieff, J. Matys et al., "Photobiomodulation-underlying mechanism and clinical applications," *Journal of Clinical Medicine*, vol. 9, no. 6, p. 1724, 2020.

[22] P. Ebrahimi, M. Hadilou, F. Naserneysari et al., "Effect of photobiomodulation in secondary intention gingival wound healing-a systematic review and meta-analysis," *BMC Oral Health*, vol. 21, no. 1, p. 258, 2021.

[23] A. Butera, S. Gallo, M. Pascadopoli, G. Luraghi, and A. Scribante, "Ozonized water administration in peri-implant mucositis sites: a randomized clinical trial," *Applied Sciences*, vol. 11, no. 17, p. 7812, 2021.

[24] A. Butera, S. Gallo, C. Maiorani et al., "Management of gingival bleeding in periodontal patients with domiciliary use of toothpastes containing hyaluronic acid, lactoferrin, or paraprobiotics: a randomized controlled clinical trial," *Applied Sciences*, vol. 11, no. 18, p. 8586, 2021.

[25] A. Butera, S. Gallo, M. Pascadopoli, D. Taccardi, and A. Scribante, "Home oral care of periodontal patients using antimicrobial gel with postbiotics, lactoferrin, and Aloe barbadensis leaf juice powder vs. conventional chlorhexidine gel: a split-mouth randomized clinical trial," *Antibiotics*, vol. 11, no. 1, p. 118, 2022.

[26] N. Ghasemi, M. Behnezhad, M. Asgharzadeh, E. Zeinalzadeh, and H. S. Kafil, "Antibacterial properties of aloe vera on intracanal medicaments against Enterococcus faecalis biofilm at different stages of development," *International Journal of Dentistry*, vol. 2020, no. 2020, p. 8855276, 2020.

8

Effect of Oral Care in a Patient with Depression and Burning Mouth Syndrome during the COVID-19 Pandemic

Yumiko Nagao,[1,2] **Hitomi Nakagaki**,[2] **and Masahide Tsuji**[2]

[1]*Department of Public Health, Graduate School of Medicine, Juntendo University, Bunkyo-ku, Tokyo 113-8421, Japan*
[2]*Tsuji Dental & Oral Surgery Clinic, Shiragane Machi, Omuta, Fukuoka 836-0052, Japan*

Correspondence should be addressed to Yumiko Nagao; y.nagao.qd@juntendo.ac.jp

Academic Editor: Vlaho Brailo

Burning mouth syndrome (BMS) is a burning sensation that occurs in the mouth without any underlying cause. There is no satisfactory treatment for BMS, so far. Herein, we report the case of a 74-year-old female with untreated depression who presented with BMS. Despite taking antidepressants, she developed suicidal thoughts, particularly due to the increasing number of coronavirus disease 2019 (COVID-19) cases and suicides in Japan. The symptoms of BMS and the oral discomfort were eliminated using a multifaceted approach, which included the following: continuous application of the oral care gel "REFRECARE-H®" to the mucous membranes, regular dental visits, collaboration with medical and dental professionals, and administration of zinc preparations. Her suicidal thoughts had disappeared, and her quality of life, assessed using the visual analogue scale, was improved following the treatment. Dentists should strive to provide oral care, while providing treatment in collaboration with specialists, for the early detection of depression and zinc deficiency in patients with BMS.

1. Introduction

The International Association for the Study of Pain (IASP) described burning mouth syndrome (BMS) as a chronic disease characterized by a burning sensation in the oral mucosa for which the cause cannot be identified [1]. In 2018, the IASP defined the diagnostic criteria for BMS as follows [2]: (a) oral pain fulfilling criteria (b) and (c); (b) recurring daily for >2 hours/day for >3 months; (c) pain has both of the following characteristics: (1) burning quality and (2) felt superficially in the oral mucosa; (d) oral mucosa is of normal appearance and clinical examination including sensory testing is normal; and (e) not better accounted for by another diagnosis.

The burning pain is often accompanied by a tingling sensation, numbness, and dryness in the mouth [3–6]. The prevalence of BMS in the general population is estimated to range from 0.7% to 15%, with a male-to-female ratio of 1 : 7; women are more affected during the peri- and postmenopausal periods [7, 8]. The etiology of BMS is unclear, but it has been suggested that it has a neuropathic origin involving the central and peripheral nerves [9, 10]. According to Feller et al., the pathogenesis of BMS is complex because it involves several psychogenic factors and dysregulated peripheral and central pain pathways [11]. BMS can be treated with clonazepam, a medication used to treat neuropathic pain [12]; vitamin, zinc, and hormone replacement therapy [13–15]; and behavioral cognitive therapy [16].

On the other hand, according to the Ministry of Health, Labor, and Welfare, the number of suicides in Japan in 2020 had increased by 4.5% ($n = 912$) compared to the previous year, marking the first increase in 11 years [17]. While the number of male suicides had decreased for the 11th consecutive year to 14,055, the number of female suicides had increased to 7,026. The Ministry of Health, Labor, and Welfare has indicated that the increase in the number of female suicides might be due to the worsening of factors such as domestic violence (DV) under the extraordinary circumstances of the severe acute respiratory syndrome coronavirus 2 (SARS-CoV-2) epidemic. Tanaka and Okamoto reported that effective prevention of suicide among vulnerable populations is an important public health issue in response to the increase in suicide rates among women and children and adolescents during the COVID19 pandemic [18].

Previously, we reported that the use of REFRECARE-H® (EN Otsuka Pharmaceutical Co. Ltd., Tokyo, Japan), a hinokitiol-containing oral care gel, improved the symptoms of BMS [19] and the quality of life (QOL) of patients with oral lichen planus [20]. Herein, we report a case of a 74-year-old woman who developed suicidal thoughts during treatment for BMS and was treated with REFRECARE-H® in collaboration with other medical professionals.

2. Case Presentation

In September 2019, a 74-year-old Japanese woman visited the Tsuji Dental and Oral Surgery Clinic (Fukuoka, Japan) complaining of a tingling pain and dryness in the tongue and a salty taste in the mouth when at rest; the symptoms had begun about five to six years ago (2013–2014). She had frequently consulted her family physician and dentist before visiting our clinic but did not receive any proper advice or treatment for the symptoms. No organic abnormalities were observed in the oral cavity. Evaluation of the tongue dryness using an oral moisture-checking device (Mucus®; Life Co. Ltd., Saitama, Japan) [21] resulted in normal values (30.1). In the taste test using the salt-impregnated test paper, SALSAVE® (Advantec Toyo Co. Ltd., Tokyo, Japan), which was prepared with various salt concentrations (0.6, 0.8, 1.0, 1.2, 1.4, and 1.6 mg/cm^2), she was unable to distinguish the saltiness, even at high concentrations. The patient was not in the habit of drinking or smoking. No signs of gingival inflammation, oral lichen planus, Sjögren's syndrome, *Candida albicans*, or oral cancer were found in the mouth. Serum anti-SS-A and anti-SS-B antibodies were negative, and there were no clinical signs of Candidiasis which was also confirmed with mycological swab and fungal culture. Subsequently, the patient was diagnosed with BMS by an oral surgeon at our clinic. Table 1 shows the medications that the patient was taking at the time of the first visit to our clinic. Some of these drugs had been reported to have oral side effects, but the drugs could not be systemically changed or discontinued.

She had developed depression, hypertension, angina pectoris, and idiopathic atrial fibrillation about 25 years ago (at the age of 50), cervical and lumbar stenosis at the age of 55, and reflux esophagitis at the age of 65, for which she was treated by various specialists. Her depression was triggered by the illness and death of her mother when she was 50 years old and later exacerbated by the illness and death of her son when she was 57 years old. The depression was left untreated since February 2019 due to relocation. Furthermore, the patient had undergone cholecystectomy for a benign gallbladder tumor at the age of 39 and an endoscopic polypectomy for colon cancer at 66 years of age.

The pathogenesis of BMS was explained to the patient in detail. She was instructed to brush her teeth after meals and apply REFRECARE-H® to the oral mucosa. Additionally, preventive treatment for periodontal disease and denture prosthesis for the missing teeth were provided at the clinic. The patient had not been treated for depression for over six months; hence, she was referred to a psychiatric clinic and started on antidepressants. In October 2019, the following three medications were administered by the psychiatrist: escitalopram oxalate, a selective serotonin reuptake inhibitor (SSRI), triazolam, and flunitrazepam as benzodiazepine.

The visual analogue scale (VAS) is a simple and frequently used method to evaluate variations in pain intensity [22]. It is represented by a horizontal line, 100 mm in length, anchored by word descriptors at each end, as illustrated in Figure 1; the patients marked the point that they felt most accurately represented their perception of their current state. The VAS score was determined by measuring in mm from the left end of the line to the point that was marked by the patient. The VAS was measured 5 months prior to the patient's visit to our clinic (April 2019) and periodically between September 6, 2019, when the patient first visited our clinic, and May 21, 2021. The mean and changes in the score are shown in Table 2 and Figure 2, respectively. Application of REFRECARE-H® improved the QOL such as dry mouth, breath odor, refreshing mouth, oral pain during rest, oral pain at a mealtime, taste disorder, loss of appetite, sleep disorder, depressive moodiness, and jitteriness.

In October 2019, the patient's tongue pain symptoms had decreased and regular monthly follow-up showed an improving trend. However, since the beginning of 2020, following the prevalence of SARS-CoV-2 infection in the country, a nationwide state of emergency was declared in April and news of the suicides of several celebrities was reported in July. Consequently, she began to admit to suicidal ideation by August 2020, saying "I want to die too" every time she had a dental revisit. Therefore, the frequency of visits to our clinic was increased, information was shared with the psychiatrist and gastroenterologist, and oral care was implemented through medical cooperation. At each visit, we, the dentists, made sure that there were no physical problems in the oral cavity or head and neck areas and explained these to the patient, as well as instructed her to eat, sleep, and exercise regularly. We also listened to and supported the psychosocial issues behind the patient's symptoms. At each visit, we displayed the VAS score visualized over time and explained the clear improvement in BMS and depressive symptoms compared to that before treatment. The application of REFRECARE-H® to the oral mucosa was continued daily. Eventually, the suicidal thoughts disappeared in December 2020. On December 26, she suffered a thoracic vertebrae fracture in a traffic accident and was required to undergo rest therapy but she never complained of wanting to die. In March 2021, the symptoms of BMS completely disappeared and have not recurred since.

From the initial visit to the present, the results of the tongue dryness assessments were normal. However, in the taste test using SALSAVE®, she was still unable to distinguish the saltiness in December 2020. Subsequently, about two months later (February 2021), she was able to recognize the taste naturally (value, 1.4), and in March, she could recognize the saltiness at low concentrations (value, 0.8). She presented with a low serum zinc level (67 μg/dL) on March 26, 2021 (Table 3), and was treated with zinc acetate dihydrate (NOBELZIN®, Nobelpharma Co. Ltd., Tokyo, Japan)

TABLE 1: Medications that the patient was taking at the time of the first visit.

Generic names	Japan trade names	Treatment in this case	Side effect		
			Oropharyngeal discomfort (yes/no)	Dry mouth (yes/no)	Taste disorders (yes/no)
Irbesartan and amlodipine besilate	ILUAMIX combination tablets	Hypertension	No	Yes (frequency: unknown)	Yes (frequency: unknown)
Bepridil hydrochloride hydrate	BEPRICOR tablets	Angina pectoris, and idiopathic atrial fibrillation	No	Yes (frequency: less than 0.1–0.5%)	No
Dabigatran etexilate methanesulfonate	PRAZAXA capsules	Idiopathic atrial fibrillation	Yes (frequency: less than 1%)	No	No
Limaprost alfadex	Limaprost alfadex	Cervical and lumbar stenosis	No	Yes (frequency: less than 0.1%)	Yes (frequency: less than 0.1%)
Mecobalamin	Methycobal	Cervical and lumbar stenosis	No	No	No
Tocopherol acetate	Juvela	Cervical and lumbar stenosis	No	No	No

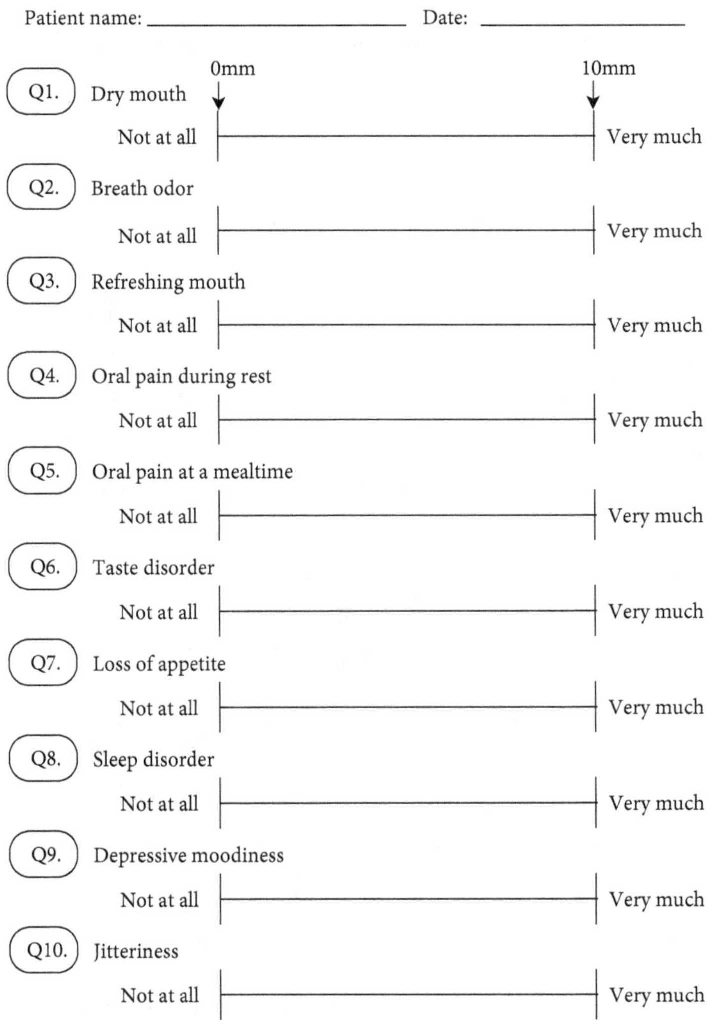

FIGURE 1: The VAS of 10 items. The VAS is a horizontal line, 100 mm in length, anchored by word descriptors at each end.

in April. The normal range of serum zinc concentration is from 80 μg/dL to 130 μg/dL. However, oral administration of NOBLEZIN was discontinued after 3 weeks due to adverse drug reactions such as diarrhea and itching. On May 7, the serum zinc level had been reduced to 70 μg/dL (below normal) but the taste sensitivity remained improved and she was able to recognize low concentrations of saltiness (value, 0.6). As shown in Table 3, free thyroxine 4 (FT4),

Table 2: VAS score before the dental visit and during REFRECARE-H application.

Subjective symptoms	Before visit (before application) April 2019	After visit (during of application) Mean ± SD
Dry mouth (mm)	100	5.76 ± 10.29
Breath odor (mm)	78	1.07 ± 4.06
Refreshing mouth (mm)	83	7.01 ± 10.40
Oral pain during rest (mm)	60	6.14 ± 4.90
Oral pain at a mealtime (mm)	54	0.46 ± 3.92
Taste disorder (mm)	79	0.94 ± 4.33
Loss of appetite (mm)	73	12.17 ± 19.78
Sleep disorder (mm)	75	48.17 ± 24.07
Depressive moodiness (mm)	89	16.92 ± 24.53
Jitteriness (mm)	63	10.92 ± 16.75

SD: standard deviation.

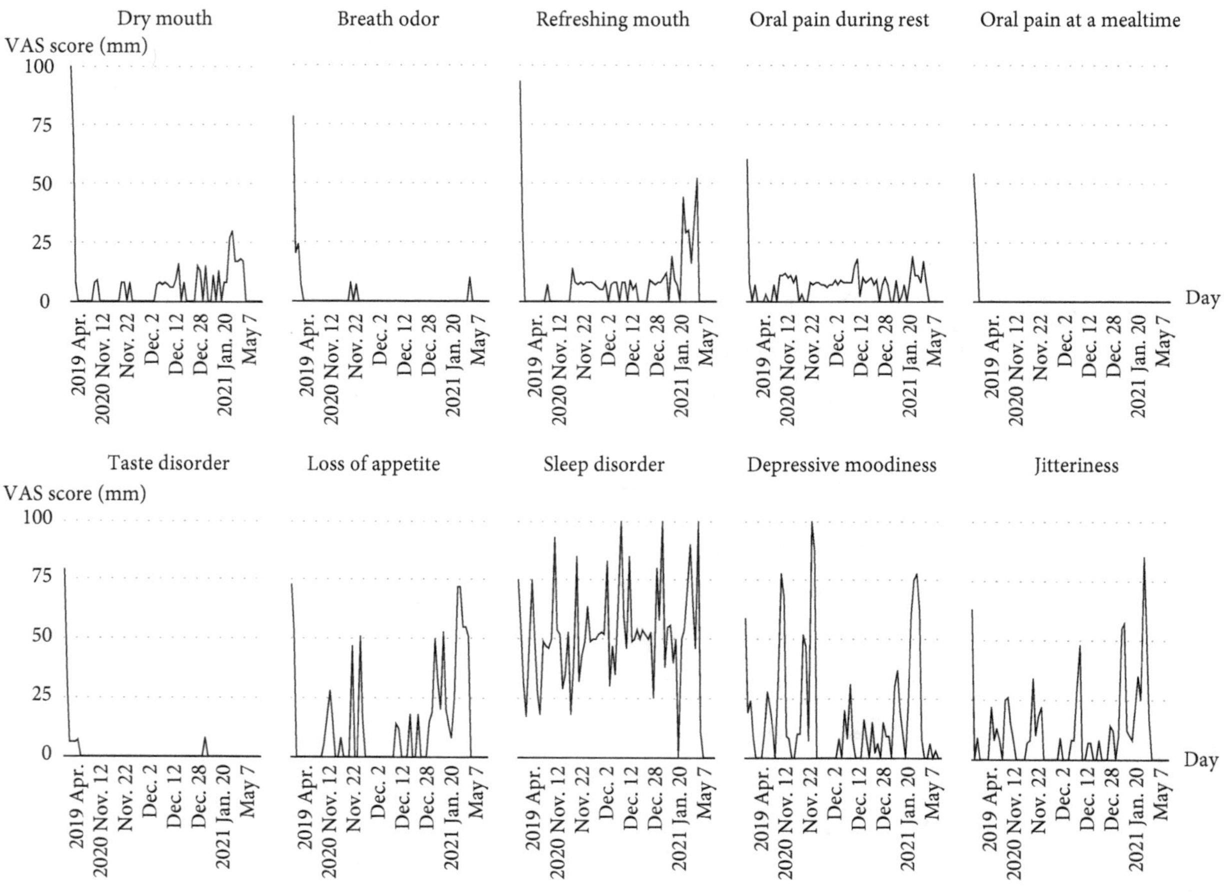

Figure 2: The distributions of the VAS scores before the dental visit and during the application of REFRECARE-H.

thyroid-stimulating hormone (TSH), HbA1c, and blood glucose levels were normal, indicating no abnormal thyroid function or diabetes mellitus in this patient.

3. Discussion

The tongue pain symptoms in this case showed a tendency to improve after SSRI and benzodiazepines were administered to treat comorbid depression, indicating that BMS may be due to psychological factors. As for the zinc deficiency, since no blood test was performed at the time of the first visit, it is impossible to evaluate whether the patient had zinc deficiency from the time of the first visit or from March 2021. However, since the patient later showed improvement in taste disorder even though the zinc level was below normal, it is considered that the underlying cause

Table 3: Summary of laboratory data.

	Normal range	213 days after the first visit	1 year and 201 days after the first visit	1 year and 243 days after the first visit	1 year and 304 days after the first visit
Date		April 6, 2020	March 26, 2021	May 7, 2021	July 7, 2021
Age		75 years old	76 years old	76 years old	76 years old
Taste disorder by taste test		Positive	Negative	Negative	Negative
Dry mouth using an oral moisture-checking device		Negative	Negative	Negative	Negative
White blood cell (μL)	3,500–9,200	5,400	4,400	5,100	2,410
Red blood cell ($10^4/\mu$L)	370–490	482	460	496	467
Hemoglobin (g/dL)	11.5–15.5	13.9	13.3	14.0	13.3
Hematocrit (%)	35.0–45.0	41.0	40.8	43.6	41.1
Platelet count ($10^4/\mu$L)	10.0–40.0	20.3	24.4	28.7	20.6
Fasting blood glucose (mg/dL)	70–110	Unknown	Unknown	Unknown	90
HbA1c (%)	4.6–6.2	5.8	Unknown	Unknown	Unknown
Total protein (g/dL)	6.7–8.3	Unknown	Unknown	6.8	6.1
Albumin (g/dL)	4.0–5.0	Unknown	Unknown	4.4	4.1
Total bilirubin (mg/dL)	0.3–1.2	Unknown	Unknown	0.4	0.6
ALP (U/L)	38–113	Unknown	Unknown	101	67
LDH (U/L)	124–222	Unknown	189	226	165
AST (U/L)	13–33	17	16	20	18
ALT (U/L)	6–30	16	14	16	14
γ-GTP (U/L)	10–47	15	18	16	15
Total cholesterol (mg/dL)	128–219	Unknown	239	225	226
HDL, mg/dL	40–96	48	Unknown	Unknown	36
LDL (mg/dL)	80–139	162	117	Unknown	137
Triglyceride (mg/dL)	30–149	208	501	Unknown	133
CK (U/L)	45–163	Unknown	80	Unknown	55
BUN (mg/dL)	8.0–20.0	Unknown	17.1	12.8	12.5
Creatinine (mg/dL)	0.40–0.70	0.70	0.68	0.76	0.75
Na (mEq/L)	138–146	Unknown	140	144	140
K (mEq/L)	3.6–4.9	Unknown	4.3	4.0	4.2
Cl (mEq/L)	99–109	Unknown	102	104	105
Ca (mg/dL)	8.7–10.3	Unknown	9.1	Unknown	8.9
Zinc (μg/dL)	80–130	Unknown	67	70	64
Copper (μg/dL)	66–130	Unknown	Unknown	147	Unknown
FT4 (ng/dL)	0.90–1.70	Unknown	1.03	Unknown	Unknown
TSH (μIU/mL)	0.500-5.000	Unknown	3.440	Unknown	Unknown

ALP: alkaline phosphatase; LDH: lactic dehydrogenase; AST: aspartate aminotransferase; ALT: alanine aminotransferase; γ-GTP: gamma-glutamyl transpeptidase; HDL: high-density lipoprotein; LDL: low-density lipoprotein; FT4: free thyroxine 4; TSH: thyroid-stimulating hormone.

of the painful tongue symptoms was not zinc deficiency. In other words, both tongue pain and taste disorder have a great possibility of being a series of symptoms associated with depression. Four of the medications (irbesartan and amlodipine besilate, bepridil hydrochloride hydrate, dabigatran etexilate methanesulfonate, and limaprost alfadex) that the patient was taking when she was diagnosed with BMS have side effects of oropharyngeal discomfort, dry mouth, and taste disorders as shown in Table 1. However, even though these medications are still being taken, the oral symptoms have disappeared, and therefore, the possibility of drug side effects is very low.

The diagnosis of BMS is defined by IASP as "can only be made when the oral mucosa is clinically normal and all systemic and local causes for a burning sensation have been ruled out" [11]. Because it is important to examine systemic and local causes of burning sensations in the mouth, blood tests to screen for comorbidities and other chronic pain should be performed in addition to performing a basic oral examination at the initial visit.

BMS patients often complain of taste abnormalities [23–25]. It has been reported that 69% of BMS patients ($n = 49$) had taste disorders [23]. Of 276 BMS patients, 74 (26.8%) were reported to have hypozincemia and zinc replacement therapy, which improved the symptoms of BMS [14]. Zinc is essential for many metabolic and enzymatic functions [26]. These findings suggest that zinc measurement should be performed at least once in patients with BMS.

The number of patients with taste disorders in Japan is increasing [27]. In 2003, it was reported that the number of patients with taste disorders in Japan was 240,000 per year, having a 1.8-fold increase from a survey in 1990 [27]. One of the reasons for this is the annual increase in the elderly population in the country [28].

The death of the mother due to terminal cancer triggered the onset of depression in the patient in this report. Subsequently, the death of her eldest son due to illness and the fact that she was currently living alone may have aggravated her depression and led to the development of BMS. The patient had not received any explanation regarding the pathogenesis of the tongue condition despite visiting several medical institutions over a period of 4–5 months. Knowledge and understanding of BMS in medical and dental clinics are necessary in order to be able to treat this condition at an early stage.

We had previously reported a case in which an oral care gel was effectively used in a patient with BMS [19]. In this case of the current study, oral care gel was used as an adjunct to relieve the pain in the tongue. Our findings indicate that, although the mechanism remains unknown, the application of an oral care gel might be effective in treating burning sensation in the mouth.

As of May 31, 2021, the number of people infected with SARS-CoV-2 in Japan was 746,745 and the number of deaths was 13,060. It was pointed out that the impact of COVID-19 on people is immeasurable, with significant psychological, social, and economic damage leading to increased mental illness, suicide, DV, and abuse of children and the elderly [29]. The number of BMS patients is expected to increase with the outbreak of SARS-CoV-2.

In conclusion, in this study, the adjunctive use of an oral care gel was effective in improving the subjective symptoms and QOL of the patient with burning sensation in the mouth. When patients with burning sensation in the mouth visit the dental clinic, it is important to check for the presence of hypozincemia and a history of depression and to provide collaborative treatment with the family physician or specialist. During the COVID-19 pandemic, dentists need to provide medical interventions and emotional support while listening to the patient's complaints and concerns.

Abbreviations

BMS: Burning mouth syndrome
SARS-CoV-2: Severe acute respiratory syndrome coronavirus 2
COVID-19: Coronavirus disease 2019
QOL: Quality of life
DV: Domestic violence
VAS: Visual analogue scale.

Consent

Informed written consent was obtained from the patient for the publication of this case report.

Authors' Contributions

YN, HN, and MT contributed to the clinical analyses of the case studied. YN contributed to the study design, review of the literature, final data analyses, and manuscript writing. All authors have read and approved the final manuscript.

Acknowledgments

We would like to thank Dr. Oka K (director of Oka Clinic), Dr. Tomiyasu N (director of Kohama Clinic), and Dr. Tsukamoto Y (director of Kurumi Clinic) for providing us with medical information. This study was supported in part by the Japan Society for the Promotion of Science (JSPS) KAKENHI Grant-in-Aid for Scientific Research (C), Grant numbers JP17K12012 and JP21K10263.

References

[1] "IASP orofacial pain fact sheet. Burning mouth syndome," September 2016, https://www.iasp-pain.org/files/Content/ContentFolders/GlobalYearAgainstPain2/20132014OrofacialPain/FactSheets/Burning_Mouth_Syndrome_2016.pdf.

[2] Headache Classification Committee of the International Headache Society (IHS), "The International Classification of Headache Disorders, 3rd edition," *Cephalalgia*, vol. 38, pp. 1–211, 2018.

[3] A. Scala, L. Checchi, M. Montevecchi, I. Marini, and M. A. Giamberardino, "Update on burning mouth syndrome: overview and patient management," *Critical Reviews in Oral Biology and Medicine*, vol. 14, pp. 275–291, 2003.

[4] L. L. Patton, M. A. Siegel, R. Benoliel, and A. De Laat, "Management of burning mouth syndrome: systematic review and management recommendations," *Oral Surgery, Oral Medicine, Oral Pathology, Oral Radiology, and Endodontology*, vol. 103, no. suppl. 39, pp. e1–13, 2007.

[5] J. A. Buchanan and J. M. Zakrzewska, "Burning mouth syndrome," *BMJ Clinical Evidence*, vol. 2010, p. 1301, 2010.

[6] G. E. Gurvits and A. Tan, "Burning mouth syndrome," *World Journal of Gastroenterology*, vol. 19, pp. 665–672, 2013.

[7] A. Sun, K. M. Wu, Y. P. Wang, H. P. Lin, H. M. Chen, and C. P. Chiang, "Burning mouth syndrome: a review and update," *Journal of Oral Pathology & Medicine*, vol. 42, pp. 649–655, 2013.

[8] J. M. Zakrzewska, H. Forssell, and A. M. Glenny, "Interventions for the treatment of burning mouth syndrome," *Cochrane Database of Systematic Reviews*, vol. 1, article Cd002779, 2005.

[9] L. Charleston, "Burning mouth syndrome: a review of recent literature," *Current Pain and Headache Reports*, vol. 17, p. 336, 2013.

[10] S. K. Jääskeläinen, "Pathophysiology of primary burning mouth syndrome," *Clinical Neurophysiology*, vol. 123, pp. 71–77, 2012.

[11] L. Feller, J. Fourie, M. Bouckaert, R. A. G. Khammissa, R. Ballyram, and J. Lemmer, "Burning Mouth Syndrome: Aetiopathogenesis and Principles of Management," *Pain Research and Management*, vol. 2017, Article ID 1926269, 6 pages, 2017.

[12] S. M. Heckmann, E. Kirchner, M. Grushka, M. G. Wichmann, and T. Hummel, "A double-blind study on clonazepam in patients with burning mouth syndrome," *Laryngoscope*, vol. 122, pp. 813–816, 2012.

[13] A. Sun, H. P. Lin, Y. P. Wang, H. M. Chen, S. J. Cheng, and C. P. Chiang, "Significant reduction of serum homocysteine level and oral symptoms after different vitamin-supplement treatments in patients with burning mouth syndrome," *Journal of Oral Pathology & Medicine*, vol. 42, pp. 474–479, 2013.

[14] G. S. Cho, M. W. Han, B. Lee et al., "Zinc deficiency may be a cause of burning mouth syndrome as zinc replacement therapy has therapeutic effects," *Journal of Oral Pathology & Medicine*, vol. 39, pp. 722–727, 2010.

[15] A. Forabosco, M. Criscuolo, G. Coukos et al., "Efficacy of hormone replacement therapy in postmenopausal women with oral discomfort," *Oral Surgery, Oral Medicine, and Oral Pathology*, vol. 73, pp. 570–574, 1992.

[16] O. Komiyama, H. Nishimura, Y. Makiyama et al., "Group cognitive-behavioral intervention for patients with burning mouth syndrome," *Journal of Oral Science*, vol. 55, no. 1, pp. 17–22, 2013.

[17] "Ministry of Health, Labour and Welfare, Suicide situation in 2020," 2020, https://www.mhlw.go.jp/content/R2kakutei-01.pdf.

[18] T. Tanaka and S. Okamoto, "Increase in suicide following an initial decline during the COVID-19 pandemic in Japan," *Nature Human Behaviour*, vol. 5, pp. 229–238, 2021.

[19] Y. Nagao, Y. Kawahigashi, K. Kimura, and M. Sata, "Effect of oral care gel for burning mouth syndrome in a patient with hepatitis C: a case report," *Case Reports in Gastroenterology*, vol. 11, pp. 480–487, 2017.

[20] Y. Nagao and M. Sata, "Effect of oral care gel on the quality of life for oral lichen planus in patients with chronic HCV infection," *Virology Journal*, vol. 8, p. 348, 2011.

[21] Y. Fukushima, T. Yoda, S. Kokabu et al., "Evaluation of an oral moisture-checking device for screening dry mouth," *Open Journal of Stomatology*, vol. 3, no. 8, pp. 440–446, 2013.

[22] C. R. Chapman, K. L. Casey, R. Dubner, K. M. Foley, R. H. Gracely, and A. E. Reading, "Pain measurement: an overview," *Pain*, vol. 22, pp. 1–31, 1985.

[23] M. Grushka, "Clinical features of burning mouth syndrome," *Oral Surgery, Oral Medicine, and Oral Pathology*, vol. 63, pp. 30–36, 1987.

[24] O. Hershkovich and R. M. Nagler, "Biochemical analysis of saliva and taste acuity evaluation in patients with burning mouth syndrome, xerostomia and/or gustatory disturbances," *Archives of Oral Biology*, vol. 49, pp. 515–522, 2004.

[25] B. K. Formaker and M. E. Frank, "Taste function in patients with oral burning," *Chemical Senses*, vol. 25, pp. 575–581, 2000.

[26] R. S. MacDonald, "The role of zinc in growth and cell proliferation," *The Journal of Nutrition*, vol. 130, pp. 1500s–1508s, 2000.

[27] M. Ikeda, T. Aiba, A. Ikui et al., "Taste disorders: a survey of the examination methods and treatments used in Japan," *Acta Oto-Laryngologica*, vol. 125, pp. 1203–1210, 2005.

[28] M. Ikeda, A. Ikui, A. Komiyama, D. Kobayashi, and M. Tanaka, "Causative factors of taste disorders in the elderly, and therapeutic effects of zinc," *The Journal of Laryngology and Otology*, vol. 122, pp. 155–160, 2008.

[29] J. Shigemura, S. Takahashi, and M. Kurosawa, "Toward the understanling of the psychosocial effect of COVID-19 pandemic (in Japanese)," *JSTSS Society Journal*, vol. 18, pp. 71–79, 2020.

9

Pemphigus Vulgaris in Old Patient

Bassel Tarakji

Department of Oral and Maxillofacial Surgery and Diagnostic Sciences, College of Dentistry Prince Sattam Bin Abdulaziz University, Al-Kharj, Saudi Arabia

Correspondence should be addressed to Bassel Tarakji; denpol@yahoo.co.uk

Academic Editor: Giuseppe Alessandro Scardina

Pemphigus vulgaris (PV) is a chronic, autoimmune, intraepidermal blistering disease of the skin and mucous membranes. The first clinical manifestation is often the development of intraoral lesions, and later, the lesions involve the other mucous membranes and skin. The etiological factors of this disease still remain unknown, although the presence of autoantibodies is consistent with an autoimmune disease. A 73-year-old man had bullous lesions on gingiva, oral mucosa first, then scalp, trunk, and face. An oral medicine specialist suspects the lesion in differential diagnosis in the first presentation of oral lesions and follows up the patient, and then these bullous lesions presented on the skin. In this article, a patient had received oral prednisolone (80 mg/kg/day) and azathioprine, then tapered oral prednisolone to 40 mg/day, with a reduction of 5 mg/day every three weeks. The patient shows remission of these lesions, and complication of this treatment includes osteoporosis, hyperglycemia, and hypertension.

1. Introduction

Pemphigus vulgaris (PV) is an autoimmune vesiculobullous skin disease in that the immune system produces autoantibody against the specific proteins of the desmosomal adhesion complex that led to the intraepidermal blister formation [1]. Pemphigus vulgaris is seen between third and sixth decades of life [2]. Blisters are associated with the binding of IgG autoantibodies of keratinocyte cell surface molecules [1, 2]. PV antibodies bind to keratinocyte desmosomes and to desmosome-free areas of the keratinocyte cell membrane [3]. Pemphigus vulgaris is slightly predominate in women and manifests in adults during fifth and sixth ages of life [3]. This case is very rare in Syria because most cases identified in literature are middle-aged, not elderly [3]. Most patients complain of painful mucous membrane erosions and may be the only sign of PV of average few months before skin lesions develop [3, 4]. Lesions may occur anywhere on the oral mucosa [4, 5], but the buccal mucosa is the most commonly affected site [4, 5]. Erosive or desquamative gingivitis is a common manifestation of the disease [4–6]. Early oral lesions of PV are difficult to diagnose, and dentists and oral medicine specialists have the main role in early detection.

2. Case Presentation

A 73-year-old male patient from Aleppo city in Syria referred to a dermatology private clinic and oral medicine clinic in Aleppo University.

The patient complains of bullous lesions on gingiva, oral mucosa first, then on scalp, trunk, and face (Figures 1–3). The patient indicates no history of medication. I have followed up the patient to detect bullous lesions if it develops on the skin. Crusted plaques were identified on the scalp, trunk, and face. In oral medicine clinic, clinical intraoral examination indicated to erosions and erythematous on gingiva and buccal mucosa. The patient indicated in the medical history that the oral erosion lesions started few months before the presentation of bullous lesions on his skin. I have referred the patient to a dermatology clinic for evaluation as well. Clinical examination of his skin indicates that the hyperpigmented circular patches were identified over the chest and abdomen as well as a sequel of rupture of bullae.

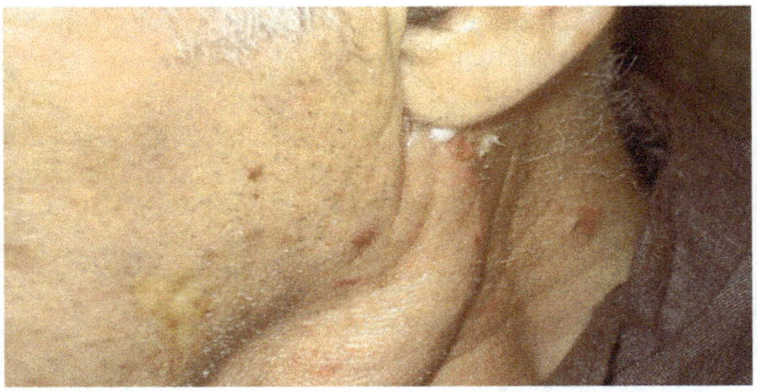

Figure 1: Bullous blisters on the face.

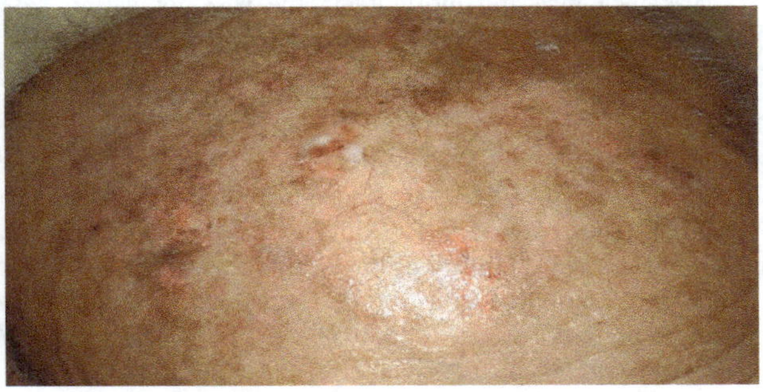

Figure 2: Bullous blisters on the scalp.

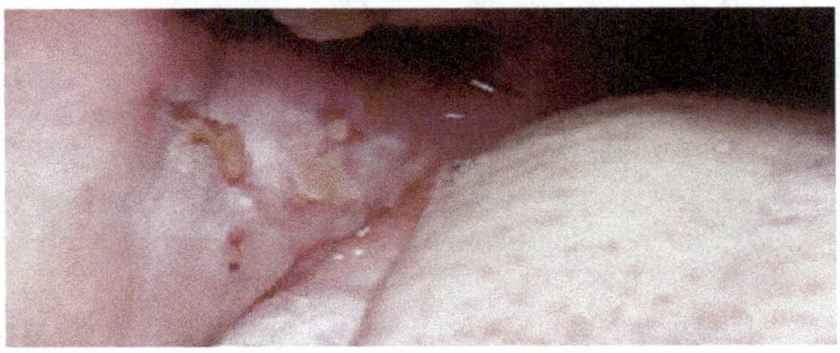

Figure 3: Erosions on the buccal mucosa.

Biopsy of skin lesions from fresh vesicles showed a suprabasal cleft formation and a row of "tomb-stone" appearance of basal cells. Direct immunofluorescence showed deposition of IgG in epidermis (Figure 4). The diagnosis confirmed as pemphigus vulgaris (Table 1).

The patient received oral prednisolone (80 mg/kg/day) and azathioprine. The consent form was signed by the patient, and ethical approval was taken from Aleppo University. The dose of prednisolone was slowly tapered down to 40 mg/day (then decrease to 5 mg every three weeks). Specialists in dermatology and oral medicine follow the lesions on his skin and mouth, respectively. All lesions show complete recovery. The patient had received the high doses of prednisolone in hospital at the beginning of treatment. The daily evaluation for this case by specialists in dermatology, oral medicine, and internal medicine is very strict. The patient has complication such as diabetic, fasting blood sugar showing 160 mg/dL, depression, and osteoporosis. The patient remained under the treatment of 5 mg/day and 100 mg/day of prednisolone and azathioprine, respectively. The patient shows complete remission achieved three years

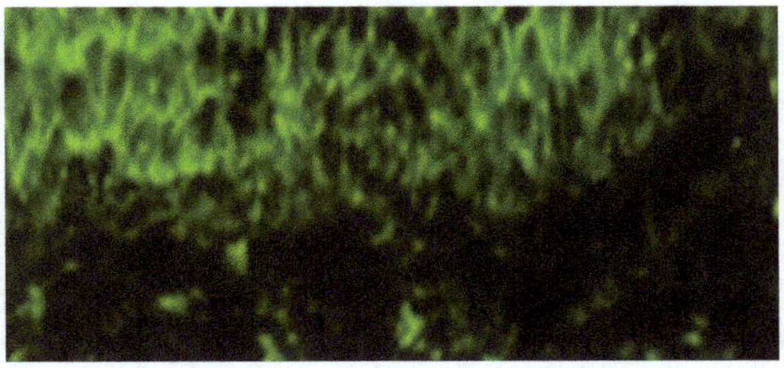

Figure 4: Immunofluorescence showed deposition of IgG in the epidermis.

Table 1: The description of this case.

Main variables	Description
Age	73
Gender	Male
Patient history	No medication
Clinical features and oral examination	Bullous lesions on his head, trunk, and face; erosions on buccal mucosa, erythematous areas on the gingiva (desquamative gingivitis); and oral mucosa
Diagnosis	Pemphigus vulgaris
Treatment	80 mg/d oral prednisolone, then reduced to 40 mg/day, and subsequently a 5 mg reduction of the prednisolone every three weeks to complete the remission of the lesion. Patient remained under treatment of 5 mg/d prednisolone and 100 mg/d azathioprine

from diagnosis. The patient shows side effects such as osteoporosis hyperglycemia and hypertension.

3. Discussion

I have indicated in this case that a 73-year-old patient with pemphigus vulgaris, complaining of mucocutaneous lesions, has fully recovered from the lesions. This case is consistent with Patvekar and Sadana [6] who reported a 94-year-old woman diagnosed with pemphigus vulgaris. Langan et al. [7] have reported that the median age at presentation in the UK is 71 years old (range, 21-102). Martel et al. [8] reported that PV incidence occurs in the third and sixth decades of life. PV occurs most often at the fifth decade of life and not in the elderly [9, 10]. Although the development of blisters and erosions in elderly patients is not fully understood, but this could be of immunologic dysregulation which occurs with aging. Also, it might be that there are differences in the skin between young and elderly patients. Parker and Kelfresh [11] indicated that the development of early blisters is more readily in the elderly skin compared to young patients. Pemphigus vulgaris is a high-risk disease and needs urgent treatment, and its prognosis is not good if the patient left without treatment. Treatment includes corticosteroids and/or immunosuppressor medication such as azathioprine and methotrexate. The patient received the initial low-dose oral prednisolone at the concentration of 80 mg/day for two weeks while he was hospitalized. The prednisolone dose was reduced to 40 mg/day. The reason for this decrease was to minimize the risk of potential side effects [2]. Based on the clinical examinations and laboratory tests, the physicians decided to reduce the dose of prednisolone to 40 mg/day, then reduced to 5 mg/day every three weeks as they evaluate the patient daily, most blisters and erosions show good improvement, and the general health of the patient was good. Herman et al. [2] have suggested a reduction of 5 to 10 mg of prednisolone per week and more slowly less than 20 mg prednisolone per day; however, the dosing schedules are experimental and can modify it depending on the practical experience and patients' situation [2]. The treatment may be withdrawn if there is prolonged clinical healing. The use of high doses of systemic corticosteroids is associated with complication such as osteoporosis and hyperglycemia [12–14]. In this case, the patient shows osteoporosis due to the aging and long use of prednisolone. Also, my patient shows hyperglycemia due to a high dosage of corticosteroids, but his blood sugar before start treatment was borderline, 125 mg/dL. The patient had hypertension due to depression and long-term treatment for pemphigus vulgaris.

This complicated case needs strict joint consultation to find the treatment plan. The role of oral medicine physician is so important to detect the early lesions in the mouth in cooperation with a dermatologist and internal medicine to follow up the patient. I believe that dentists and especially oral medicine can evaluate the abnormal lesions related to autoimmunity disease, and that can help the patient to detect these lesions as early as possible. Assessment of pemphigus vulgaris in literature especially in elderly patients is so limited.

It is recommended to highlight the difficulties in this complicated disease especially in elderly patients over 70 years old. I conclude that the disease has subsided in my case due to the age-related immune suppression.

Consent

Written informed consent was obtained from the patient for publication of this case report and accompanying images. A copy of the written consent is available for review by the Editor-in-Chief of this journal on request.

Acknowledgments

I would like to thank the Deanship of Scientific Research at Prince, Sattam Bin Abdulaziz University.

References

[1] S. A. Grando, "Pemphigus autoimmunity: hypotheses and realities," *Autoimmunity*, vol. 45, no. 1, pp. 7–35, 2012.

[2] K. E. Harman, S. Albert, and M. M. Black, "Guidelines," *The British Journal of Dermatology*, vol. 149, no. 5, pp. 926–937, 2003.

[3] A. Ali, Y. AliReza, and F. Gita, "Pemphigus vulgaris in Iran: epidemiology and clinical profile," *SKINmed*, vol. 5, no. 2, pp. 69–71, 2006.

[4] S. Dagistan, M. Goregen, O. Miloglu, and B. Çakur, "Oral pemphigus vulgaris: a case report with review of the literature," *Journal of Oral Science*, vol. 50, no. 3, pp. 359–362, 2008.

[5] A. Karagir, S. G. Ranpise, and T. Ranpise, "Oral pemhigus vulgaris-a case report," *JIDA*, vol. 6, p. 2012, 2012.

[6] M. A. Patvekar and D. Sadana, "Pemphigus vulgaris in an elderly patient," *Indian Journal of Dermatology*, vol. 59, no. 1, p. 105, 2014.

[7] S. M. Langan, L. Smeeth, R. Hubbard, K. M. Fleming, C. J. P. Smith, and J. West, "Bullous pemphigoid and pemphigus vulgaris–incidence and mortality in the UK: population based cohort study," *BMJ*, vol. 337, no. jul09 1, p. a180, 2008.

[8] P. Martel, N. Cordel, P. Courville, D. Gilbert, P. Musette, and P. Joly, "Pemphigus with clinical, histological and immunological features of both vulgaris and foliaceus subtypes," *The British Journal of Dermatology*, vol. 147, no. 6, p. 1263, 2002.

[9] S. Ikeda, S. Imamura, I. Hashimoto, S. Morioka, M. Sakuma, and H. Ogawa, "History of the establishment and revision of diagnostic criteria, severity index and therapeutic guidelines for pemphigus in Japan," *Archives of Dermatological Research*, vol. 295, no. S1, pp. S12–S16, 2003.

[10] T. Shamim, V. I. Varghese, P. M. Shameena, and S. Sudha, "Pemphigus vulgaris in oral cavity: clinical analysis of 71 cases," *Medicina Oral, Patología Oral y Cirugía Bucal*, vol. 13, pp. E622–E626, 2008.

[11] S. R. Parker and J. MacKelfresh, "Autoimmune blistering diseases in the elderly," *Clinics in Dermatology*, vol. 29, no. 1, pp. 69–79, 2011.

[12] M. Kasperkiewicz, E. Schmidt, and D. Zillikens, "Current therapy of the pemphigus group," *Clinics in Dermatology*, vol. 30, no. 1, pp. 84–94, 2012.

[13] S. Ljubojevic, J. Lipozencic, S. Brenner, and D. Budimcic, "Pemphigus vulgaris: a review of treatment over a 19-year period," *Journal of the European Academy of Dermatology and Venereology*, vol. 16, no. 6, pp. 599–603, 2002.

[14] R. Chovatiya and J. I. Silverberg, "Association of pemphigus and pemphigoid with osteoporosis and pathological fractures," *Archives of Dermatological Research*, vol. 312, no. 4, pp. 263–271, 2020.

10

Jaw Manipulation using Ultrasound-Guided Inferior Alveolar Nerve Block for Trismus in Temporomandibular Disorders

Yuki Kojima[1] **and Ryozo Sendo**[2]

[1]*Department of Anesthesiology, Asahi General Hospital, Chiba, Japan*
[2]*Department of Anesthesiology, Imakiire General Hospital, Kagoshima, Japan*

Correspondence should be addressed to Yuki Kojima; cojicoji1109@gmail.com

Academic Editor: Pia L. Jornet

Temporomandibular disorders are a group of disorders with symptoms that include pain and clicking sounds in the temporomandibular joint and restricted mouth opening. For the treatment of temporomandibular disorders with trismus, herein, we suggest a new approach: "jaw manipulation using the ultrasound-guided inferior alveolar nerve block technique." A woman in her 60s developed temporomandibular disorders and presented with severe trismus owing to pain in the temporomandibular joint. Ultrasound-guided inferior alveolar nerve block was performed with ropivacaine, which relieved the pain in the patient. Furthermore, we performed jaw manipulation for trismus. Since the analgesic effect lasts for 3 days, self-training can be performed while the pain is relieved. After five sessions of "jaw manipulation using the ultrasound-guided inferior alveolar nerve block technique," trismus significantly improved in this patient. Ultrasound-guided inferior alveolar nerve block can be effective in relieving temporomandibular disorder-related pain and trismus.

1. Introduction

Temporomandibular disorder (TMD) is a collective term for functional and structural disorders involving the temporomandibular joint (TMJ), masticatory muscles, head and neck muscles, and/or related tissue components [1, 2]. Its symptoms include pain and clicking sounds in the TMJ and restricted mouth opening, with pain being the most common symptom and frequent reason for seeking treatment [3–5]. Several anatomical, biological, behavioural, biomechanical, and emotional factors affect the masticatory system, contributing to the development of signs and symptoms and/or perpetuation of TMDs. Therefore, TMDs can be considered multifactorial diseases [4]. Restricted jaw movement causes trismus, which leads to difficulty in eating and receiving dental treatments. If the symptoms do not improve with treatment, the patient's mental health can be adversely affected. Moreover, if the condition becomes chronic, the symptoms may become too severe to manage and improve. Therefore, the effective treatment of TMDs associated with trismus can significantly improve the quality of life [1, 5].

The manipulation of the jaw has been the cornerstone of TMD treatment. However, this procedure elicits severe pain in patients with chronic TMD. Ultrasound-guided trigeminal nerve block has been administered for perioperative analgesia in maxillofacial surgery [6, 7]. Ultrasound-guided inferior alveolar nerve block (IANB) with ropivacaine achieves effective long-term pain relief in the trigeminal nerve's region of distribution. We hypothesized that the use of ultrasound-guided IANB would facilitate painless jaw manipulation.

Herein, we report the case of a patient who underwent a novel approach for treating severe trismus due to TMDs.

2. Case Presentation

A woman in her 60s presented with a medical history of hypothyroidism, rheumatoid arthritis, and ulcerative colitis. Six months prior to presentation, she had experienced severe

Table 1: Changes in the maximum mouth opening, visual analogue scale, and hospital anxiety and depression scale scores.

	The maximum mouth opening (mm) Case 1	Visual analogue scale Case 1	Hospital anxiety and depression scale Case 1
Before treatment	15	100/100	24
After 1st treatment	28	21/100	—
After 2nd treatment	30	—	—
After 3rd treatment	30	—	—
After 4th treatment	33	—	—
After 5th treatment	40	21/100	9

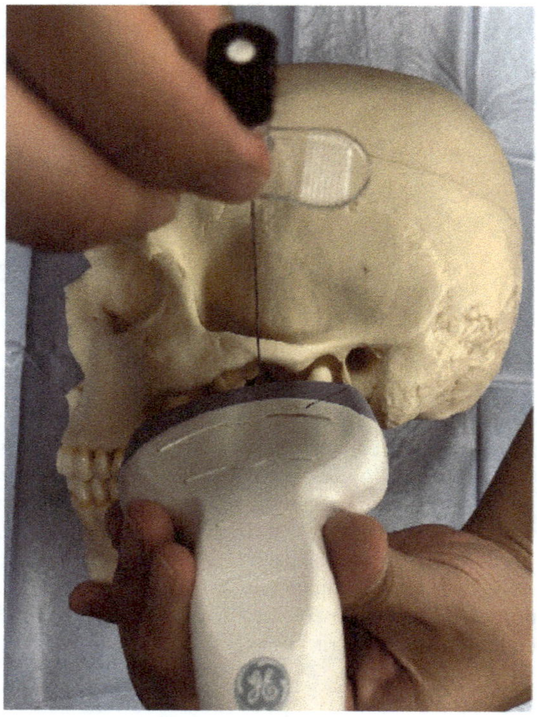

Figure 1: The technique of ultrasound-guided inferior alveolar nerve block.

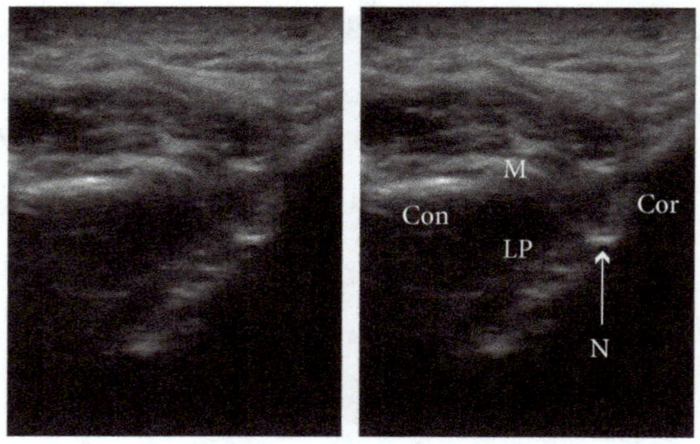

Figure 2: Intraprocedural image of ultrasound-guided IANB. We confirmed the spread of the local anaesthetics (6 ml of 0.375% ropivacaine). Cor: coronoid; Con: condyle; M: masseter; LP: lateral pterygoid muscle; N: needle.

pain when she attempted to open her mouth wide. Subsequently, she had been experiencing pain on mouth opening wide. Physical as well as imaging examinations did not reveal any abnormality in the morphology of the TMJ. Bite splint therapy did not result in any improvement, and the intensity of pain prevented training for mouth opening. She was referred to an outpatient pain clinic, where five trigger point local anaesthesia injections were administered, but without any improvement. Furthermore, Chinese herbal medicine did not alleviate her symptoms. Therefore, she was referred to our clinic, which specialises in dental anaesthesiology.

When pain on mouth opening is relieved, the fear of opening the mouth to eat is reduced. To evaluate the effect of treatment, the maximum mouth opening and visual analogue scale (VAS) scores were measured for the quantification of pain. Since TMDs are also associated with emotional factors, we used the hospital anxiety and depression scale (HADS) scores for her mental evaluation (Table 1).

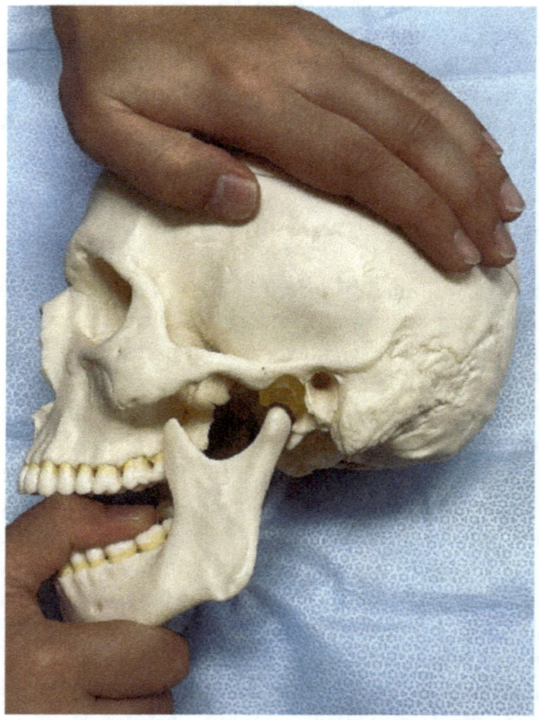

Figure 3: The technique of jaw manipulation.

The patient was treated using this novel approach. The patient was seated in the dental chair, and the vital signs were verified to be normal. The head was turned away from the clinician, and a linear ultrasonic probe was placed just

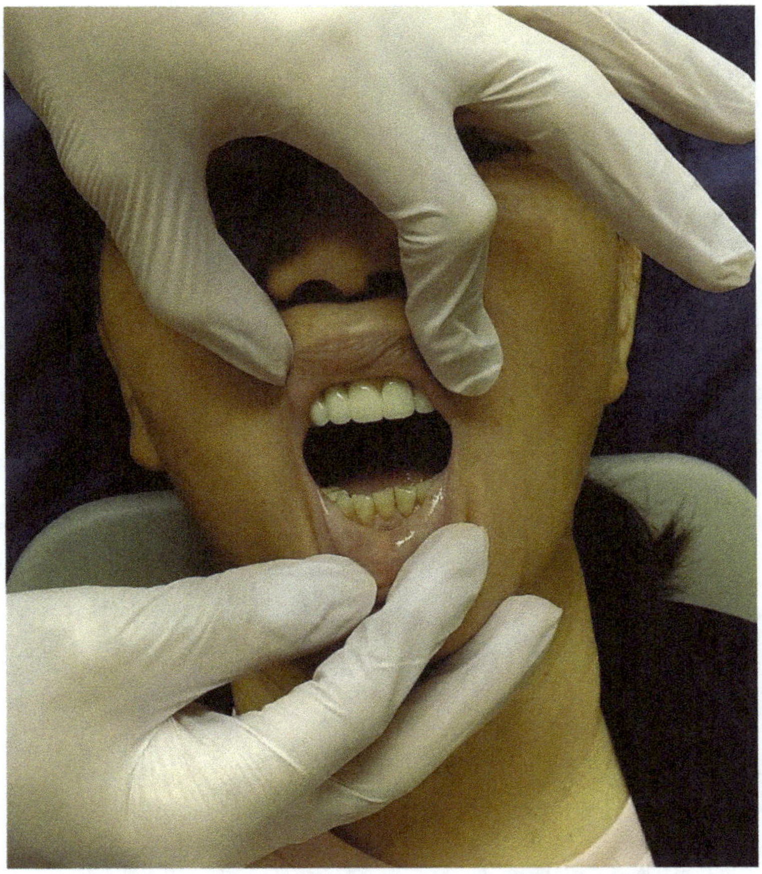

FIGURE 4: Before the JMUI technique.

caudad to the zygomatic arch. Thereafter, the masseter and lateral pterygoid muscles were observed. The space between them is the pterygomandibular space (PMS), which contains the inferior alveolar nerve and the peripheral branches of the mandibular nerve [8]. A 22 G needle was inserted to reach the PMS near the inferior alveolar nerve using the extraoral approach (Figure 1). Ultrasound-guided IANB was performed bilaterally with 6 ml of 0.375% ropivacaine on each side. An ultrasound can confirm the spread of the local anaesthetic (Figure 2), and the needle can be inserted while avoiding blood vessels [6]. Jaw manipulation was performed using the conventional method [9]. The patient's forehead was held to stabilise the head, and the thumb was placed on the mandibular posterior teeth. Thereafter, the patient was instructed to open the mouth with maximum effort while being aided in this movement (Figure 3). We have designated this method the "jaw manipulation using the ultrasound-guided IANB (JMUI)" technique. Since the analgesic effect lasts for 3 days, self-training can be performed in the absence of pain. The patient was instructed to use her fingers for self-training in opening the mouth.

At presentation, her maximum mouth opening was 15 mm, and the pain on wide mouth opening was assigned a VAS score of 100/100 (Figure 4). Since no morphological changes were evident in the TMJ, pain in the masticatory muscles and disc dislocation was suspected. Hence, we applied the "JMUI technique." The maximum mouth opening increased to 28 mm, and the pain reduced to a VAS score of 21/100 (Figure 5). The procedure was performed once a week, and after 5 weeks, the maximum mouth opening was 40 mm and the VAS score was 21/100. The HADS score was also improved significantly (Table 1).

3. Discussion

The normal range of mouth opening varies individually, but a maximum mouth opening of 38-40 mm is required for the normal functioning of routine activities. Our patient had a chronic TMD. All standard treatments for TMD were administered; however, there was no improvement in pain when opening the mouth. The trismus persisted due to severe pain on mouth opening.

Ultrasound-guided IANB alleviated the trismus caused by TMD-related pain in our patient, who exhibited satisfactory recovery after five sessions. Furthermore, the training for mouth opening was continued (daily, 30 min/day), and maximum mouth opening was maintained. No complications were reported. A recent study showed that ultrasound-guided IANB is useful in the perioperative management of patients who undergo mandibular sequestrectomy for medication-related osteonecrosis of the jaw [6]. The results demonstrated that IANB provides effective pain control for 72 h. In our case, the improvement in mouth opening lasted for 3 days after the procedure, which is consistent with the previous report.

The "JMUI technique" may be effective in cases wherein the traditional treatment modalities are unsuccessful. Jaw

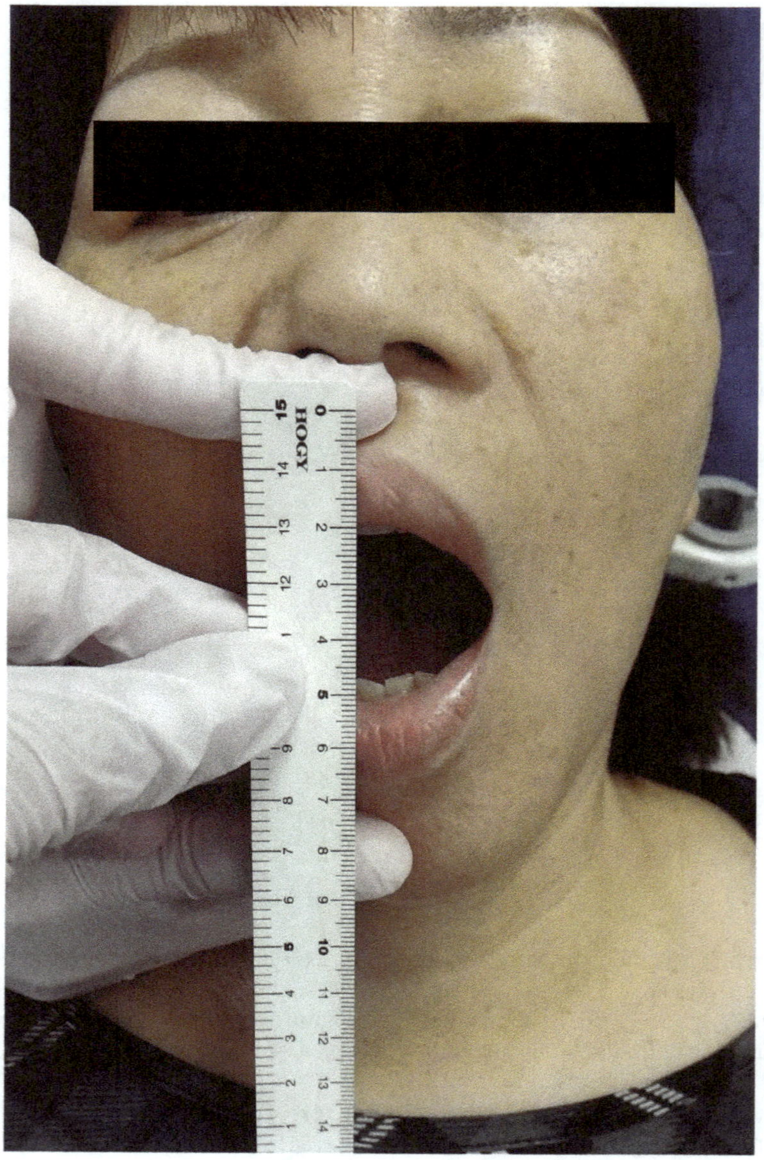

FIGURE 5: After the first session of JMUI technique.

manipulation and home training for mouth opening are difficult in patients who experience severe pain during mouth opening. The pain hinders self-motivation for treatment. The "JMUI technique" has the advantage of achieving a longer duration of analgesia than other methods. If the pain is relieved, self-motivation for treatment can also be improved. It is noteworthy that mental stress is also an exacerbating factor for TMDs. Therefore, we evaluated the associated mental factors using the HADS score. In our patient, these scores improved after five sessions. Negative cognition can be corrected by making the patient aware that the pain has been relieved and mouth opening has been increased by the JMUI technique, thus highlighting the technique's therapeutic effect. Such novel treatment methods improve mouth opening and reduce pain, ultimately addressing anxiety and depression-related pain. TMDs can be treated by addressing mental stress, as it is an important contributing factor. Additionally, ultrasound can also be used for blocking the masseteric nerve, which can relax the muscles of mastication. Aside from pain relief, addressing their mental health is equally important.

This approach to clinical practice can apply to refractory severe chronic TMD, even if dentists have provided an effective treatment. As it is less invasive and reversible than surgery, it may be administrable earlier than conventional treatments. This technique was performed by a pain clinician, dentist, or anaesthesiologist, who requires specific training for administering nerve blocks with ultrasound devices.

Because this is a case report, we cannot conclude that the technique would be effective in all types of TMDs. Further long-term studies with a greater number of participants are needed to clarify its definitive indications and effectiveness.

4. Conclusion

The JMUI technique involves jaw manipulation after ultrasound-guided IANB. This technique may be a novel approach for the effective treatment of trismus due to chronic TMD. After undergoing JMUI, self-training can be performed while the pain is relieved. Moreover, after five sessions, trismus remarkably improved in our patient.

References

[1] A. B. Tuncer, N. Ergun, A. H. Tuncer, and S. Karahan, "Effectiveness of manual therapy and home physical therapy in patients with temporomandibular disorders: a randomized controlled trial," *Journal of Bodywork and Movement Therapies*, vol. 17, no. 3, pp. 302–308, 2013.

[2] V. V. G. Patnaik, B. Sanju, and S. K. Rajan, "Anatomy of temporomandibular joint: a review," *Journal of the Anatomical Society of India*, vol. 49, pp. 191–197, 2000.

[3] S. Beaumont, K. Garg, A. Gokhale, and N. Heaphy, "Temporomandibular disorder: a practical guide for dental practitioners in diagnosis and management," *Australian Dental Journal*, vol. 65, no. 3, pp. 172–180, 2020.

[4] R. Ohrbach, E. Bair, R. B. Fillingim et al., "Clinical orofacial characteristics associated with risk of first-onset TMD: the OPPERA prospective cohort study," *The Journal of Pain*, vol. 14, no. 12, pp. T33–T50, 2013.

[5] S. F. Dworkin, K. H. Huggins, L. LeResche et al., "Epidemiology of signs and symptoms in temporomandibular disorders: clinical signs in cases and controls," *Journal of the American Dental Association*, vol. 120, no. 3, pp. 273–281, 1990.

[6] Y. Kojima, T. Murouchi, M. Akiba, and T. Oka, "Ultrasound-guided inferior alveolar nerve block for postoperative analgesia after mandibular sequestrectomy: a single-center retrospective study," *Journal of Clinical Anesthesia*, vol. 60, pp. 39-40, 2020.

[7] Y. Kojima, K. Furuse, T. Murouchi, K. Hirabayashi, M. Kato, and T. Oka, "Ultrasound-guided local anesthetic nerve blocks in a forehead flap reconstructive maxillofacial procedure," *Anesthesia Progress*, vol. 67, no. 3, pp. 164–169, 2020.

[8] S. Kumita, T. Murouchi, and J. Arakawa, "Ultrasound-guided maxillary and inferior alveolar nerve blocks for postoperative analgesia in gnathoplasty," *Asian Journal of Anesthesiology*, vol. 55, no. 4, pp. 89-90, 2017.

[9] K. Nagata, S. Hori, R. Mizuhashi et al., "Efficacy of mandibular manipulation technique for temporomandibular disorders patients with mouth opening limitation: a randomized controlled trial for comparison with improved multimodal therapy," *Journal of Prosthodontic Research*, vol. 63, no. 2, pp. 202–209, 2019.

11

Evaluation of Therapeutic Benefits of a Novel Herbal Ingredient-Based Hyaluronic Acid Gel as Monotherapy for Inflammatory Enlargement of a Patient with Diabetes Mellitus

Jaahnavi Lanka and Santhosh Kumar

Department of Periodontology, Manipal College of Dental Sciences, Manipal, Manipal Academy of Higher Education, Manipal, 576104, Udupi, Karnataka, India

Correspondence should be addressed to Santhosh Kumar; santhosh.kumar@manipal.edu

Academic Editor: Giuseppe Alessandro Scardina

The reason for the destruction of the attachment apparatus in patients with periodontal disease is the supra- and the subgingival microflora. Hence, the treatment of this inflammatory gingival disease is primarily focused on eliminating the cause. The present case report assessed the therapeutic benefit of adjunctive use of a commercially available topical agent containing 1% hyaluronic acid gel combined with nonsurgical periodontal therapy. A patient aged 64 years with type 2 diabetes mellitus reported to the Department of Periodontology. He complained of gum enlargement and frequent bleeding during brushing. The patient was not under any medication for his diabetes control. On examination, there was a localized papillary gingival enlargement. Therefore, Klirich gel containing hyaluronic acid was applied on the surface of the gingiva during the first visit of the patient. During the follow-up visit, he continued with this adjunctive use of the gel along with the nonsurgical periodontal therapy. In addition, he controlled his blood sugar level with diet and exercise. During the follow-up visit after one year, there was a noticeable clinical change in the overall health of his gingiva.

1. Introduction

Gingival enlargements occur due to excessive proliferation of gingival soft tissues [1]. The abnormal increase in the size of the gingiva can cause functional and aesthetic concerns to the patient. The etiology can be local factors like plaque and calculus or systemic diseases [2]. Malignant etiologies like hematological and squamous cell carcinoma should be ruled out. Other etiologies include periodontal disease, genetic diseases, conditioned enlargements like puberty, pregnancy, and systemic diseases, and drug-induced and iatrogenic causes [3]. A few drugs that are studied to cause gingival enlargement are cyclosporin, phenytoin, and calcium channel blockers [4]. Bondon-Guitton and colleagues [5] in 2012 studied that a few other drugs like immunosuppressants, anticonvulsants, antibiotics, and contraceptive pills also caused gingival enlargement.

In cases of drug-induced gingival enlargement, replacing the causative drug resolves the enlargement [6] in most cases. In other cases presenting with unknown etiology, thorough scaling and root planing will be needed to manage the local factors. If the enlargement does not subside after nonsurgical therapy, surgical procedures like gingivoplasty and gingivectomy can eliminate pockets and improve oral hygiene [7, 8].

Evidence from human studies suggests that gingival enlargement is mainly influenced by the microbial aspect [9, 10], which forms the basis for the use of antimicrobial therapy as an adjunct in the management of gingival enlargement. The outcomes of periodontal debridement have been enhanced by the adjunctive use of systemic antibiotics, topical antibiotics, and topical antiseptics [10]. However, adverse reactions, hypersensitivity, superinfection, and antibiotic resistance have been widely reported with antibiotic use. Considering the various shortcomings of antimicrobial therapy, the need for the development of therapeutic agents which are safe and biocompatible is undoubtedly high. Hence, research on plant-based herbal agents came into existence. Natural therapeutic agents such as antioxidants, micronutrients, and herbal medications have been proposed and tested [11, 12]. Herbal agents are very effective and comparable to antimicrobial therapy in managing various periodontal conditions.

In the present case report, the therapeutic benefit of Klirich® (Itena Clinical products, France) containing 1% high molecular weight hyaluronic acid gel in combination with herbal ingredients like alchemilla leaf extract, calendula flower extracts, avocado oil, clove essential oil, and grapefruit seed extract given as monotherapy is briefly illustrated and examined in a subject with gingival inflammation and diffuse enlargement secondary to uncontrolled diabetes mellitus.

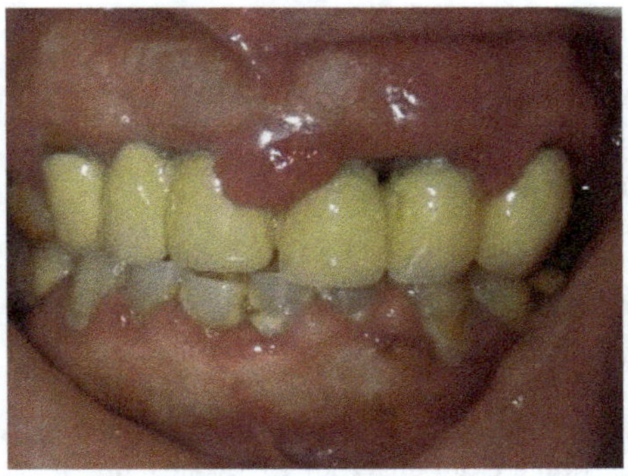

FIGURE 1: Presentation of gingival enlargement at baseline.

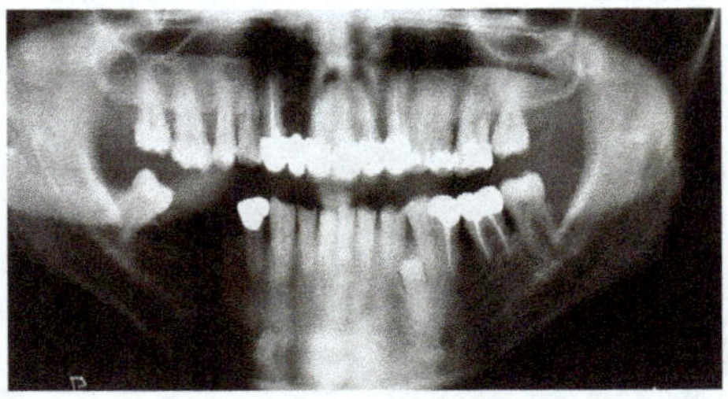

FIGURE 2: Preoperative radiograph.

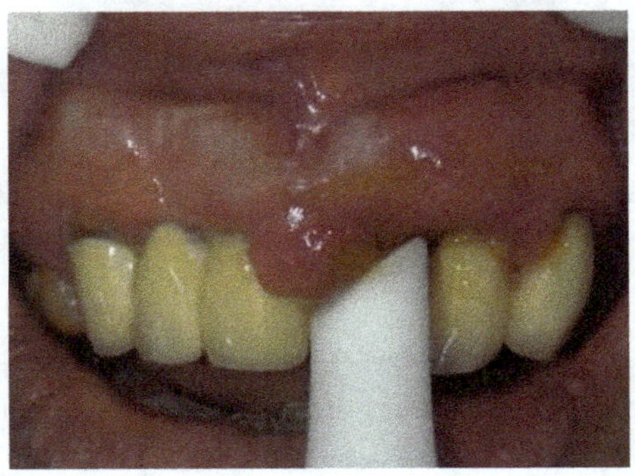

FIGURE 3: Application of Klirich gel on the inflamed areas as monotherapy.

2. Case Report

In 2019, a male patient aged 65 years reported to the Department of Periodontology, Dental Outpatient ward, with a chief complaint of swelling around the gums and bleeding during brushing. Upon clinical examination, gingival enlargement was observed in the upper and lower anterior tooth regions (Figure 1), and there was a generalized, moderate (up to the coronal third of the root) to severe (up to the middle third of the root) bone loss in the panoramic radiograph (Planmeca Promax, Finland, Romexis software) (Figure 2). The patient gave a history of bleeding gums while brushing his teeth and discomfort due to swollen gums. His systemic health history was recorded, and the patient was a known case of diabetes mellitus which was not under medication at the initial visit. All the possible etiologies were ruled out by a thorough case history, blood investigations, and biopsy. The fasting blood glucose level was 145 mg/dl at the initial visit. The patient's past dental history was uneventful, where he underwent procedures ranging from oral prophylaxis and periodontal flap surgery four years from the presenting complaint. The patient presented with a prosthesis in the upper anterior region from 13 to 23. The enlargement could be easily distinguished from the surrounding gingiva. The patient had difficulty in oral hygiene maintenance due to the enlargement. The proper placement of restorative margins and cleanability were evaluated to rule out any possible irritation from the restorative materials from the fixed prosthesis [13]. Periodontal pocket was recorded using the Hufriedy (Chicago, United States) University of North Carolina-15 (UNC-15) probe. The pocket charting showed persistent pocket depths ranging from 5 mm to 6 mm, in the upper anterior and the posterior region suggesting moderate attachment loss. Poor oral hygiene maintenance by the patient and the overhang surrounding the fixed prosthesis could have resulted in the accumulation of the deposits. The case was diagnosed as generalized stage II grade B periodontitis, currently unstable with a risk factor of diabetes mellitus. The gingival inflammation and the enlargement were secondary to uncontrolled diabetes mellitus, plaque, and calculus deposits.

2.1. Treatment Planning. The treatment plan was a comprehensive periodontal therapy comprising a nonsurgical phase, maintenance phase, and surgical therapy. However, in the first visit, scaling was postponed due to increased blood sugar levels (fasting blood sugar:145 mg/dl), and the application of Klirich gel, a patented formula of *Itena Clinical products, France (EP2954902 A1)*, was performed as monotherapy, as seen in Figure 3. The application of the novel gel as monotherapy was made considering the available evidence from studies reporting management of oral lesions in uncontrolled diabetic patients by using plant-based gels like aloe vera as monotherapy, which showed beneficial results [14]. The instructions of use are illustrated in Table 1. The patient was referred to a physician for a review of diabetes mellitus and suggested to come back after the blood sugar levels returned to normal. In addition, the patient was educated about the importance of oral hygiene,

Table 1: Ingredients of Klirich gel.

Nonanimal-based herbal ingredients	Main ingredient
Grapefruit seed extract Alchemilla leaf extract Clove essential oil Avocado oil Calendula flower extract	1% high molecular weight hyaluronic acid
Instructions for usage (i) Massage once daily after brushing (ii) Apply a pea-sized amount of gel on the inflamed areas and massage the gel with a clean finger for 15 seconds until it gets absorbed (iii) Let the gel stay in the mouth for another 15 seconds without massaging (iv) Recommended period of use can range from 1 to 2 weeks and may vary depending upon the severity of inflammation	

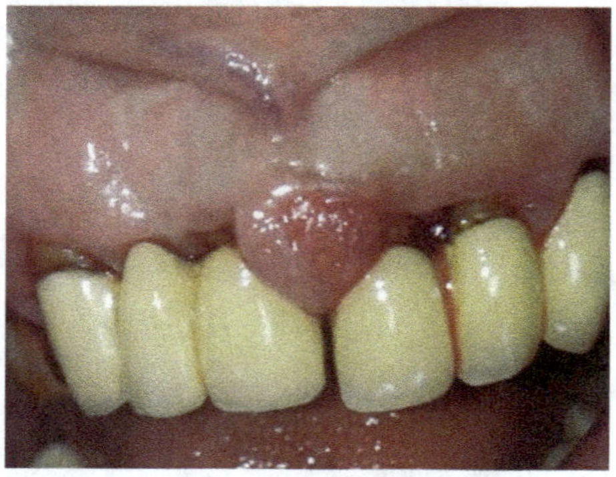

Figure 4: Review at 2 weeks: subsided inflammation, except for the interdental area.

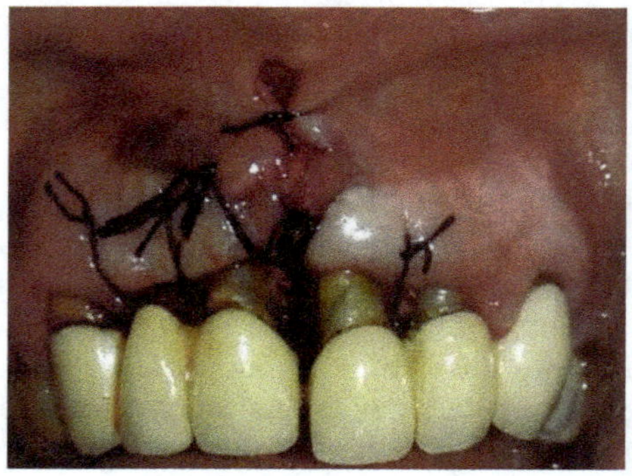

Figure 5: Surgical phase: 4 weeks: gingivectomy and open flap debridement.

and brushing technique was demonstrated. A review after two weeks was scheduled. At this review, fasting blood sugar levels were found to be 128 mg/dl.

2.2. Nonsurgical Therapy. After two weeks of monotherapy, with Klirich gel (no scaling has been performed during the first two weeks), grade II (Bökenkamp and Bohnhorst index 1994 [15]) overgrowth resolved, as seen in Figure 4. However, the enlargement in the interdental area between the two upper central was persistent, and when palpated, it was a fibrous nodular overgrowth, which was later diagnosed as pyogenic granuloma after a biopsy.

At the second visit, supragingival, subgingival scaling, root planing, and curettage were performed. Klirich gel was given for topical application again as described previously, and the patient was recalled for review after two weeks.

2.3. Surgical Therapy. At the four-week review, as the upper anterior region showed persistent probing pocket depths, it required surgical intervention. For the surgical excision of the gingival enlargement, an internal bevel gingivectomy of the fibrotic overgrowth and open flap debridement were planned. Initial probing and the marking of the periodontal pocket depth were done using the pocket marker (Crane Kaplan, Hufriedy). Then, an internal bevel gingivectomy was performed using the Kirkland knife and Orban's interdental knives. Residual tissue tags were cleaned, and the margins were smoothened using the no. 15 B. P. blade and handle (Figure 5). The 4-0 silk sutures were used for approximation of the flaps. There was a high frenal attachment and needed management. Hence, conventional frenotomy was performed to remove the aberrant frenum. Analgesic ibuprofen 400 mg (Brufen®) was prescribed and instructed to be taken thrice daily for two days till the pain subsided, and postoperative instructions were given.

During the postoperative visit, the healing was uneventful, the enlargement was eliminated, and pocket-depth reduction was noted when evaluated at a one-month review (Figure 6). The postoperative radiograph after one year is shown in Figure 7.

3. Discussion

Periodontal disease management has always been challenging in diabetic patients. Research in these aspects indicated that periodontal disease and diabetes have a synergistic relationship [16–19]. The risk of periodontal disease aggravated systemic disorders like diabetes mellitus [19]. Difficulties posed by wound healing patterns in diabetic patients also restricted periodontal management to nonsurgical therapy [16–19]. However, the fact that deeper bone defects or residual pockets cannot be eliminated by nonsurgical therapy alone makes surgical intervention necessary in these areas. Hence, adjuvants to surgical therapies that enhance wound healing are invaluable for better prognosis and long-term

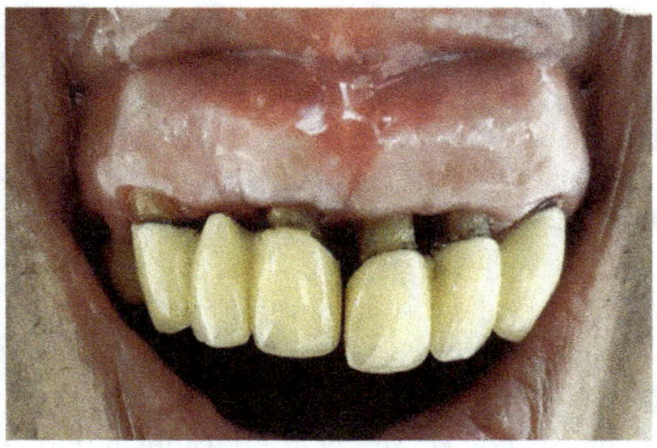

FIGURE 6: Postoperative clinical presentation after complete healing; resolved gingival enlargement and reduced pocket depths at 1-month postoperative review.

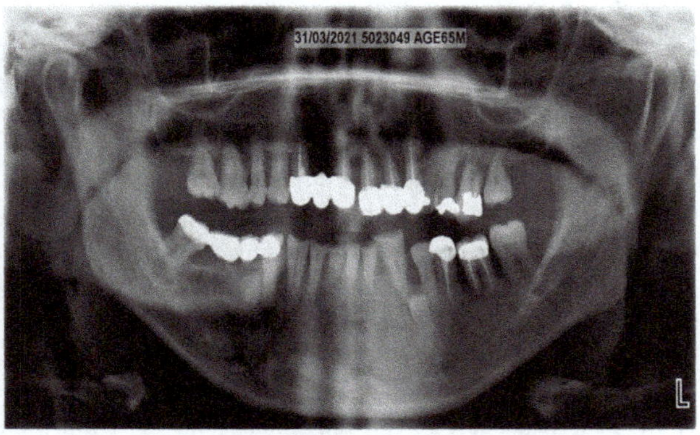

FIGURE 7: Postoperative radiograph after one year.

success in periodontal management. Zhang et al. [20] observed that hyaluronic acid-based hydrogel shows anti-inflammatory effects and promotes angiogenesis in chronic diabetic wounds. The use of hyaluronic acid in combination with nanofibers for enhanced wound healing was studied by El-Aassar and his colleagues in January 2021 [21].

The bacteriostatic property of hyaluronic acid is also well established by a study conducted by Zamboni et al. [22]. In a recent animal study by Shirakata et al. [23], periodontal management of infrabony defects using hyaluronic acid has shown beneficial results. Mamajiwala and coworkers [24] have seen improved clinical and radiographic outcomes using 0.8% hyaluronic acid as an adjunct in treating periodontal infrabony defects by open flap debridement.

Besides the excellent wound-healing abilities of hyaluronic acid, its bacteriostatic activity, biocompatibility, non-immunogenic property, and safety were confirmed by Becker et al. [25] and various other studies [20–26], suggesting that hyaluronic acid is an ideal adjuvant in periodontal surgical and nonsurgical therapy.

The FDA approved it in 2005, which also published a summary of the safety and effectiveness data in the same year [27]. Hence, in the present case report, the use of herbal ingredients in combination with hyaluronic acid has been evaluated. The combination of all the herbal agents with hyaluronic acid in the present case showed a remarkable reduction in inflammation and swelling. However, biochemical analysis of inflammatory biomarkers would have added more scientific evidence to the case report.

A larger group randomized trial could provide evidence of the effectiveness of this gel. Further comparison with new alternative treatment options, like probiotics [28], antioxidants [29], and plant-based therapy [30], could be assessed in patients with periodontal disease. Apart from these alternatives, using lasers to manage gingival inflammation and enlargement is currently being studied as an effective treatment option [31].

4. Conclusion

The use of Klirich ® in the present case has shown a therapeutic benefit as an adjunct to scaling and root planing. It is clinically safe and effectively manages inflammatory gingival enlargement due to periodontal disease in diabetes. Furthermore, the present study's findings should be confirmed in future randomized controlled clinical trials, including microbial and biochemical analysis.

Consent

We affirm that the patient is explained about the complete treatment protocol, and consent for surgical intervention and use of clinical images was taken. The identity of the patient is completely concealed in the interest of privacy of the patient.

References

[1] O. A. Korczeniewska, T. C. Hart, and S. R. Diehl, "The role of genetics in oral medicine," *Burket's Oral Medicine.*, vol. 30, pp. 1009–1035, 2021.

[2] A. Punj and M. Chaturvedi, "Diagnosis and treatment plan for gingival diseases and conditions," in *Oral Diseases*, Intech Open, 2020.

[3] A. A. Agrawal, "Gingival enlargements: differential diagnosis and review of literature," *World Journal of Clinical Cases*, vol. 3, no. 9, pp. 779–788, 2015.

[4] H. Hatahira, J. Abe, Y. Hane et al., "Drug-induced gingival hyperplasia: a retrospective study using spontaneous reporting system databases," *Journal of Pharmaceutical Health Care and Sciences*, vol. 3, no. 1, p. 19, 2017.

[5] E. Bondon-Guitton, H. Bagheri, and J. L. Montastruc, "Drug-induced gingival overgrowth: a study in the French Pharmacovigilance Database," *Journal of Clinical Periodontology*, vol. 39, no. 6, pp. 513–518, 2012.

[6] V. Bharti and C. Bansal, "Drug-induced gingival overgrowth: the nemesis of gingiva unravelled," *Journal of Indian Society of Periodontology*, vol. 17, no. 2, pp. 182–187, 2013.

[7] T. M. Feijó Miguelis, K. von Ahn Pinto, L. E. Rilling Nova Cruz, J. P. Aitken Saavedra, and J. Martos, "Systemic and clinical treatment of gingival hyperplasia associated with use of anticonvulsant," *Revista Clínica de Periodoncia, Implantología y Rehabilitación Oral*, vol. 12, no. 1, pp. 50–52, 2019.

[8] P. Khera, M. J. Zirwas, and J. C. English III, "Diffuse gingival enlargement," *Journal of the American Academy of Dermatology*, vol. 52, no. 3, pp. 491–499, 2005.

[9] L. Bontemps, F. Gaultier, F. Anagnostou, A. L. Ejeil, and S. M. Dridi, "Drug-induced gingival overgrowth," in *Drug-Induced Oral Complications*, Springer, Cham, 2021.

[10] H. Mawardi, A. Alsubhi, N. Salem et al., "Management of medication-induced gingival hyperplasia: a systematic review," *Oral Surgery, Oral Medicine, Oral Pathology, Oral Radiology*, vol. 131, no. 1, pp. 62–72, 2021.

[11] S. Muralidharan, M. Giri, S. Patankar, A. P. Kamble, D. A. Kamble, and N. Ismail, "The effect of triphala and chlorhexidine mouthwash on dental plaque and gingival inflammation: an open labelled clinical study," *Natural Volatiles and Essential Oils*, vol. 8, no. 5, pp. 6848–6860, 2021.

[12] M. Mazur, A. Ndokaj, M. Jedlinski, R. Ardan, S. Bietolini, and L. Ottolenghi, "Impact of green tea (*Camellia sinensis*) on periodontitis and caries. Systematic review and meta-analysis," *Japanese Dental Science Review*, vol. 57, no. 57, pp. 1–11, 2021.

[13] A. Avetisyan, M. Markaryan, D. Rokaya et al., "Characteristics of periodontal tissues in prosthetic treatment with fixed dental prostheses," *Molecules*, vol. 26, no. 5, p. 1331, 2021.

[14] N. Ghasemi, M. Behnezhad, M. Asgharzadeh, E. Zeinalzadeh, and H. S. Kafil, "Antibacterial properties of Aloe vera on intracanal medicaments against *Enterococcus faecalis* biofilm at different stages of development," *International Journal of Dentistry*, vol. 2020, 6 pages, 2020.

[15] A. Bökenkamp, B. Bohnhorst, C. Beier, N. Albers, G. Offner, and J. Brodehl, "Nifedipine aggravates cyclosporine A-induced gingival hyperplasia," *Pediatric Nephrology*, vol. 8, no. 2, pp. 181–185, 1994.

[16] C. M. Santoso, F. Ketti, T. Bramantoro, J. Zsuga, and A. Nagy, "Association between oral hygiene and metabolic syndrome: a systematic review and meta-analysis," *Journal of Clinical Medicine*, vol. 10, no. 13, p. 2873, 2021.

[17] W. A. Soskolne and A. Klinger, "The relationship between periodontal diseases and diabetes: an overview," *Annals of Periodontology*, vol. 6, no. 1, pp. 91–98, 2001.

[18] F. Q. Pirih, S. Monajemzadeh, N. Singh et al., "Association between metabolic syndrome and periodontitis: the role of lipids, inflammatory cytokines, altered host response, and the microbiome," *Periodontology 2000*, vol. 87, no. 1, pp. 50–75, 2021.

[19] J. W. Albright, P. H. Woo, S. Ji, B. Sun, K. Lang, and J. F. Albright, "Synergism between obesity and poor oral health associated with diabetes in an elderly human population," *The Southeast Asian Journal of Tropical Medicine and Public Health*, vol. 44, no. 2, pp. 318–331, 2013.

[20] L. Yang, L. Zhang, J. Hu, W. Wang, and X. Liu, "Promote anti-inflammatory and angiogenesis using a hyaluronic acid-based hydrogel with miRNA-laden nanoparticles for chronic diabetic wound treatment," *International Journal of Biological Macromolecules*, vol. 166, pp. 166–178, 2021.

[21] M. R. el-Aassar, N. G. el-Beheri, M. M. Agwa et al., "Antibiotic-free combinational hyaluronic acid blend nanofibers for wound healing enhancement," *International Journal of Biological Macromolecules*, vol. 167, pp. 1552–1563, 2021.

[22] F. Zamboni, C. Okoroafor, M. P. Ryan et al., "On the bacteriostatic activity of hyaluronic acid composite films," *Carbohydrate Polymers*, vol. 260, no. 260, article 117803, 2021.

[23] Y. Shirakata, T. Imafuji, T. Nakamura et al., "Periodontal wound healing/regeneration of two-wall intrabony defects following reconstructive surgery with cross-linked hyaluronic acid-gel with or without a collagen matrix: a preclinical study in dogs," *Quintessence International*, vol. 1, no. 52, pp. 2–10, 2021.

[24] A. S. Mamajiwala, K. S. Sethi, C. P. Raut, P. A. Karde, and B. S. Mamajiwala, "Clinical and radiographic evaluation of 0.8% hyaluronic acid as an adjunct to open flap debridement in the treatment of periodontal intrabony defects: randomized controlled clinical trial," *Clinical Oral Investigations*, vol. 25, no. 9, pp. 5257–5271, 2021.

[25] L. C. Becker, W. F. Bergfeld, D. V. Belsito et al., "Final report of the safety assessment of hyaluronic acid, potassium hyaluronate, and sodium hyaluronate," *International Journal of Toxicology*, vol. 28, 4_suppl, pp. 5–67, 2009.

[26] A. Pilloni, B. Zeza, D. Kuis et al., "Treatment of residual periodontal pockets using a hyaluronic acid-based gel: a 12 month multicenter randomized triple-blinded clinical trial," *Antibiotics*, vol. 10, no. 8, p. 924, 2021.

[27] FDA, *Nutrition C for FS and A. Cosmetic ingredients*, FDA, 2020.

[28] A. Butera, S. Gallo, C. Maiorani et al., "Management of gingival bleeding in periodontal patients with domiciliary use of toothpastes containing hyaluronic acid, lactoferrin, or paraprobiotics: a randomized controlled clinical trial," *Applied Sciences*, vol. 11, no. 18, p. 8586, 2021.

[29] Y. T. Chin, H. P. Tu, C. Y. Lin et al., "Antioxidants protect against gingival overgrowth induced by cyclosporine A," *Journal of Periodontal Research*, vol. 56, no. 2, pp. 397–407, 2021.

[30] M. Rudrapal, N. Hussain, and C. Egbuna, "Diabetes mellitus and it management with plant-based therapy," in *Dietary Phytochemicals*, Springer, Cham, 2021.

[31] M. Pal, A. Saokar, P. Gopalkrishna, H. R. Rajeshwari, and S. Kumar, "Diode laser-assisted management of intraoral soft tissue overgrowth: a case series," *General Dentistry*, vol. 68, no. 4, pp. 28–31, 2020.

12

Continuous Professional Oral Health Care Intervention Improves Severe Aspiration Pneumonia

Wakako Nawata,[1,2] Yojiro Umezaki,[1,3] Masahiro Yamaguchi,[1,3] Masato Nakajima,[1,4] Michiko Makino,[1] Masahiro Yoneda,[4] Takao Hirofuji,[4] Takafumi Yamano,[5] Hiroaki Ooboshi,[6] and Hiromitsu Morita[1]

[1]*The Center for Visiting Dental Service, Fukuoka Dental College Medical and Dental General Hospital, Fukuoka, Japan*
[2]*Division of Dental Hygiene, Fukuoka Dental College Medical and Dental General Hospital, Fukuoka, Japan*
[3]*Section of Geriatric Dentistry, Department of General Dentistry, Fukuoka Dental College, Fukuoka, Japan*
[4]*Section of General Dentistry, Department of General Dentistry, Fukuoka Dental College, Fukuoka, Japan*
[5]*Section of Otorhinolaryngology, Department of General Medicine, Fukuoka Dental College, Fukuoka, Japan*
[6]*Section of Internal Medicine, Department of General Medicine, Fukuoka Dental College, Fukuoka, Japan*

Correspondence should be addressed to Hiromitsu Morita; morita@college.fdcnet.ac.jp

Academic Editor: Sonja Pezelj-Ribarić

Professional oral health care (POHC) is known to prevent aspiration pneumonia in patients with dysphagia and/or those at the perioperative stage of surgery. However, the effect of POHC on patients suffering from aspiration pneumonia remains unknown. Here, we report a case where continual POHC intervention improved severe aspiration pneumonia. A 74-year-old male patient with a brain infarction suffered from severe aspiration pneumonia (PSI: IV, A-DROP: 3) complicated by vascular dementia and severe dysphagia. Because an antimicrobial approach following the treatment guidelines for pneumonia was not effective, we started a POHC intervention to improve his poor oral condition at the request of the attending doctor and the patient's family. The severe pneumonia markedly improved after continual POHC by the dental team. This case suggests that continual POHC intervention by a dental hygienist may improve severe aspiration pneumonia.

1. Introduction

Professional oral health care (POHC) prevents aspiration pneumonia caused by aspiration in older adults, especially when it is associated with dysphagia [1–6]. However, there is little evidence that POHC intervention after illness improves severe aspiration pneumonia.

Here, we report a case in which continual POHC intervention improved severe aspiration pneumonia caused by *Klebsiella pneumoniae* and/or multidrug-resistant *Pseudomonas aeruginosa* (MDRP) in a patient with a brain infarction complicated by vascular dementia and dysphagia.

2. Case Report

A 74-year-old male residing in a nursing home was hospitalized with a diagnosis of aspiration pneumonia. *Klebsiella pneumoniae* was detected by sputum culture. He was treated with tazobactam/piperacillin (TAZ/PIPC) following the guidelines for the treatment of respiratory infectious diseases including community-acquired pneumonia (CAP) in Japan. The patient's medical history was as follows: multiple cerebral infarctions, hypertension, diabetes mellitus, and chronic kidney disease. Vascular dementia with parkinsonism and severe dysphagia were also diagnosed. He took nutrition by

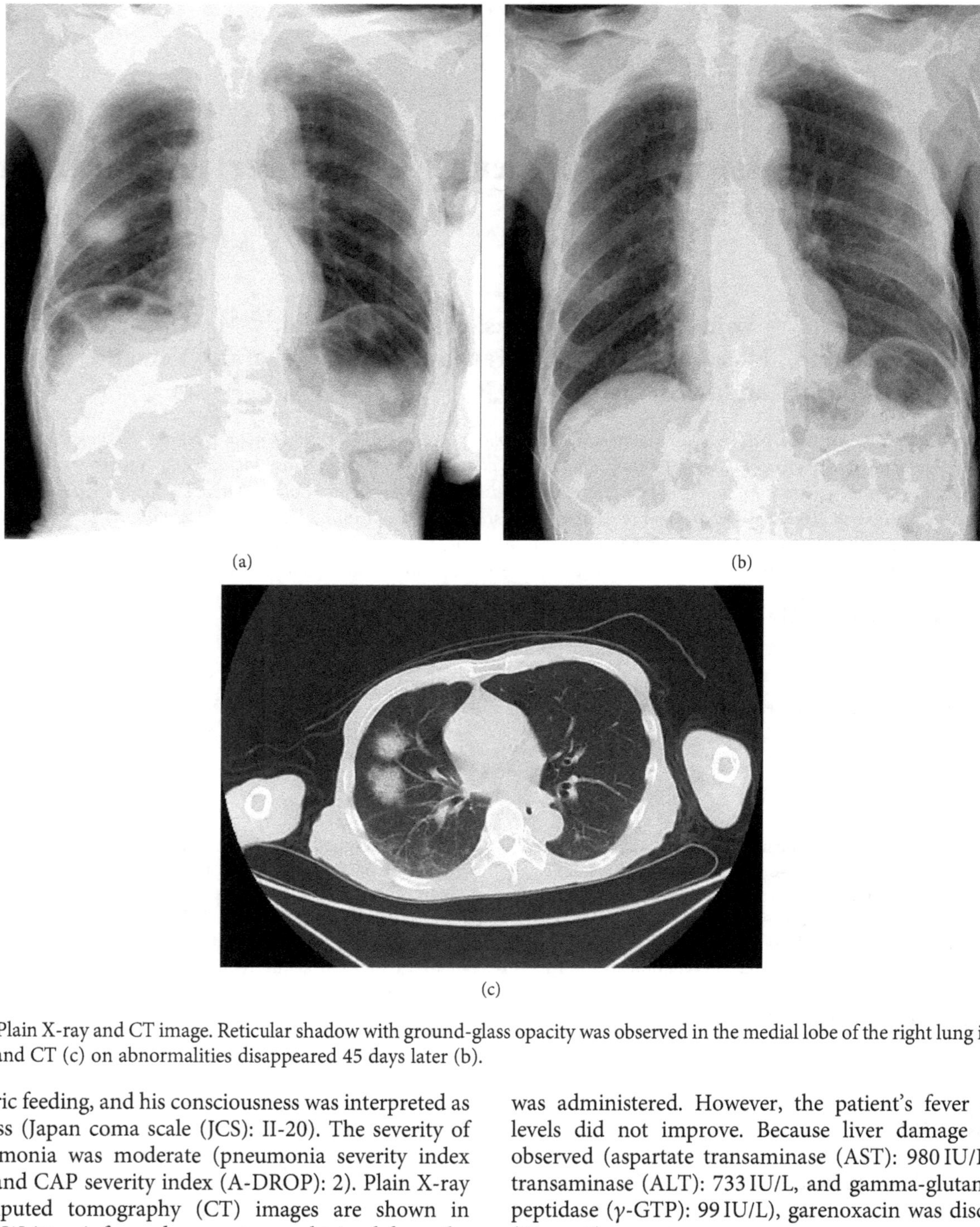

FIGURE 1: Plain X-ray and CT image. Reticular shadow with ground-glass opacity was observed in the medial lobe of the right lung in the plain X-ray (a) and CT (c) on abnormalities disappeared 45 days later (b).

nasoenteric feeding, and his consciousness was interpreted as drowsiness (Japan coma scale (JCS): II-20). The severity of the pneumonia was moderate (pneumonia severity index (PSI): II and CAP severity index (A-DROP): 2). Plain X-ray and computed tomography (CT) images are shown in Figure 1. Written informed consent was obtained from the patient's family for publication of this case report following the Ethical Guidelines of Fukuoka Dental College, and this case study was approved by the ethical committee of Fukuoka Dental College (#370).

The patient transiently recovered from the fever, and the elevated C-reactive protein (CRP) levels returned to normal after TAZ/PIPC and acetaminophen therapy. However, exacerbation of the fever and elevated CRP levels occurred within a couple of days. MDRP was detected in his sputum culture (Figure 2) and the severity of the pneumonia increased (PSI: IV and A-DROP: 3). Because the MDRP isolate was only sensitive to fluoroquinolone and cephem, garenoxacin was administered. However, the patient's fever and CRP levels did not improve. Because liver damage was then observed (aspartate transaminase (AST): 980 IU/L, alanine transaminase (ALT): 733 IU/L, and gamma-glutamyl transpeptidase (γ-GTP): 99 IU/L), garenoxacin was discontinued (Figure 2).

POHC was requested by the attending physician and the patient's family to improve his oral condition, along with physical rehabilitation. His intraoral condition was poor and quite dry. He had only three remaining natural teeth, which were all missing their crowns (13, 21, and 23; Figure 3). Multiple membranous substances were found to be adhering to the surface of the tongue, palate, and buccal mucosa at the initial oral examination (Figure 3(a), Table 1, Oral Health Assessment Tool (OHAT) score: 13). We performed twice daily POHC to clean multiple membranous substances carefully using disposable sponge brushes and moisturizing gel (Refrecare®, EN Otsuka Pharmaceutical

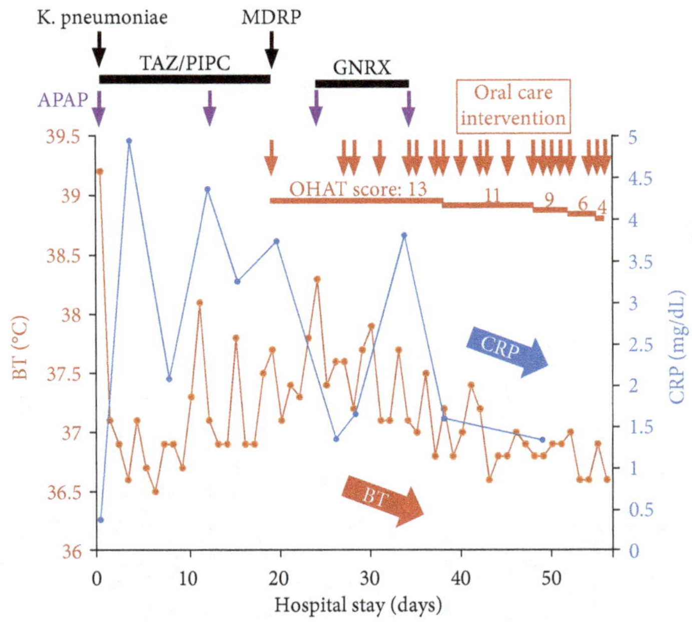

FIGURE 2: Time course of body temperature (BT) and C-reactive protein (CRP). BT and CRP are indicated by red closed circles and a solid line and blue closed circles and a solid line, respectively. Detection of bacteria by sputum culture, administration of acetaminophen (APAP), and professional oral health care intervention are indicated by black, purple, and red arrows, respectively. Treatment durations of tazobactam/piperacillin (TAZ/PIPC) and garenoxacin (GNRX) are indicated by solid bars. Oral Health Assessment Tool (OHAT) scores, assessed by the patient's oral condition at each timepoint, are indicated by red colored and red underlined text in the upper part of the figure.

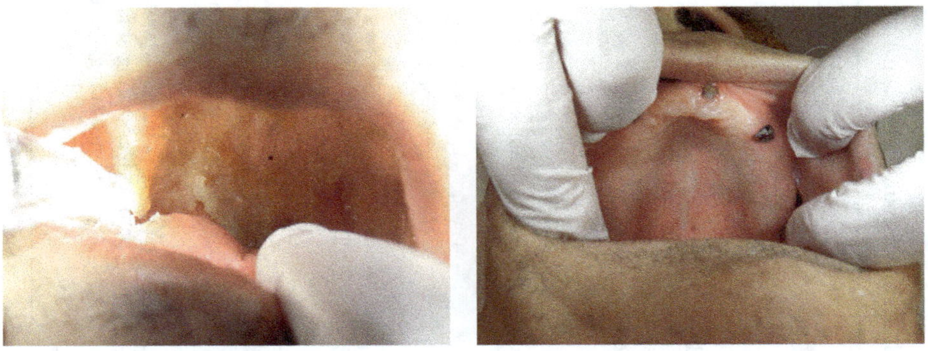

(a) (b)

FIGURE 3: Oral condition at (a) initial dental examination and (b) after receiving professional oral health care.

Co., Ltd., Tokyo, Japan), which also provided moisture for stabilizing the oral mucosa and tongue dorsum. In the early stages of POHC intervention, the patient's oral condition worsened and became dry 1 day after POHC. An oral-candidiasis-like redness on his oral mucosa and the dorsum of the tongue was also observed after removal of multiple membranous substances. The patient seemed to feel pain when we touched his oral mucosa despite our gentle procedure using moisturizing gel. However, our persistent POHC gradually became effective in achieving a healthy oral condition 2 weeks after starting the POHC intervention. Additionally, the patient ceased expressing pain vocally and through facial expression during POHC, and the redness of the oral mucosa totally disappeared (Figures 2 and 3, Table 1). Following recovery of his oral health, the patient's fever subsided and CRP levels returned to within the normal range. The X-ray abnormality and his consciousness (JCS: I-3) also improved (Figures 1(b) and 2). Finally, he was moved to another hospital for recuperation almost 1 month after starting POHC.

3. Discussion

Here, we report a case in which the patient recovered from severe aspiration pneumonia after continual POHC intervention. The main cause of pneumonia was thought to be aspiration of oral bacteria under poor oral conditions complicated by dysphagia. This case suggests that, in addition to antimicrobial treatment, the POHC intervention should have commenced at the initial stages of pneumonia. In fact,

Table 1: Evaluation results by Oral Health Assessment Tool: category scores at initial day and last day of oral care.

Category	0 = healthy	1 = changes	2 = unhealthy	Category scores (initial day)	Category scores (last day)
Lips	Smooth, pink, moist	Dry, chapped, or red at corners	Swelling or lump, white/red/ulcerated patch; bleeding/ulcerated at corners	1	0
Tongue	Normal, moist roughness, pink	Patchy, fissured, red, coated	Patch that is red and/or white, ulcerated, swollen	1	0
Gums and tissues	Pink, moist, smooth, no bleeding	Dry, shiny, rough, red, swollen, one ulcer/sore spot under dentures	Swollen, bleeding, ulcers, white/red patches, generalized redness under dentures	1	0
Saliva	Moist tissues, watery and free flowing saliva	Dry, sticky tissues, little saliva present, resident thinks they have a dry mouth	Tissues parched and red, very little/no saliva present, saliva is thick, resident thinks they have a dry mouth	2	0
Natural teeth Yes/no	No decayed or broken teeth/roots	1-3 decayed or broken teeth/roots or very worn down teeth	4+ decayed or broken teeth/roots, or very worn down teeth, or less than 4 teeth	2	2
Dentures Yes/no	No broken areas or teeth, dentures regularly worn, and named	1 broken area/tooth or dentures only worn for 1-2 h daily, or dentures not named, or loose	More than 1 broken area/tooth, denture missing or not worn, loose and needs denture adhesive, or not named	2	2
Oral cleanliness	Clean and no food particles or tartar in mouth or dentures	Food particles/tartar/plaque in 1-2 areas of the mouth or on small area of dentures or halitosis (bad breath)	Food particles/tartar/plaque in most areas of the mouth or on most of the dentures or severe halitosis (bad breath)	2	0
Dental pain	No behavioural, verbal, or physical signs of dental pain	Verbal and/or behavioural signs of pain such as pulling at face, chewing lips, not eating, aggression	Physical pain signs (swelling of cheek or gum, broken teeth, ulcers), as well as verbal and/or behavioural signs (pulling at face, not eating, aggression)	2	0
Total score (maximum: 16)	—	—	—	13	4

pneumonia did not improve until the POHC intervention began. However, persistent POHC intervention effectively contributed to improving the OHAT score (from 13 to 4) as well as lessening the severity of the pneumonia [7]. The Japanese guidelines for respiratory infectious diseases and CAP treatment also recommend that when antibiotics are not effective, physicians should consider systemic etiologic factors, including the presence of antibiotic-resistant bacteria, although the side effects of the antibiotics themselves can also include a rising fever and an elevated CRP level [8–10]. Another possible mechanism of recurrent inflammation observed in this case is repetitive aspiration of oral pathogens. Our results suggest that POHC involving the mechanical removal of oral pathogens may prevent the exacerbation of aspiration pneumonia in patients with dysphagia, notwithstanding the effects of antibiotics. Interestingly, several reports have shown evidence that *Candida albicans*, a commensal and opportunistic pathogen, forms a biofilm when cocultured with *K. pneumoniae* and other oral bacteria as pathogens of bacterial pneumonia [11]. Biofilms are often intrinsically resistant to conventional antifungal and antibiotic therapeutics. POHC can reduce the number of oral and oropharyngeal bacteria by mechanically removing bacterial biofilms, including respiratory pathogens [12]. We did not perform a culture test for the diagnosis of oral candidiasis in this case, although some clinical features of oral candidiasis, such as redness of the oral mucosa and sore mouth, were observed [13, 14]. It is therefore reasonable to presume that the antibiotic treatment was ineffective, but mechanical POHC was effective, in the recovery from aspiration pneumonia in this case.

Currently, POHC is recommended for the prevention of fever and aspiration pneumonia in older adults; however, no clear evidence exists that it can suppress the exacerbation of aspiration pneumonia [1–6]. There is some evidence that POHC can contribute to a better quality of life by improving oral complications such as halitosis, xerostomia, and oral infectious diseases in the terminal stages of systemic diseases [15]. Moreover, mechanical stimulation of the oral mucosa by POHC leads to brain stimulation and improvements in dysphagia, latency time of the swallowing response, and the cough reflex [16–18]. While further study is needed, POHC may become a supportive therapy for patients with severe aspiration pneumonia even if they are in the terminal stages of disease.

In conclusion, POHC may contribute to preventing both the occurrence and exacerbation of aspiration pneumonia by improving patients' oral condition.

Acknowledgments

We thank Helen Jeays, BDSc AE, from Edanz Group (http://www.edanzediting.com/ac) for editing a draft of this manuscript. This study was supported by JSPS KAKENHI (#16K11713 to HM and #17K12035 to TH and HM) and the Private University Research Branding Project (to Fukuoka Dental College) from the Ministry of Education, Culture, Sports, Science and Technology of Japan.

References

[1] T. Yoneyama, M. Yoshida, T. Matsui, and H. Sasaki, "Oral care and pneumonia," *The Lancet*, vol. 354, no. 9177, p. 515, 1999.

[2] T. Yoneyama, M. Yoshida, T. Ohrui et al., "Oral care reduces pneumonia in older patients in nursing homes," *Journal of American Geriatrics Society*, vol. 50, no. 3, pp. 430–433, 2002.

[3] C. Liu, Y. Cao, J. Lin et al., "Oral care measures for preventing nursing home-aquired pneumonia," *Cochrane Database Systematic Reviews*, vol. 9, article CD012416, 2018.

[4] P. E. Marik and D. Kaplan, "Aspiration pneumonia and dysphagia in the elderly," *Chest*, vol. 124, no. 1, pp. 328–336, 2003.

[5] S.-T. Huang, C.-C. Chiou, and H.-Y. Liu, "Risk factors of aspiration pneumonia related to improper oral hygiene behavior in community dysphagia persons with nasogastric tube feeding," *Journal of Dental Sciences*, vol. 12, no. 4, pp. 375–381, 2017.

[6] T. Nakashima, K. Maeda, K. Tahira et al., "Silent aspiration predicts mortality in older adults with aspiration pneumonia admitted to acute hospitals," *Geriatrics and Gerontology International*, vol. 18, no. 6, pp. 828–832, 2018.

[7] J. M. Chalmers, P. L. King, A. J. Spencer, F. A. Wright, and K. D. Carter, "The oral health assessment tool—validity and reliability," *Australian Dental Journal*, vol. 50, no. 3, pp. 191–199, 2005.

[8] K. Mikasa, N. Aoki, Y. Aoki et al., "JAID/JSC guidelines for the treatment of respiratory infectious diseases: the Japanese Association for Infectious Diseases/Japanese Society of Chemotherapy - the JAID/JSC guide to clinical management of infectious disease/guideline-preparing committee respiratory infectious disease WG," *Journal of Infection and Chemotherapy*, vol. 22, 7 Suppl, pp. S1–S65, 2016.

[9] Committee for The Japanese Respiratory Society guidelines in management of respiratory infections, "Guidelines for the management of community acquired pneumonia in adults, revised edition," *Respirology*, vol. 11, pp. S79–S133, 2006.

[10] S. Kohno, M. Seki, A. Watanabe, and CAP Study Group, "Evaluation of an assessment system for the JRS 2005: A-DROP for the management of CAP in adults," *Internal Medicine*, vol. 50, no. 11, pp. 1183–1191, 2011.

[11] M. Gulati and C. J. Nobile, "*Candida albicans* biofilms: development, regulation, and molecular mechanisms," *Microbes and Infection*, vol. 18, no. 5, pp. 310–321, 2016.

[12] A. Ishikawa, T. Yoneyama, K. Hirota, Y. Miyake, and K. Miyatake, "Professional oral health care reduces the number of oropharyngeal bacteria," *Journal of Dental Research*, vol. 87, no. 6, pp. 594–598, 2008.

[13] S. Patil, R. S. Rao, B. Majumdar, and S. Anil, "Clinical appearance of oral candida infection and therapeutic strategies," *Frontiers in Microbiology*, vol. 6, p. 1391, 2015.

[14] M. Nakajima, Y. Umezaki, S. Takeda et al., "Association between oral candidiasis and bacterial pneumonia, a retrospective study," *Oral Diseases*, 2019, in press.

[15] R. Fitzgerald and J. Gallagher, "Oral health in end-of-life patients: a rapid review," *Special Care in Dentistry*, vol. 38, no. 5, pp. 291–298, 2018.

[16] T. Kikutani, T. Yoneyama, K. Nishiwaki, F. Tamura, M. Yoshida, and H. Sasaki, "Effect of oral care on cognitive function in patients with dementia," *Geriatrics and Gerontology International*, vol. 10, no. 4, pp. 327-328, 2010.

[17] A. Yoshino, T. Ebihara, S. Ebihara, H. Fuji, and H. Sasaki, "Daily oral care and risk factors for pneumonia among elderly nursing home patients," *JAMA*, vol. 286, no. 18, pp. 2235-2236, 2001.

[18] A. Watando, S. Ebihara, T. Ebihara et al., "Daily oral care and cough reflex sensitivity in elderly nursing home patients," *Chest*, vol. 126, no. 4, pp. 1066–1070, 2004.

13

Five-Year Recall after Treatment of External Cervical Resorption

Fahd A. Aljarbou

Department of Restorative Dental Sciences, Division of Endodontics, College of Dentistry, King Saud University, Riyadh, Saudi Arabia

Correspondence should be addressed to Fahd A. Aljarbou; faljarbou@ksu.edu.sa

Academic Editor: Leandro Napier de Souza

The management of external cervical resorption can be challenging. This study described a two-step procedure for the treatment of external cervical resorption. It involved nonsurgical root canal treatment and a dental amalgam core buildup, followed by a surgical approach to restore the root structure using resin-modified glass ionomer (Geristore®). The patient was recalled for a period of five years, and the overall outcome was successful.

1. Introduction

Root resorption is a physiological process in primary teeth and a pathological process in permanent teeth. It is a rare and undesirable occurrence in permanent roots. On the contrary, bone undergoes constant remodeling, including periods of resorption and deposition [1]. The process of root resorption involves two major events: injury to the protective dental tissue and activation of an inflammatory response [2]. It can affect the internal or external part of the root. It may be transient or progressive [3]. External cervical resorption (ECR) is an example of progressive external root resorption. It is been studied extensively by Heithersay, who termed it as invasive cervical resorption (ICR) [4, 5]. The defect appears extensive clinically and occurs at the cervical third of the root, possibly with a pinkish discoloration of the crown. It is classified into four classes depending on its severity, in which the more the class, the worse in clinical outcome it gets. The aim of this study was to report the management of a case of ECR involving the maxillary left canine.

2. Case Report

A 70-year-old man of European descent, with controlled type II diabetes, was referred to us by the periodontics clinic. He took 81 mL of aspirin orally, once a day, and 10 mEq of potassium citrate orally, thrice a day. He had no known allergies to dental materials. The patient was asymptomatic. He was referred to us, after the intraoperative observation of resorption in the palatal half of the coronal one-third of the root of tooth #23, during periodontal surgery related to an implant placed in the region of tooth #24. The invasive resorbing tissues were deep and confined to the coronal third and it is classified as Heithersay class III. Root repair was attempted using Fuji IX GIC (GC Corp, Japan), with poor results. Tooth number 23 was an abutment in joint crowns of multiple units, extending from canine to canine. Informed consent was obtained upon the patient's arrival. The cold test was normal for 22 and was negative for 23. Percussion and palpation were normal in this area. Palatal recession, measuring 2 mm, was observed with 23. The probing depth was within 2-3 mm on the buccal aspect and 7-8 mm on palatal aspect, which felt soft on tactile perception, along the inner part of the tooth indicating the presence of granulation tissue and confirming the diagnosis of ECR. Nonsurgical root canal treatment was planned, followed by surgical repair of the defect.

One carpule of 1.8 mL solution of lidocaine 2% with 1 : 80,000 epinephrine (Lidocaine HCl, Huons Co., Seoul, Korea) was used for buccal and palatal infiltration anesthesia for 23. Rubber dam was used to isolate the operating field. An access opening (into the canal) was created, using a long shank round-ended tapered diamond bur at a 45° angle for about 4 mm, while preserving the lingual triangle. Isolation was difficult to achieve, and electronic determination of working length was not feasible. The working length (29 mm) was obtained radiographically, using size 15 K-hand file (Dentsply Co., Munich, Germany) from

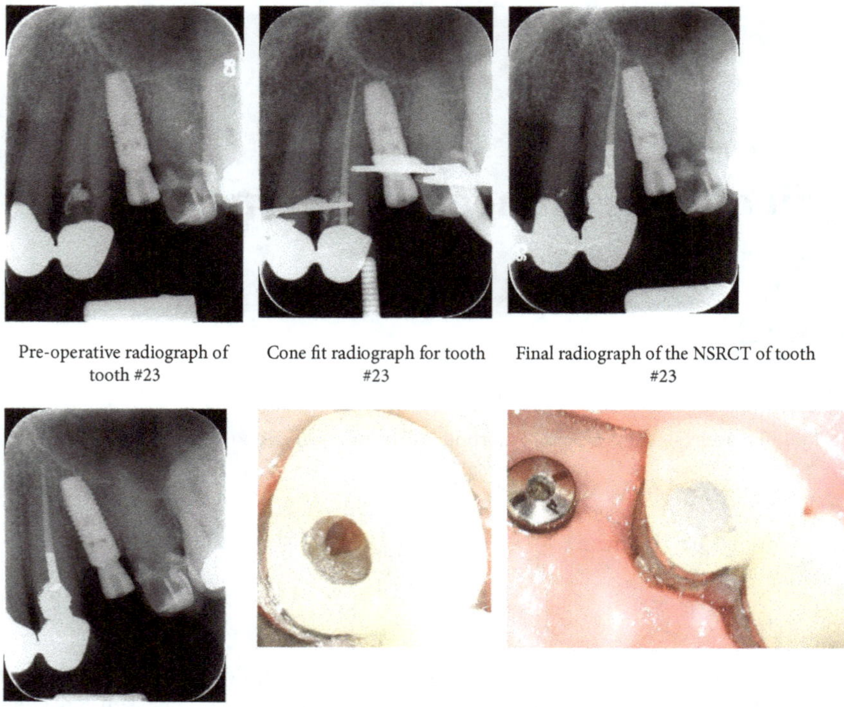

Pre-operative radiograph of tooth #23

Cone fit radiograph for tooth #23

Final radiograph of the NSRCT of tooth #23

Mesial shift for the final radiograph of the NSRCT of tooth #23

Clinical photo of the access for tooth #23

Clinical photo of the finished NSRCT of tooth #23

FIGURE 1: Radiographs and clinical photos showing the steps of nonsurgical root canal treatment of tooth #23 with amalgam post and core buildup.

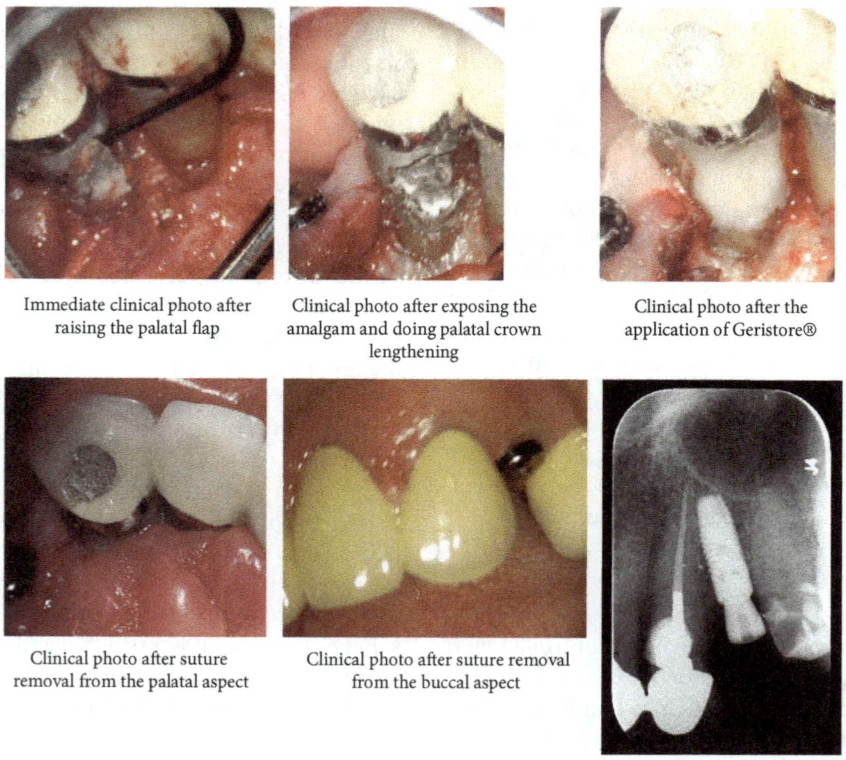

Immediate clinical photo after raising the palatal flap

Clinical photo after exposing the amalgam and doing palatal crown lengthening

Clinical photo after the application of Geristore®

Clinical photo after suture removal from the palatal aspect

Clinical photo after suture removal from the buccal aspect

Post-surgical radiograph for tooth #23

FIGURE 2: Clinical photos and postsurgical radiograph showing the whole steps for managing the resorptive defect surgically in tooth #23.

the cusp tip. Rotary instrumentation was performed up to size 35, using the entire sequence of ProTaper® Universal (Dentsply Tulsa Dental Specialties, Tulsa, OK, USA) up to size F3, followed by ProFile Ni-Ti files (size: 35, 0.04 taper) (Maillefer, Ballaigues, Switzerland). Irrigation was performed with 12 cc of 5.25% sodium hypochlorite between each file and as a final rinse after 17% EDTA (5 mL) (Meta Biomed Co. Ltd., Mandaluyong, Korea). The canal was dried with sterile paper points and obturated with the warm vertical compaction technique, 3 mm short of the apical margin of the resorption, using Kerr Pulp Canal Sealer EWT (Kerr, Orange, CA) and gutta-percha cones (size: 35, 0.04 taper) (Meta Biomed Co. Ltd., Cheongju City, Chungbuk, Korea). The palatal access opening in the crowned tooth was filled with dental amalgam (Valliant ™, Ivoclar Vivadent Inc., Amherst NY) and vertically adapted using a range of Schilder pluggers (Dentsply, Maillefer, Switzerland).

The patient was reassessed a week later, and no significant changes were observed. Surgery was confined to the palatal aspect and two carpules containing 3.6 mL of 2% lidocaine with 1 : 100,000 epinephrine (Lidocaine HCl, Huons Co., Seoul, Korea) were used for buccal and palatal infiltration anesthesia for 23. A triangular flap was raised, subsequent to a palatal intersulcular incision from 21 to 23, with 1 cm distal vertical release. The surgical site was exposed, and the poorly adapted repair material was removed, followed by crown lengthening along the palatal margin. Geristore® (Den-Mat, Santa Maria, CA) was used to cover the fully set dental amalgam, to preserve the palatal root contour, and enhance gingival tissue attachment. Finishing and polishing were followed by five simple interrupted sutures using silk (size 5-0, reverse cutting needle FS-2, Ethicon Inc., Somerville, NJ, USA). Postoperative instructions were given and suture removal was scheduled after three days. The patient was scheduled for a proper follow-up visits in the future. Figure 1 represents the radiographic and clinical photographs of the nonsurgical management of 23. Figure 2 represents the clinical photos of the surgical management in 23. Figure 3 shows the recall radiographs and clinical photographs for 23.

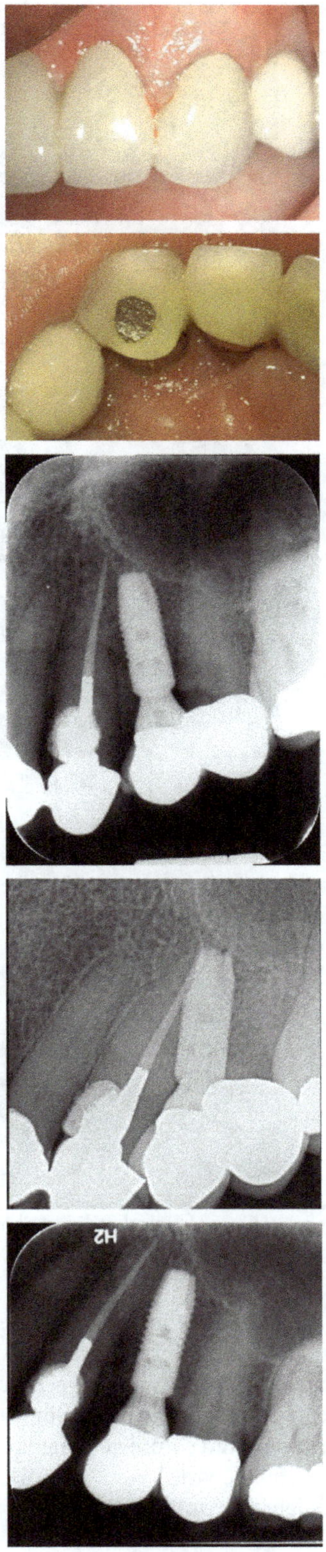

Clinical photo from the buccal aspect at two years recall

Clinical photo from the palatal aspect at two years recall

Radiograph of tooth #23 at two years recall

Radiograph of tooth #23 at four years recall

Radiograph of tooth #23 at five years recall

FIGURE 3: Recall radiographs and clinical photos for tooth #23.

3. Discussion

The ECR defect is characterized by root resorption in cervical third, which can progress rapidly. This patient was diagnosed clinically and intraoperatively by chance during a periodontal surgery in which a granulation tissue covering the whole palatal side of the coronal third and it was removed. However, in retrospection, radiographic progression of the resorptive defect was evident, as seen in Figure 4.

The management of this case involved a two-step procedure, which started with the nonsurgical approach and ended with surgery. We used dental amalgam as a post and core buildup material, followed by Geristore®. These materials had beneficial properties, which were well suited to this case, as shown by the recall visits.

The use of dental amalgam has been minimized or prohibited in some countries, mainly because of its potential health hazards, caused by mercury release [6]. We countered this drawback, by covering it with a high-sealing, periodontally compatible restorative material, which will also promote tissue attachment and maintain the proper root contour [7]. Geristore® even showed advantageous properties at inflammatory cytokine expression levels [8]. The advantages of

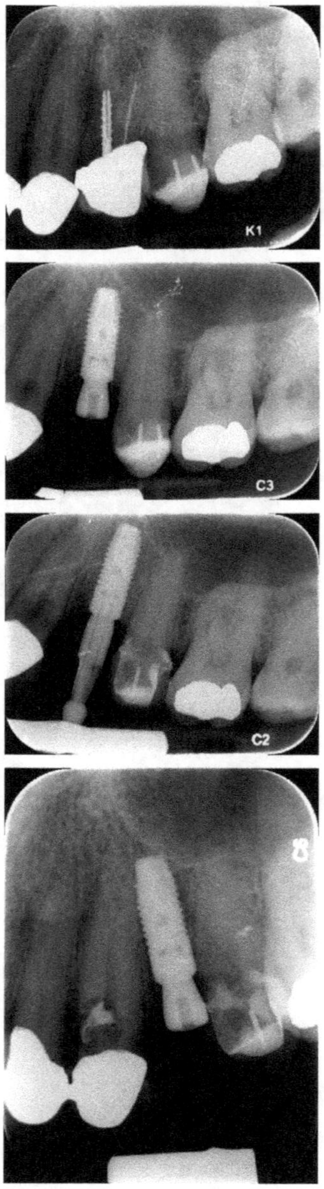

Radiograph taken after cementation of the fixed partial prosthesis connecting tooth #13 to #23 while there was discussion about the prognosis of tooth #24

1 year after, tooth #24 was extracted and endosseous implant was placed. Radiographically, notice the initiation of the cervical resorption in tooth #23.

3 months after, the resorption defect was not addressed and there was significant increase in the size of defect.

A month after, the case received in endodontic clinic to be managed and the resorption size is significantly increased.

FIGURE 4: Chronological radiographic evaluation of the resorptive defect in tooth #23.

amalgam over resin-bonded restorations include the ease of manipulation, good seal, and lower cost. Its principal property that informed our clinical decision was the technique insensitivity, as contamination is expected when dealing with such a large defect. Therefore, we could complete the nonsurgical root canal treatment in a single visit.

Surgical exposure of the defect permitted direct observation of the resorptive lesion. Cone beam computed tomography (CBCT) imaging can reveal such lesions preoperatively, thus aiding in treatment planning and management [9]. Limited access to CBCT at that time prevented its use in this case. We strongly recommend performing CBCT before treatment.

Acknowledgments

I would like to thank Dr. Ibrahim Alaugaily for his great help in collecting patient records.

References

[1] L. Hammarstrom and S. Lindskog, "General morphological aspects of resorption of teeth and alveolar bone," *International Endodontic Journal*, vol. 18, no. 2, pp. 93–108, 1985.

[2] M. Trope, "Root resorption of dental and traumatic origin: classification based on etiology," *Practical Periodontics and Aesthetic Dentistry*, vol. 10, no. 4, pp. 515–522, 1998.

[3] L. Tronstad, "Root resorption — etiology, terminology and clinical manifestations," *Endodontics & Dental Traumatology*, vol. 4, no. 6, pp. 241–252, 1988.

[4] G. S. Heithersay, "Invasive cervical resorption: an analysis of potential predisposing factors," *Quintessence International*, vol. 30, no. 2, pp. 83–95, 1999.

[5] G. S. Heithersay, "Clinical, radiologic, and histopathologic features of invasive cervical resorption," *Quintessence International*, vol. 30, no. 1, pp. 27–37, 1999.

[6] S. M. Koral, "Mercury from dental amalgam: exposure and risk assessment," *Compendium of Continuing Education in Dentistry*, vol. 34, no. 2, pp. 138–40, 142, 144 passim, 2013.

[7] S. K. Gupta, P. Saxena, V. A. Pant, and A. B. Pant, "Adhesion and biologic behavior of human periodontal fibroblast cells to resin ionomer Geristore: a comparative analysis," *Dental Traumatology*, vol. 29, no. 5, pp. 389–393, 2013.

[8] R. R. Oliveira, W. L. F. Tavares, A. L. Reis, V. A. Silva, L. Q. Vieira, and A. P. Ribeiro Sobrinho, "Cytokine expression in response to root repair agents," *International Endodontic Journal*, vol. 51, no. 11, pp. 1253–1260, 2018.

[9] S. Patel, A. M. Mavridou, P. Lambrechts, and N. Saberi, "External cervical resorption-part 1: histopathology, distribution and presentation," *International Endodontic Journal*, vol. 51, no. 11, pp. 1205–1223, 2018.

14

Extremely Rare Intraoral Presentation of Localized Amyloidosis

Luka Morelato[1], **Igor Smojver**[2], **Sven Seiwerth**[3], **and Dragana Gabrić**[4]

[1]*Department of Oral Surgery, Faculty of Dental Medicine, University of Rijeka, Croatia*
[2]*Special Hospital, St. Catherine, Zagreb, Croatia*
[3]*Department of Pathology, School of Medicine, University of Zagreb, Croatia*
[4]*Department of Oral Surgery, School of Dental Medicine, University of Zagreb, Croatia*

Correspondence should be addressed to Dragana Gabrić; dgabric@sfzg.hr

Academic Editor: Kenji Yamagata

Purpose. To present an extremely rare case of localized amyloidosis of the mucosa of the maxillary alveolar ridge. *Case Report.* A 71-year-old man was referred to the Department of Oral Surgery, School of Dental Medicine, University of Zagreb, for a persistent nodular formation in the edentulous ridge of the anterior maxillary region. The nodular formation had a reddish color, solid consistency, and an approximate size of 40×15 mm. Orthopantomographic imaging excluded bone resorption and defects. Histopathological assessments of the biopsy specimen showed that the stroma was occupied by a multiplied, partially hyalinized connective tissue. The samples were subsequently stained with Congo red, and collagen accumulation under polarized light showed an apple-green birefringence indicating amyloid. Subsequently, the nodular formation was completely excised and a maxillary total denture was made. The patient showed normal tissue healing with no sign of recurrence at a follow-up assessment 1.5 years after the procedure. *Conclusion.* This is only the third reported case of localized amyloidosis of the alveolar ridge mucosa. Histopathological analysis is the first step for diagnosis, but systemic tests, blood counts, urinalysis, bone marrow biopsy, electrocardiography, and digestive endoscopy are recommended to rule out a systemic disease.

1. Introduction

The term "amyloidosis" is used to describe a progressive metabolic disease with abnormal amyloid protein deposits in one or more organs [1, 2]. To date, 36 human proteins have been shown to possess the potential to form extracellular amyloid aggregates that precipitate in the extracellular spaces of different organ tissues, causing functional damage. Of these, 14 proteins are associated with systemic amyloidosis and 19 are known to cause localized forms of the disease, whereas the remaining three cause both localized and systemic forms of amyloidosis [2, 3]. These different types of proteins are currently named after the specific protein that is precipitated, using the prefix "A" for "amyloid," followed by the letters indicating the protein type.

Amyloidosis may be acquired or hereditary, and the disease presentation may be primary or secondary. It may be restricted to a single organ (localized form), or it may affect many organs (systemic form) [4]. The cause of primary amyloidosis is unknown, and it has not yet been linked to any primary disease. Monoclonal immunoglobulin amyloid is deposited in organs such as the liver, heart, kidney, and spleen, leading to systemic manifestations such as congestive heart failure and unexplained proteinuria [5]. In patients with systemic forms of amyloidosis, the prognosis depends on the type and stage of the disease in the affected organs [6]. Secondary amyloidosis is the most common form of systemic amyloidosis, accounting for approximately 45% of the cases of systemic amyloidosis [7]. It occurs secondarily to a series of primary diseases involving chronic inflammation, such as rheumatoid arthritis, sarcoidosis, Crohn's disease, ulcerative colitis, and tuberculosis. Chronic oral periodontitis has also been suggested to lead to secondary amyloidosis [8]. Proper periodontal treatment can effectively reduce the formation of inflammatory mediators caused by amyloidosis [9]. Intraoral amyloidosis is a rare and usually benign condition. The most commonly affected areas in the oral cavity are the tongue and buccal mucosa, and the involvement of other areas is considered to be extremely rare [10].

Localized amyloidosis is a rare type of disease characterized by the deposition of amyloid in the localized tissue of a particular anatomical region. It manifests as a tissue mass that can mimic a growing tumor [11]. If head and neck structures are involved, localized amyloidosis is usually a benign condition with a good prognosis [7]. The incidence of amyloidosis is approximately nine to twelve cases per million people per year [6, 12]. The diagnosis of amyloidosis is not difficult, since the lesions of the localized forms are mostly superficial and easy to observe and require a biopsy. Congo red staining is the gold standard for histological confirmation; it is used with polarized light microscopy under which amyloid deposits show a characteristic apple-green birefringence [12].

The aim of the present study was to report a rare case of intraoral localized amyloidosis discovered as an incidental finding due to the patient's inability to wear a maxillary total denture.

2. Case Presentation

A 71-year-old man was referred by his general dentist to the Department of Oral Surgery, School of Dental Medicine, University of Zagreb, in July 2019 because of a persistent nodular formation in the vestibular intercanine region of the edentulous ridge of the maxilla. The nodular formation was reddish-pink in color, had a solid consistency, and measured approximately 40 × 15 mm with a periodontal probe (Deppeler SA, Rolle, Switzerland) (Figure 1). The patient reported noticing this small and painless mass growing for the first time approximately 15 years ago, after his general dentist made a maxillary total denture. After time, denture was adapted to avoid the nodular mass. He had been wearing the total denture using a denture adhesive (Figure 2).

The patient had a history of type II diabetes mellitus and arterial hypertension. He had also undergone several medical procedures, including penile amputation due to planocellular carcinoma T2NxMx in February 2018, and lymphadenectomy in May of the same year. In August 2018, he broke his femoral neck and underwent left hip total endoprosthesis replacement. He also had cardiovascular disease in the form of aortic stenosis and ischemic cardiomyopathy and had undergone surgery for aortic valve replacement with a biological prosthesis (Dokimos 23 mm, Labcor, Calafate, Belo Horizonte) and a double coronary bypass in June 2019. He was regularly taking nebivolol 2.5 mg, trimetazidine 2 × 35 mg, indapamide 1.5 mg, acetylsalicylic acid 100 mg, ramipril 1.25 mg, atorvastatin 40 mg, and gliclazide 60 mg.

After recovering from the cardiac surgery, the patient decided to get a new maxillary total denture when the nodular formation was observed. The preoperative differential diagnosis concluded a suspect epulis fissuratum due to irritation caused by a worn upper dental prosthesis or a growing neoplasm. Orthopantomographic imaging was performed, and underlying bone resorption and defects were excluded (Figure 3). Extraoral examination did not show enlarged lymph nodes in the head and neck area.

Consistent with the ethical requirements of the School of Dental Medicine, University of Zagreb, Croatia, written informed consent for the publication of this study was obtained from the patient prior to the surgery. In the first stage, biopsy material was obtained under local anesthesia (1.7 mL articaine 4%; 1:100000) by performing wedge incisions along the long side of the nodule formation; two tissue samples obtained with this procedure were sent for histopathological assessment. Excisional biopsy findings were analyzed after fixation in 6% buffered formalin, dehydration, and paraffin embedding of the tissue samples, after which 4 μm thick sections were cut and stained with hematoxylin-eosin for diagnostic purposes. The histopathological assessments revealed a slightly mottled, multilayered squamous epithelium over a stroma occupied by a multiplied, partially hyalinized binder (Figure 4). The samples were subsequently stained with Congo red, following which collagen accumulations were observed with the apple-green birefringence of amyloid under polarized light (Figure 5). The histopathological findings indicated a case of amyloidosis.

Laboratory tests for blood and urine showed that proteinuria was absent and the complete blood count was normal. Lung radiography and brain computed tomography did not reveal any pathology. Electrocardiogram monitoring also showed normal findings after aortic valve replacement.

In the second stage of the procedure, after the application of local anesthesia (1.7 mL of articaine 4%; 1:100000), the formation was completely excised using electrocauterization (ART Electrosurge, Bonart Co., New Taipei City, Taiwan) with a wire electrode.

After a healing period of two weeks, a new, complete upper denture was made.

The whole ductile formation measuring 3.2 × 1.3 × 1.1 cm was submitted for histopathological analysis, and the diagnosis of amyloidosis was confirmed (Figure 6).

Based on the normal findings of all tests such as the blood and urine assessments, electrocardiography, gastrointestinal endoscopy, lung radiography, and brain computed tomography as well as the long and slow growth period of the nodular formation, a localized amyloidosis of the mucosa of the upper alveolar ridge was diagnosed. However, due to the patient's age and medical condition, he refused to undergo bone marrow biopsy to completely rule out systemic disease. The patient was followed up for 1.5 years, during which he showed normal tissue healing and no sign of recurrence (Figure 7).

3. Discussion

Localized intraoral amyloidosis is an extremely rare disease. The most commonly affected areas in the head and neck region are the larynx, thyroid, and subglottis. In the oral cavity, usually affected is the tongue, whereas the buccal mucosa is affected less often [13]. Amyloidosis in other locations is extremely rare. To the best of our knowledge, this is the third case of localized amyloidosis of the maxillary alveolar mucosa ever reported in the literature [14].

The etiology of localized amyloidosis itself is not completely clear; the first step in the development could be the reaction of plasma cells to environmental antigens and

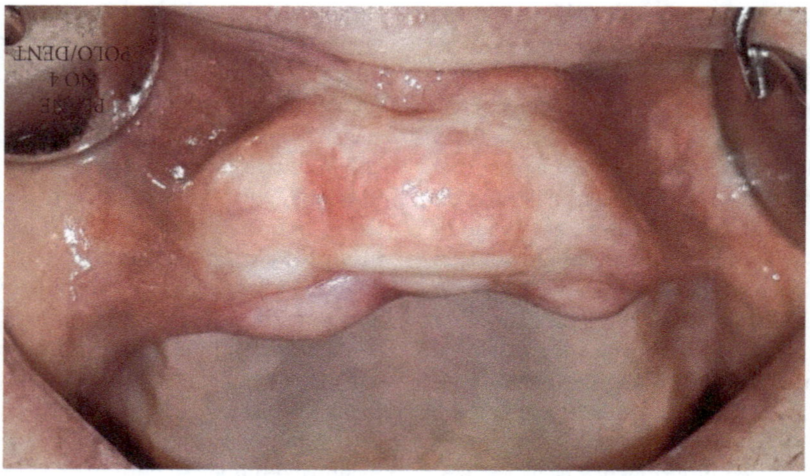

FIGURE 1: Slow-growing painless mass.

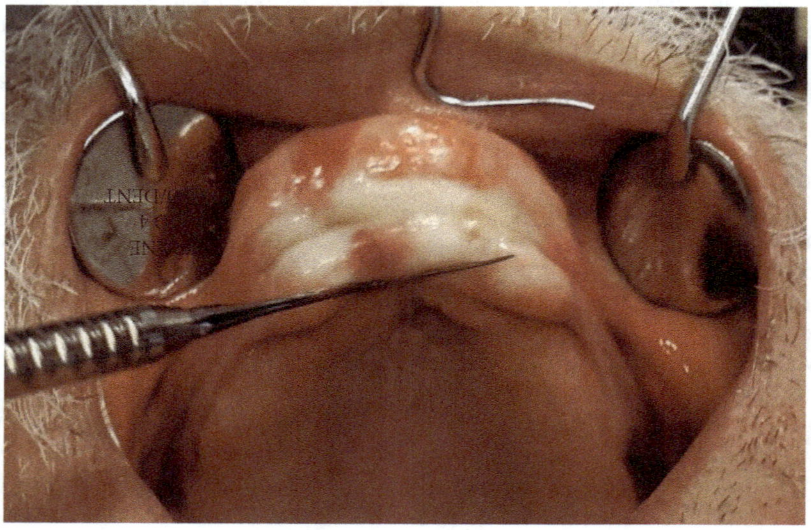

FIGURE 2: Intraoral findings.

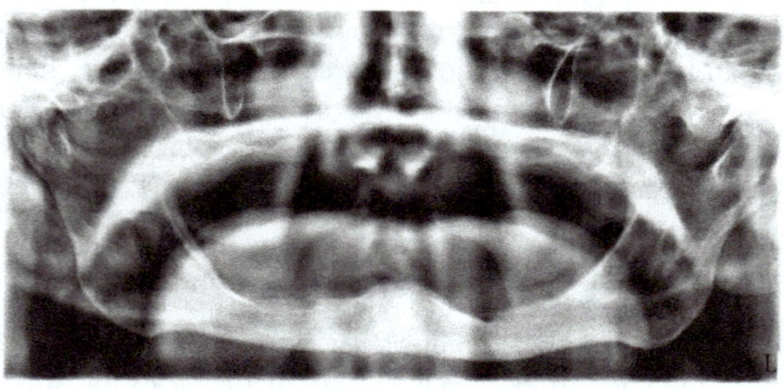

FIGURE 3: Orthopantomographic image showing no underlying bone resorption or defect.

chronic inflammation, followed by abundant production of light chains of immunoglobulins that transform into insoluble fibrils and locally deposit in tissues [15]. Nevertheless, only a few plasma cells could be identified in the biopsy material, leading to the "suicidal neoplasm" theory [16].

In the present case, the chronic local irritation could be caused by an improperly adjusted upper removable prosthesis. The same was suggested in a second case reported in the literature by Bucci et al. [14, 17].

During the period of 15 years, painless mass was slowly growing without bleeding, ulceration, or acute inflammation periods. Due to the localization and retarded growth of the nodular formation during the total denture-wearing period, the differential diagnosis indicated epulis fissuratum, which typically occurs in the area of chronic irritation caused by inadequately adjusted denture margin [18] or a suspected malignant neoplasm due to the nodular mass. The patient has several severe illnesses considering that the literature could not be related to oral amyloidosis and by conducting tests that excluded potential organ involvement in systemic amyloidosis form [6].

Treatment of localized amyloidosis depends on the affected organ as well as on the degree of functional impairment [19, 20]. Surgical excision of the amyloid deposits has

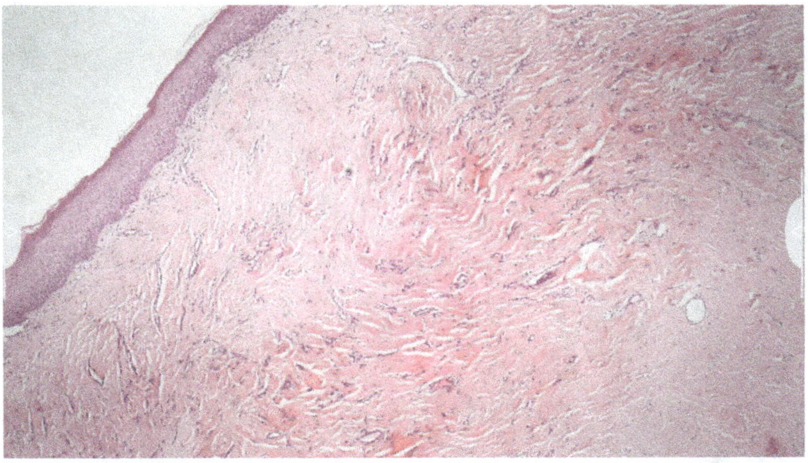

Figure 4: Slightly mottled, multilayered squamous epithelium over a stroma occupied by a multiplied, partially hyalinized binder.

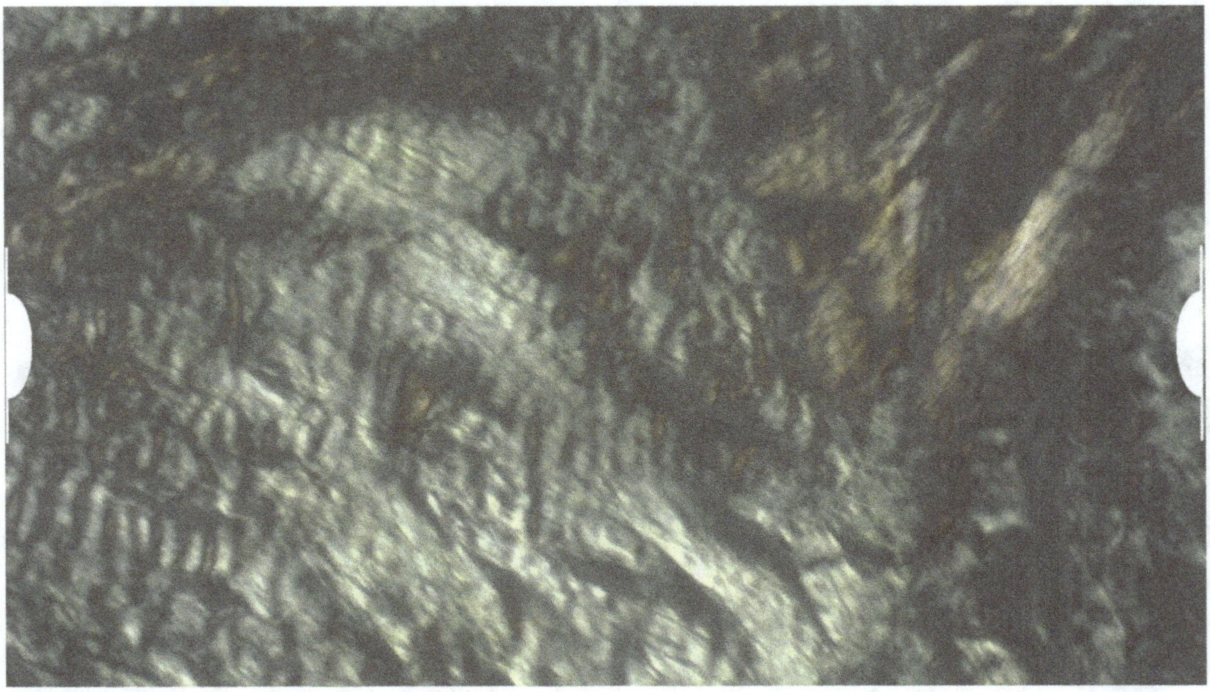

Figure 5: Collagen accumulations showing apple-green birefringence of amyloid under polarized light.

been suggested to avoid functional damage as a result of growth formation, although frequent recurrences have been described. However, there is no consensus on the optimal treatment approach, and there are no relevant surgical guidelines. No randomized controlled trials have been conducted, and the current knowledge is based mainly on the findings from a few case reports [21, 22]. In the literature, surgical excision was reported in nine cases, in which recurrence occurred in two cases. Namely, Babburi et al. performed complete surgical excision in a case of nodular tongue amyloidosis, which recurred 3 years later [23], and O'Reilly et al. reported recurrence in one case after a year, necessitating repeated excision [24]. Bleeding may be a major complication of the excision of localized amyloidosis, and it is explained by the lack of factor X and the fragility of blood vessels as a result of the interaction of blood with amyloid fibrils [18, 25]. The prognosis of localized oral amyloidosis is good. In previous retrospective studies, many authors did not report the transition of the disease from an oral localized to a systemic form [23, 26, 27]. In the present case, the patient was normally wearing the upper dental prosthesis made after the surgical excision of the lesion and showed normal tissue healing with no recurrence after 1.5 years.

Our findings are very similar to two previous cases reported in the literature, and it could be suggested that local amyloidosis of the alveolar mucosa could be caused by

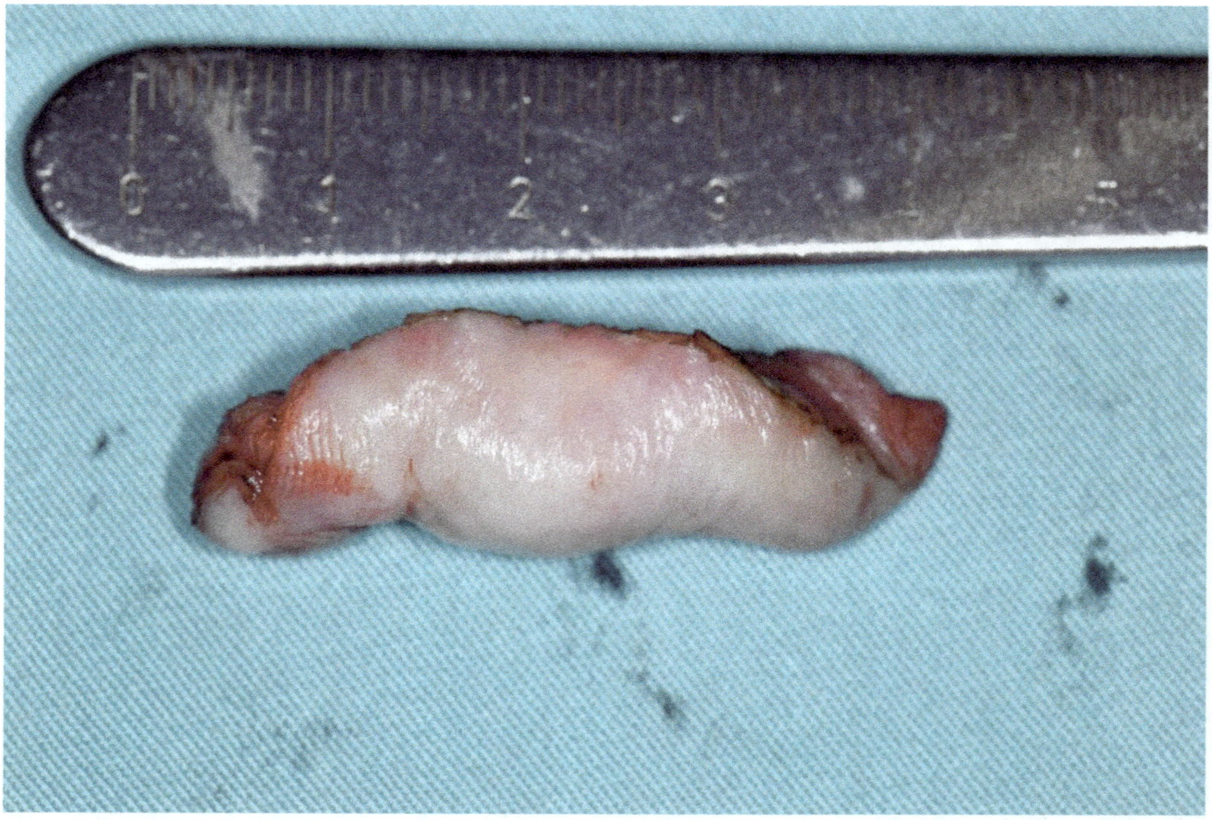

Figure 6: Ductile formation specimen after surgical excision.

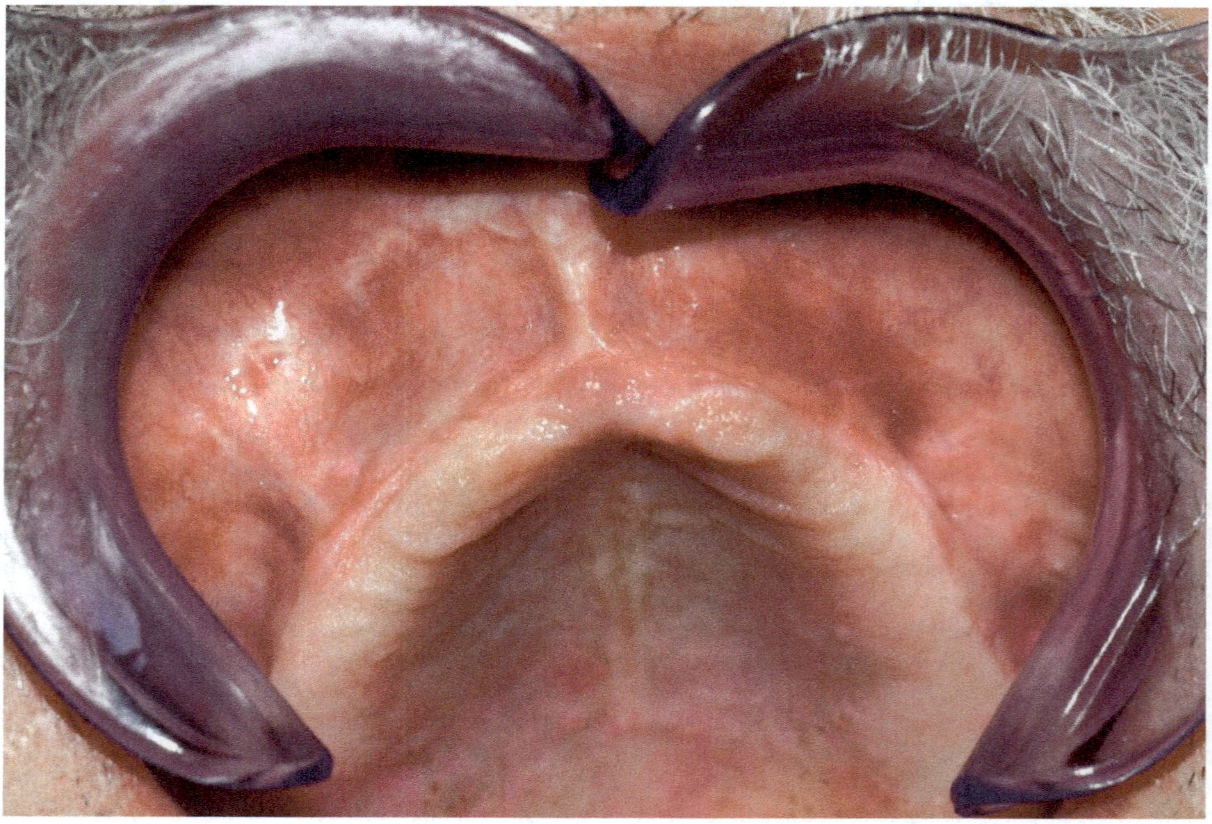

Figure 7: Normal tissue healing at the follow-up assessment after 1.5 years.

chronic irritation of ill-fitting dentures, but other studies on larger numbers of cases have to be conducted to confirm the finding.

According to mostly very clear clinical findings, with specific anamnesis in everyday practice, not all epulis fissuratum after excision were pathohistologically analyzed. This case shows unusual findings and suggests that all even typical specimens should sustain pathohistological diagnosis and according to that should be followed up properly.

In conclusion, our findings emphasize the need for cooperation among dentists, oral and maxillofacial surgeons, pathologists, and general practitioners in the diagnosis, treatment, and lifelong follow-up of patients diagnosed with local amyloidosis. After an excisional biopsy of the lesion, histological examination is the first step toward diagnosis, followed by the exclusion of the systemic form of the disease, and immunohistochemical tests are desirable. The diagnosis of localized amyloidosis should always be accompanied by blood tests, bone marrow biopsy, echocardiography, and gastrointestinal endoscopy to rule out systemic amyloidosis or any other hematological/immune disorders or organ dysfunctions. There is no consensus on the treatment of local amyloidosis. Surgical treatment is indicated to reduce the functional damage produced by the bulky mass. In any case, lifelong follow-up of the patient is recommended.

Consent

Informed consent was obtained from the patient for the publication of this study.

References

[1] R. Virchow, "Ueber eine im Gehirn und Rückenmark des Menschen aufgefundene Substanz mit der chemischen Reaction der Cellulose," *Archiv für Pathologische Anatomie und Physiologie und für Klinische Medicin*, vol. 6, no. 1, pp. 135–138, 1854.

[2] M. D. Benson, J. N. Buxbaum, D. S. Eisenberg et al., "Amyloid nomenclature 2018: recommendations by the International Society of Amyloidosis (ISA) nomenclature committee," *Amyloid*, vol. 25, no. 4, pp. 215–219, 2018.

[3] P. Mollee, P. Renaut, D. Gottlieb, and H. Goodman, "How to diagnose amyloidosis," *Internal Medicine Journal*, vol. 44, no. 1, pp. 7–17, 2014.

[4] K. S. Fahrner, C. C. Black, and B. J. Gosselin, "Localized amyloidosis of the tongue: a review," *American Journal of Otolaryngology*, vol. 25, no. 3, pp. 186–189, 2004.

[5] M. A. Gertz, "Immunoglobulin light chain amyloidosis: 2016 update on diagnosis, prognosis, and treatment," *American Journal of Hematology*, vol. 91, no. 9, pp. 947–956, 2016.

[6] M. A. Gertz and A. Dispenzieri, "Systemic amyloidosis recognition, prognosis, and therapy: a systematic review," *Journal of the American Medical Association*, vol. 324, no. 1, pp. 79–89, 2020.

[7] T. P. Quock, T. Yan, E. Chang, S. Guthrie, and M. S. Broder, "Epidemiology of AL amyloidosis: a real-world study using US claims data," *Blood Advances*, vol. 2, no. 10, pp. 1046–1053, 2018.

[8] S. Khoury, J. J. Dusek, G. B. Anderson, and N. Vigneswaran, "Systemic amyloidosis manifesting as localized, severe periodontitis," *Journal of the American Dental Association (1939)*, vol. 135, no. 5, pp. 617–623, 2004.

[9] M. İ. Cengiz, N. Yayla, K. Cengiz, H. Bagci, and E. Taşkın, "Interaction between periodontal disease and systemic secondary amyloidosis: from inflammation to amyloidosis," *Journal of Periodontology*, vol. 82, no. 4, pp. 566–574, 2011.

[10] S. Elad, R. Czerninski, S. Fischman et al., "Exceptional oral manifestations of amyloid light chain protein (AL) systemic amyloidosis," *Amyloid*, vol. 17, no. 1, pp. 27–31, 2010.

[11] L. Turiak, B. Kaszás, K. Katona et al., "Localized amyloidosis of the upper aerodigestive tract: complex analysis of the cellular infiltrate and the amyloid mass," *Anal. Cell. Pathol*, vol. 2019, article 6165140, 9 pages, 2019.

[12] J. Deng, Q. Chen, P. Ji, X. Zeng, and X. Jin, "Oral amyloidosis: a strategy to differentiate systemic amyloidosis involving the oral cavity and localized amyloidosis," *Oral Diseases*, vol. 25, no. 3, pp. 670–675, 2019.

[13] E. T. Stoopler, T. P. Sollecito, and S. Y. Chen, "Amyloid deposition in the oral cavity: a retrospective study and review of the literature," *Oral Surgery, Oral Medicine, Oral Pathology, Oral Radiology, and Endodontics*, vol. 95, no. 6, pp. 674–680, 2003.

[14] T. Bucci, E. Bucci, A. M. P. Rullan, P. Bucci, and P. Nuzzolo, "Localized amyloidosis of the upper gingiva: a case report," *Journal of Medical Case Reports*, vol. 8, no. 1, p. 198, 2014.

[15] P. Westermark, M. D. Benson, J. N. Buxbaum et al., "Amyloid: toward terminology clarification. Report from the nomenclature committee of the International Society of Amyloidosis," *Amyloid*, vol. 12, no. 1, pp. 1–4, 2005.

[16] P. Westermark, "Localized AL amyloidosis: a suicidal neoplasm?," *Upsala Journal of Medical Sciences*, vol. 117, no. 2, pp. 244–250, 2012.

[17] R. P. S. Mohan, S. Verma, U. Singh, and N. Agarwal, "Epulis fissuratum: consequence of ill-fitting prosthesis," *Case Reports*, vol. 2013, no. jul17 1, p. bcr2013200054, 2013.

[18] P. R. Greipp, R. A. Kyle, and E. J. Bowie, "Factor-X deficiency in amyloidosis: a critical review," *American Journal of Hematology*, vol. 11, no. 4, pp. 443–450, 1981.

[19] M. Paccalin, E. Hachulla, C. Cazalet et al., "Localized amyloidosis: a survey of 35 French cases," *Amyloid*, vol. 12, no. 4, pp. 239–245, 2005.

[20] H. Bartels, F. G. Dikkers, H. M. Lokhorst, J. E. van der Wal, and B. P. C. Hazenberg, "Laryngeal amyloidosis: localized versus systemic disease and update on diagnosis and therapy," *The Annals of Otology, Rhinology, and Laryngology*, vol. 113, no. 9, pp. 741–748, 2004.

[21] A. Patel, S. Pambuccian, and R. Maisel, "Nasopharyngeal amyloidosis," *American Journal of Otolaryngology*, vol. 23, no. 5, pp. 308–311, 2002.

[22] G. T. Simpson 2nd, M. Skinner, M. S. Strong, and A. S. Cohen, "Localized amyloidosis of the head and neck and upper aerodigestive and lower respiratory tracts," *The Annals of Otology, Rhinology, and Laryngology*, vol. 93, no. 4, pp. 374–379, 1984.

[23] S. Babburi, B. Ramya, R. V. Subramanyam, V. Aparna, and G. Srivastava, "Amyloidosis of the tongue-report of a rare case," *Journal of Clinical and Diagnostic Research*, vol. 7, pp. 3094-3095, 2013.

[24] A. O'Reilly, A. D'Souza, J. Lust, and D. Price, "Localized tongue amyloidosis: a single institutional case series," *Otolaryn-*

gology and Head and Neck Surgery, vol. 149, no. 2, pp. 240–244, 2013.

[25] C. A. Thompson, R. Kyle, M. Gertz, J. Heit, R. Pruthi, and A. Pardanani, "Systemic AL amyloidosis with acquired factor X deficiency: a study of perioperative bleeding risk and treatment outcomes in 60 patients," *American Journal of Hematology*, vol. 85, no. 3, pp. 171–173, 2010.

[26] P. Stoor, R. Suuronen, C. Lindqvist, J. Hietanen, and P. Laine, "Local primary (AL) amyloidosis in the palate: a case report," *International Journal of Oral and Maxillofacial Surgery*, vol. 33, no. 4, pp. 402-403, 2004.

[27] R. A. Kyle and E. D. Bayrd, "Amyloidosis: review of 236 cases," *Medicine*, vol. 54, no. 4, pp. 271–299, 1975.

15

Compound Odontoma Associated with Dentigerous Cyst Incidentally Detected in an Adult Patient: Tomography and Histological Features

Mattia Manfredini,[1,2] Susanna Ferrario,[1,2] Luca Creminelli,[1,2] Elisabetta Kuhn,[2,3] and Pier Paolo Poli[1,2]

[1]*Implant Center for Edentulism and Jawbone Atrophies, Maxillofacial Surgery and Odontostomatology Unit, Fondazione IRCCS Cà Granda Ospedale Maggiore Policlinico, Milan, Italy*
[2]*Department of Biomedical, Surgical and Dental Sciences, University of Milan, Milan, Italy*
[3]*Division of Pathology, Fondazione IRCCS Ca' Granda Ospedale Maggiore Policlinico, 20122 Milan, Italy*

Correspondence should be addressed to Susanna Ferrario; ferrariosusanna@gmail.com

Academic Editor: Kenji Yamagata

Odontoma is the most common benign odontogenic tumor of epithelial and mesenchymal origin. The standard treatment involves a conservative approach. While this procedure is generally well accepted and tolerated, some difficulties may arise in case of odontomas associated with cystic lesions. In general, the expansive nature of cystic lesions requires their surgical excision, different from isolated nonsymptomatic odontomas that can be monitored radiographically. However, to the best of our knowledge, there is scarce evidence currently available reporting on the presence of odontoma-associated cystic lesions in the oral cavity. Therefore, the present case report is aimed at describing the diagnostic clinical, radiological, and histological features together with the surgical management of a dentigerous cyst associated with a compound odontoma. Following surgical removal of the lesion, no recurrence was observed after 12 months of follow-up.

1. Introduction

Odontomas are benign proliferations of odontogenic origin, characterized by a mixed histopathological composition, being formed by epithelial and mesenchymal cells with dental hard tissues [1–5]. They are considered hamartomatous malformations producing mineralized dental tissues, rather than true benign neoplasms. Although they are the most frequently detected benign tumors in the clinical practice, their aetiology remains unclear. Typical clinical signs include retention of deciduous teeth, delayed eruption, presence of inclusions, and increased gingival volume among others. Odontomas are most commonly observed in patients during their second decade of life, with no apparent gender susceptibility, being equally distributed in males and females [6, 7].

From a histomorphological standpoint, odontomas are divided into two different entities according to the latest classification of the World Health Organization [8]: compound and complex. The former is characterized by small variable formations structurally similar to teeth, while the complex form has no anatomical similarity to teeth and appears as an undefined mass of enamel and dentin [9].

Odontomas can be observed in both the jaws, are generally symptomless, and are typically discovered accidentally following routine radiological examinations performed for other oral conditions. Radiographically, they appear as radiopaque lesions, consisting of a cluster of more or less developed tooth structures. A radiolucent band is often visible around the radiopaque mass. In this context, odontomas and osteomas can be hardly distinguishable radiographically.

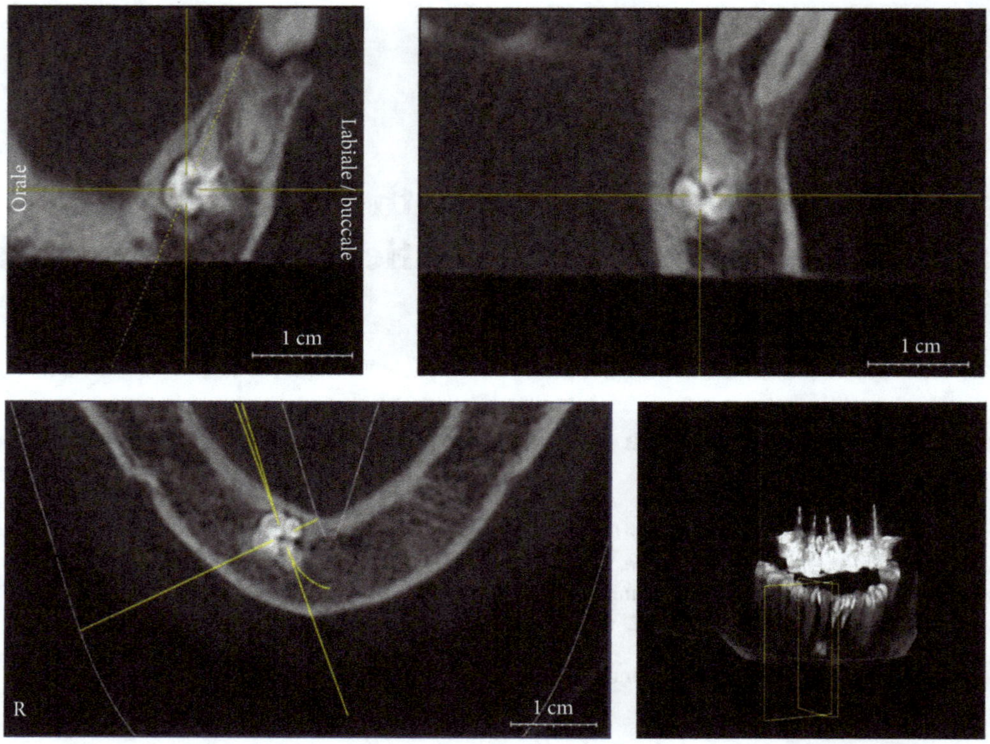

Figure 1: The image shows the size of the lesion in the CBCT scan approximately 10 years before its removal.

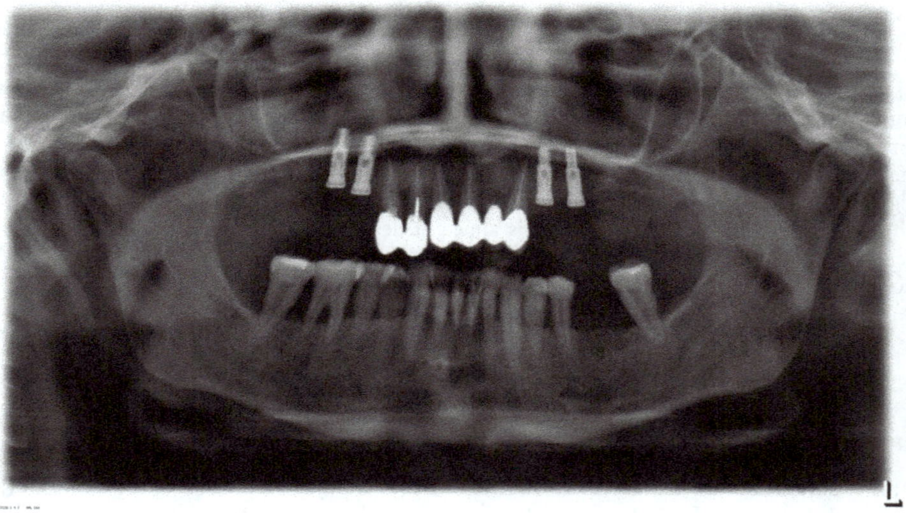

Figure 2: Orthopantomography performed in 2013.

The calcified component has a mixture of enamel, tubular or dysplastic dentine, epithelial-connective matrix producing enamel, and connective tissue [3].

If the diagnosis of odontoma is certain, it is generally not necessary to remove the lesion, unless it prevents tooth eruption or gives rise to complications, such as the development of cystic lesions. In these cases, surgical removal might be indicated.

Both odontomas and odontogenic cysts are frequently encountered in dental practice; however, the simultaneous presence of both lesions in the same anatomical region is somewhat rare. In addition, the diagnostic hypothesis is solely based on the radiographic appearance. The interpretation is therefore uncertain, as these lesions can be misdiagnosed for other radiographically similar fibro-osseous lesions, such as fibrous dysplasia and fibroma ossificans [10]. In this respect, there is still little evidence concerning the diagnostic workup of combined cystic and tumor lesions. Thus, the purpose of the present report was to describe the diagnostic and surgical aspects in a case of a compound odontoma associated with a dentigerous cyst in the mandibular interforaminal region.

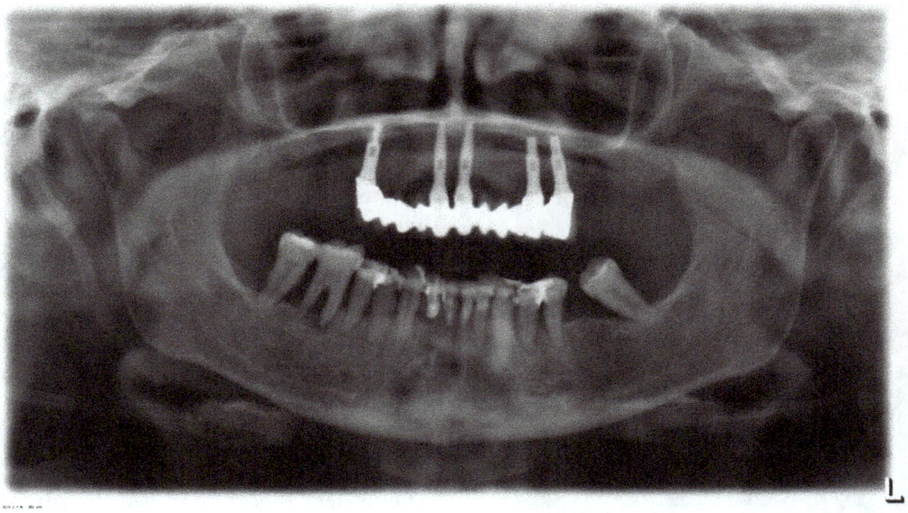

FIGURE 3: Orthopantomography performed in 2019.

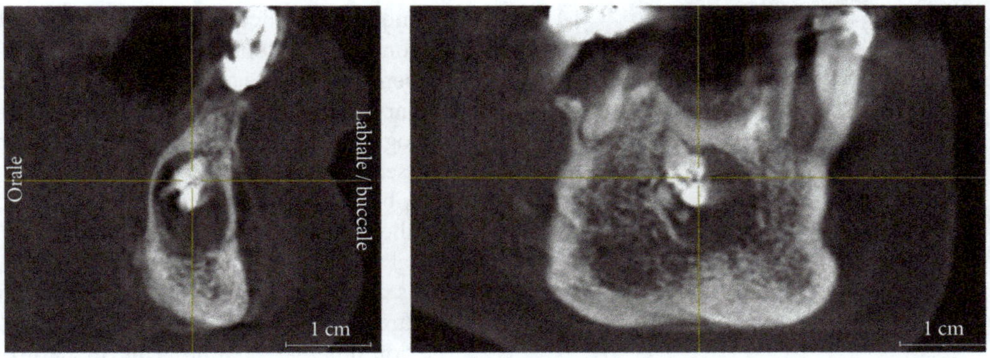

FIGURE 4: CBCT scan performed in 2020, showing the enlargement of the lesion compared to the first CBCT scan.

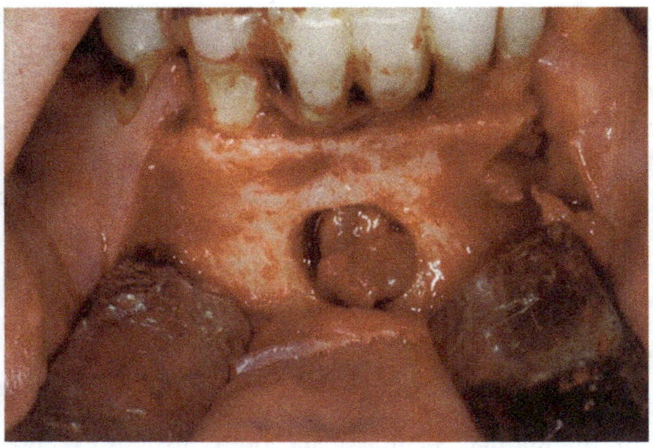

FIGURE 5: Vision of the vestibular bone hatch.

2. Case Presentation

The present clinical case is reported in accordance with the CARE guidelines (http://www.care-statement.org) for improving the quality of reporting of case reports. All treatment procedures were performed in compliance with the Declaration of Helsinki on ethical principles for medical research involving human subjects.

A 65-year-old white Caucasian woman came to the authors' attention sent by her private dentist seeking for a consultation to evaluate the removal of a lesion located in the interforaminal region of the mandible. The medical history was noncontributory.

The patient underwent an initial cone beam computed tomography (CBCT) scan in 2010 and two different orthopantomographs, in 2013 and 2019, respectively (Figures 1–3). The examination of the patient's radiological records revealed an osteolytic cystic-like lesion associated with a radiopaque solid mass delimited by radiopaque margins, involving the apices of the lower incisors. By comparing the two orthopantomographs, it was possible to appreciate an expansive growth of the lesion; therefore, a new CBCT scan was prescribed in 2020 (Figure 4). From the comparison of the multiplanar reconstructions obtained in the two CBCT scans, it was possible to confirm the enlargement of the lesion throughout the years. The expansive behavior of the lesion and the need for a histopathological analysis to confirm the final diagnosis led to the decision of a surgical approach.

Upon clinical examination, the interforaminal region showed no signs or symptoms of swelling, redness, or inflammation despite the patient's poor oral hygiene

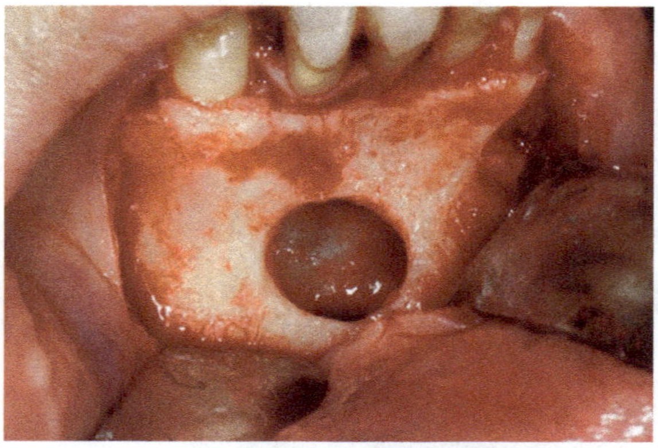

FIGURE 6: Removal of the lesion through the bone hatch.

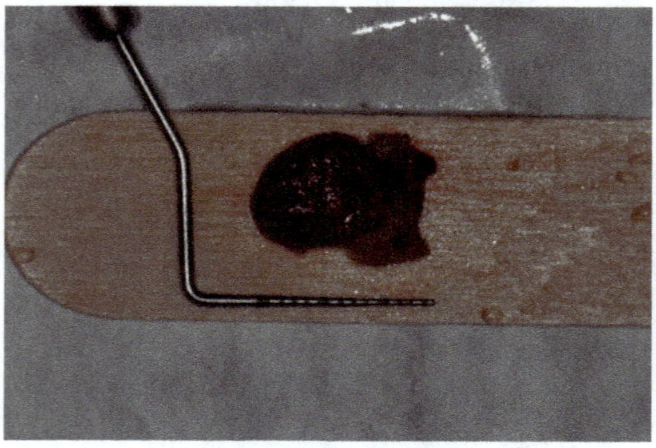

FIGURE 7: Lesion with millimeter probe.

conditions. The lower incisors presented with no mobility, although they were splinted with composite resin to the neighboring teeth. The patient was asymptomatic.

The surgical procedure was performed on an outpatient basis under local anesthesia induced with mepivacaine hydrochloride 20 mg/mL with epinephrine 1 : 100.000 (Optocain, Molteni Dental Srl, Milan, Italy) injections. Bacterial decontamination was achieved with an antiseptic rinsing solution consisting of 0.2% chlorhexidine digluconate for 1 minute. To access the lesion, an intrasulcular incision was made with divergent releasing vertical incisions distally with respect to the right canine and the left lateral incisor. After flap elevation and soft tissue debridement, a thinned and more transparent buccal cortical wall was appreciated in correspondence with the lesion. A circular osteotomy was made with a surgical handpiece under copious irrigation with sterile saline to create a bony window and expose the lesion. At this point, a careful isolation of the encapsulated lesion and complete removal were accomplished with Lucas-like surgical curettes of different sizes and shapes. The entire lesion was excised in toto with the help of mosquito surgical forceps. The surgical defect was debrided to remove any soft tissue remnants and expose macroscopically healthy bleeding bone tissue. The surgical site was irrigated vigorously with sterile saline, and the flap was finally repositioned and sutured with 4/0 silk single stitches. The lesion measuring $15 \times 10 \times 7$ mm was sent to the anatomical pathology department for histopathological examination (Figures 5–7).

From an initial macroscopic evaluation, the resected specimen consisted of a cystic lesion with a thin 1 mm diameter regular wall, associated to a tooth-like structure measuring 7 mm in its long axis. Histologically, the cyst had a thin fibrous wall with brown hemosiderin deposits, covered by a hyperplastic nonkeratinizing squamous epithelium, consistent with a dentigerous cyst. The tooth-like structure was mainly composed of dentin with a thin outer layer of cement and little inner dental pulp-like tissue, compatible with compound odontoma (Figure 8). No recurrence was observed at the 12-month follow-up recall (Figure 9).

3. Discussion

The present report described the surgical management of a compound odontoma associated with a cystic lesion in the interforaminal area. Heterogeneity can be found in literature regarding the epidemiology of odontomas. In this matter, our findings are inconsistent with other studies reporting that compound odontomas are more frequently diagnosed in patients during the first two decades of life [11] in the premaxillary region [12]. Furthermore, also the clinical and radiological features of the odontoma diagnosed herein do not resemble those commonly encountered for this type of lesion, being in intimate contact with an odontogenic cyst. Nonetheless, the radiographic evidence of the lesion allowed surgical intervention in good time, avoiding further complications and pathological expansion toward healthy structures.

Odontomas are odontogenic in nature, as they derive from the epithelial and/or mesenchymal tissues from which the teeth originate, and can induce cystic proliferation [13]. This cystic lesion results from degeneration of the enamel organ after partial or total development of the crown within the odontoma itself and arises following accumulation of fluid between reduced enamel epithelium and crown of an unerupted tooth [14]. Although these changes are mentioned as possible, they have been seldomly observed in the clinical practice. Dentigerous cyst is developmental in origin, mostly associated with an unerupted tooth or rarely with an odontoma. When they occur concurrently, it is possible to observe a combined lesion, increased in size, with the potential to expand towards noble structures [15].

Clinically, odontomas can present as intraosseous or extraosseous lesions. Intraosseous odontomas develop within mandibular or maxillary bone structures and, in some cases, may also erupt into the oral cavity. Peripheral ones arise at the level of extraosseous soft tissues, are very rare, and tend to exfoliate [16]. In the present case, the lesion was classified as intraosseous, being limited to the cortical plates of the symphysis region.

Typically, treatment of odontomas involves surgical removal, while therapeutic strategies reported for dentigerous cysts range from marsupialization to enucleation. This complies favorably with the therapeutic plan adopted in the present report, where surgical removal of the lesion was considered as the treatment of choice. Conversely,

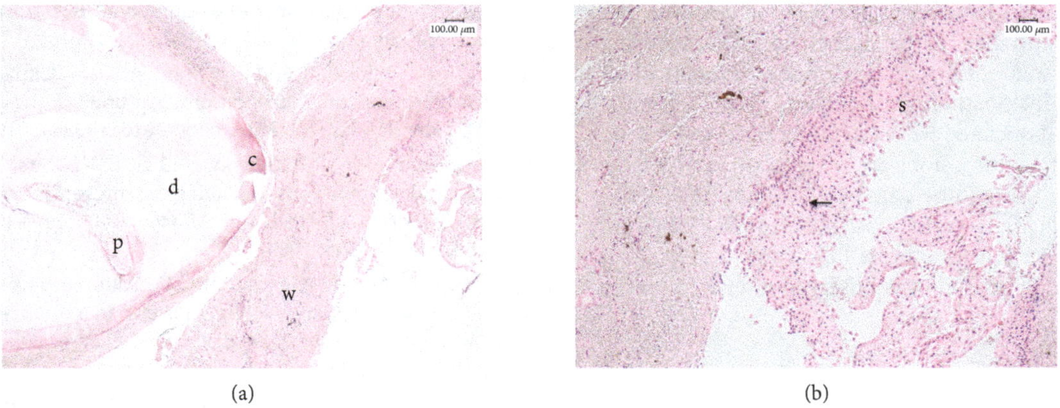

FIGURE 8: Representative histological pictures of the lesion. (a) The odontoma has a well-organized tooth-like structure composed mainly of dentin (d) with a thin outer layer of cement (c) and little inner dental pulp-like tissue (p). (b) It is appreciable a thin fibrous wall (w) with brown hemosiderin deposits of a cystic lesion ((a) 50x magnification). At higher magnification, the cyst is covered by a hyperplastic nonkeratinizing squamous epithelium (s) with exocytosis of neutrophils (arrow, (b) 100x magnification) (haematoxylin-eosin staining).

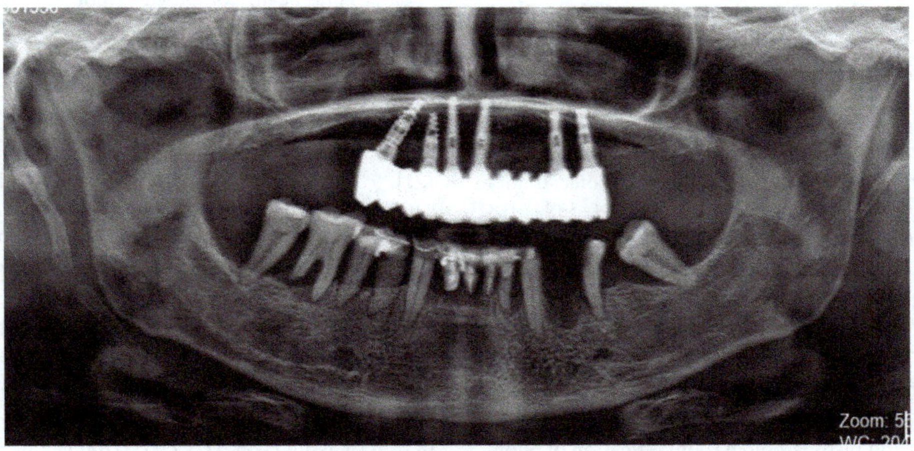

FIGURE 9: Orthopantomography performed in 2021.

marsupialization is more commonly used in children when compared to enucleation because it is surgically less invasive and preserves the eruption of permanent teeth. Other factors favoring marsupialization include young age, lack of patient compliance for more invasive surgical treatment, tooth position and development, and eruptive potential [17, 18].

In the present case, the bidimensional radiographic features of the lesion were initially inconclusive for diagnostic purposes. Additional radiographic evaluation with CBCT scan, at a relatively low radiation dose and high resolution, was necessary to determine the real extent and characteristics of the lesion. Indeed, the bidimensional limitations of periapical and panoramic images did not allow a complete three-dimensional visualization of the anatomical region. In this regard, CBCT images are necessary not only to assess the lesion itself but also to identify possible associated pathologies, the proximity to noble structures, and to formulate a correct treatment plan [19–21].

The imaging features of fibro-osseous lesions are very difficult to be distinguished among the large group of similar pathologies such as fibroma ossificans and fibrous dysplasia. In those cases, CBCT is an important tool for the differential diagnosis of such lesions [22]. In the present report, the CBCT images provided a better representation of the structures involved. In addition to the hyperdense image detected in the interforaminal region, a second area with a cystic appearance was noticed. These radiological features were critical during the therapeutic approach, allowing an ideal planning of the surgical procedure and clarification of the diagnosis. It should be noted that CBCT represents the gold standard radiological exam to exclude any suspect of inferior alveolar nerve involvement or to reveal any neurological involvement of the lesion [19, 20]. Nevertheless, histopathological analysis remains mandatory to confirm the initial diagnostic hypothesis. It is worth noting that ameloblastic odontomas and fibro-ameloblastic odontomas are rare but clinically and radiographically similar to common odontomas [23]. This strengthens the essential role of the histopathological analysis in the differential diagnosis of these lesions.

In the present report, the odontoma was associated with another lesion with cystic features. In this regard, a dentigerous cyst could have been probably the result of cystic degeneration and had to be chosen as the diagnostic hypothesis. This was confirmed after surgical removal of the lesion, as the histopathological analysis showed a compound odontoma associated with a dentigerous cyst. Despite their benign nature, these lesions are well recognized by their growth pattern and should be completely removed to avoid secondary complications and possible sequelae for the patient, with an excellent prognosis following surgery. As a matter of fact, no recurrence was observed after 12 months of follow-up.

References

[1] T. Ćabov, M. Krmpotić, J. Grgurević, B. Perić, D. Jokić, and S. Manojlović, "Large complex odontoma of the left maxillary sinus," *Wiener Klinische Wochenschrift*, vol. 117, no. 21-22, pp. 780–783, 2005.

[2] M. Hisatomi, J. I. Asaumi, H. Konouchi, Y. Honda, T. Wakasa, and K. Kishi, "A case of complex odontoma associated with an impacted lower deciduous second molar and analysis of the 107 odontomas," *Oral Diseases*, vol. 8, no. 2, pp. 100–105, 2002.

[3] P. M. Speight and T. Takata, "New tumour entities in the 4th edition of the World Health Organization Classification of Head and Neck tumours: odontogenic and maxillofacial bone tumours," *Virchows Archiv*, vol. 472, no. 3, pp. 331–339, 2018.

[4] P. P. Broca, *Traité Des Tumeurs*P. Asselin (Paris)1866.

[5] B. Neville, D. D. Damm, C. Allen, and J. Bouquot, *Oral and Maxillofacial Pathology*, Saunders, 3rd edition, 2008.

[6] A. K. El-Naggar, J. K. C. Chan, J. R. Grandis, T. Takata, and P. J. Slootweg, *WHO Classification of Head and Neck Tumours*, vol. 9, 4th edition, 2017.

[7] M. Soluk Tekkesin, S. Pehlivan, V. Olgac, N. Aksakall, and C. Alatl, "Clinical and histopathological investigation of odontomas: review of the literature and presentation of 160 cases," *Journal of Oral and Maxillofacial Surgery*, vol. 70, no. 6, pp. 1358–1361, 2012.

[8] L. Pereira Da Silva, A. De Paiva, R. Macedo et al., "Global frequency of benign and malignant odontogenic tumors according to the 2017 WHO classification," *Journal of Oral Diagnosis*, vol. 2, 2017.

[9] J. M. Wright and M. Vered, "Update from the 4th edition of the World Health Organization classification of head and neck tumours: odontogenic and maxillofacial bone tumors," *Head and Neck Pathology*, vol. 11, no. 1, pp. 68–77, 2017.

[10] J. L. Smith and R. M. Kellman, "Dentigerous cysts presenting as head and neck infections," *Otolaryngology and Head and Neck Surgery*, vol. 133, no. 5, pp. 715–717, 2005.

[11] R. Gedik and S. Müftüoglu, "Compound odontoma: differential diagnosis and review of the literature," *The West Indian Medical Journal*, vol. 63, no. 7, pp. 793–795, 2014.

[12] B. Heloisa De Oliveira and V. Campos, *Compound odontoma-diagnosis and treatment: three case reports*, Oral Pathology, 2014.

[13] M. Sales and M. G. Cavalcanti, "Complex odontoma associated with dentigerous cyst in maxillary sinus: case report and computed tomography features," *Dento Maxillo Facial Radiology*, vol. 38, no. 1, pp. 48–52, 2009.

[14] C. Jayam, A. Bandlapalli, N. Patel, and R. S. K. Choudhary, "A case of impacted central incisor due to dentigerous cyst associated with impacted compound odontome," *BMJ Case Reports.*, vol. 2014, no. mar20 1, p. bcr2013202447, 2014.

[15] K. Dagrus, S. Purohit, and B. S. Manjunatha, "Dentigerous cyst arising from a complex odontoma: an unusual presentation," *BMJ Case Reports*, vol. 2016, p. bcr2016214936, 2016.

[16] R. G. Shamaskin, J. A. Svirsky, and G. E. Kaugars, "Intraosseous and extraosseous calcifying odontogenic cyst (Gorlin cyst)," *Journal of Oral and Maxillofacial Surgery*, vol. 47, no. 6, pp. 562–565, 1989.

[17] A. B. Cankaya, K. Gencay, and O. Aktoren, "Conservative management of a large dentigerous cyst in a 6-year-old girl: a case report," *Journal of Dentistry for Children*, vol. 78, no. 3, pp. 163–167, 2011.

[18] B. C. Kirtaniya, V. Sachdev, A. Singla, and A. K. Sharma, "Marsupialization: a conservative approach for treating dentigerous cyst in children in the mixed dentition," *Journal of the Indian Society of Pedodontics and Preventive Dentistry*, vol. 28, no. 3, pp. 203–208, 2010.

[19] F. A. Quereshy, T. A. Savell, and J. M. Palomo, "Applications of cone beam computed tomography in the practice of oral and maxillofacial surgery," *Journal of Oral and Maxillofacial Surgery*, vol. 66, no. 4, pp. 791–796, 2008.

[20] K. M. Au-Yeung, A. T. Ahuja, A. S. C. Ching, and C. Metreweli, "DentaScan in oral imaging," *Clinical Radiology*, vol. 56, no. 9, pp. 700–713, 2001.

[21] S. C. Isler, S. Demircan, M. Soluk, and Z. Cebi, "Radiologic evaluation of an unusually sized complex odontoma involving the maxillary sinus by cone beam computed tomography," *Quintessence international (Berlin, Germany : 1985)*, vol. 40, no. 7, pp. 533–535, 2009.

[22] B. Anuraag, M. Choudhary, B. Choudhary, B. Motwani Mukta, and S. M. Chaudhary, "Utility of cone beam CT in maxillofacial radiology," *International Journal of Dentistry.*, vol. 3, pp. 134–145, 2013.

[23] K. S. Kim, H. G. Lee, J. H. Hwang, and S. Y. Lee, "Incidentally detected odontoma within a dentigerous cyst," *Archives of Craniofacial Surgery.*, vol. 20, no. 1, pp. 62–65, 2019.

16

A Bilocular Radicular Cyst in the Mandible with Tooth Structure Components Inside

Akari Noda,[1] Masanobu Abe,[1,2] Aya Shinozaki-Ushiku,[3] Yae Ohata,[4] Liang Zong,[5,6] Takahiro Abe,[1] and Kazuto Hoshi[1]

[1]*Department of Oral & Maxillofacial Surgery, University of Tokyo Hospital, Tokyo, Japan*
[2]*Division for Health Service Promotion, University of Tokyo, Tokyo, Japan*
[3]*Department of Pathology, Graduate School of Medicine, University of Tokyo, Tokyo, Japan*
[4]*Department of Oral Pathology, Graduate School of Medical and Dental Sciences, Tokyo Medical and Dental University, Tokyo, Japan*
[5]*Graduate School of Medicine, The University of Tokyo, Tokyo, Japan*
[6]*Department of Gastrointestinal Surgery, Peking University Cancer Hospital & Institute, Beijing, China*

Correspondence should be addressed to Masanobu Abe; ave.dance@gmail.com

Academic Editor: Tatiana Pereira-Cenci

Background. A radicular cyst is the most common odontogenic cyst of inflammatory origin. Radiographically, it commonly demonstrates clear unilocular radiolucency; radicular cysts with multilocular radiolucency are quite rare. *Case Presentation.* A 64-year-old Japanese man who presented with a bilocular radiolucent lesion in his left mandible was referred by a dental clinic to our oral and maxillofacial surgery department. He had no particular subjective symptoms. Orthopantomography and computed tomography (CT) revealed an 18 mm × 15 mm lesion with well-defined bilocular radiolucency in the left mandible expanding from the distal side of a canine tooth to the bottom of the 2nd premolar. The lesion included the roots of the 1st and 2nd premolars. The root of the 2nd premolar showed knife-edge resorption. Although the 1st premolar was nonvital, the 2nd premolar was a vital tooth. As differential diagnoses, a radicular cyst, ameloblastoma, odontogenic keratocyst, pseudocyst, and others might be considered. We performed a total resection of the bilocular lesion and diagnosed the lesion as a radicular cyst with tooth structure components inside. The tooth structure components represented lamellar structures of cementum; they were located only in the proximal part (under the 1st premolar) of the lesion. The distal part of the lesion presented distinctive inflammation without tooth structure components. *Conclusion.* We encountered a rare case of a bilocular radicular cyst with tooth structure components inside.

1. Introduction

A radicular cyst is the most common odontogenic cyst of inflammatory origin [1]. It is commonly associated with pulpal necrosis leading to inflamed periapical tissues. Radiographically, a radicular cyst presents well-defined unilocular radiolucency. However, multilocular radiolucent radicular cysts are quite rare; there are few reported cases [2–4]. For multilocular radicular cysts, a differential diagnosis with other cysts and tumors (dentigerous cyst, ameloblastoma, odontogenic keratocyst, pseudocyst, etc.) is necessary [5]. Here, we describe the rare case of a bilocular radicular cyst located periapically to the first premolar of the fourth quadrant, presenting diagnostic difficulties.

2. Case Report

A 64-year-old Japanese man who presented with a bilocular radiolucent lesion in his left mandible was referred by a dental clinic to our department of oral and maxillofacial surgery. He had no subjective symptoms. His medical history

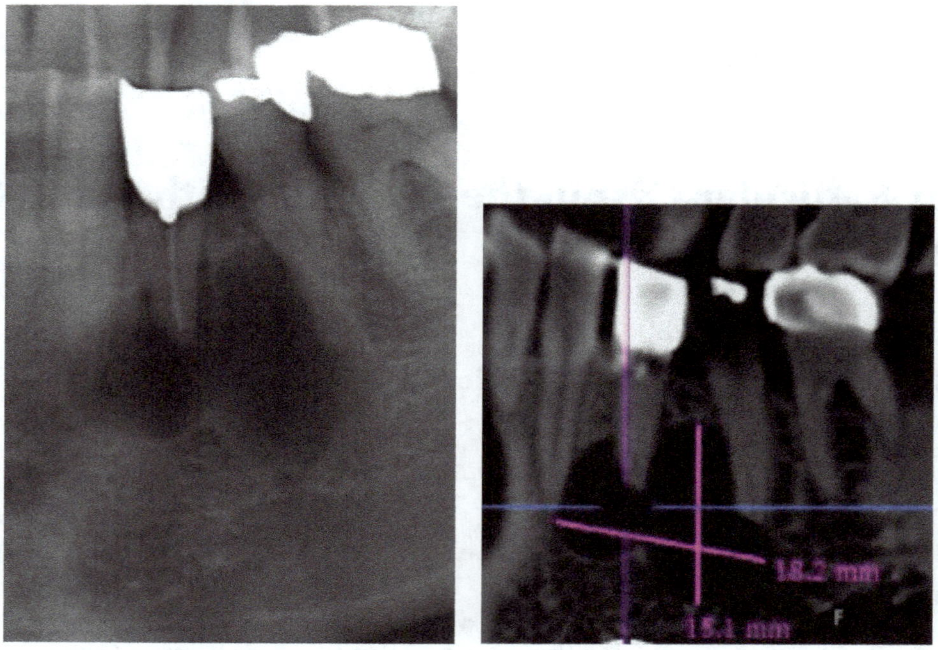

(a) (b)

Figure 1: Clinical images of the bilocular lesion in the mandible. (a) Orthopantomography. The well-defined bilocular lesion is observed in the left mandible expanding from the distal of the canine tooth to the bottom of the 2nd premolar. (b) CT findings. The size of the bilocular lesion was 18 mm × 15 mm. The root of the 2nd premolar showed knife-edge resorption.

included coronary vasospastic angina, diabetes mellitus, and hyperlipidemia.

Orthopantomography and computed tomography (CT) revealed an 18 mm × 15 mm lesion with well-defined bilocular radiolucency in the left mandible expanding from the distal side of the canine tooth to the bottom of the 2nd premolar. The roots of the 1st and 2nd premolars were included in the lesion. Knife-edge root resorption was observed in the 2nd premolar (Figures 1(a) and 1(b)). Although the 1st premolar was nonvital, the 2nd premolar was found to be a vital tooth.

As a differential diagnosis, radicular cyst, ameloblastoma, odontogenic keratocyst, ameloblastic fibroma, odontogenic fibroma, odontogenic myxoma, jawbone central hemangioma, schwannoma, giant cell granuloma pseudocysts (simple bone cyst, aneurysmal bone cyst, and latent bone cyst), and hybrid lesions were considered.

A biopsy was performed for the lesion under local anesthesia, because the knife-edge root resorption observed in the 2nd premolar suggested the possibility of ameloblastoma. When an ameloblastoma was identified in the biopsy, an adequate margin of safety was necessary for the resection. Based on the biopsy results, the lesion was diagnosed as a radicular cyst with a fibrous cystic wall and nonkeratinized squamous epithelium lining. However, there was a possibility that the incision biopsy did not reflect the entire lesion. We performed a total resection of the bilocular lesion with extraction of the 1st premolar under general anesthesia (Figures 2(a) and 2(b)). The inner surface of the entire lesion was covered by acanthotic squamous epithelium showing elongation of rete ridges. There was no clear border between the proximal and distal parts of the lesion.

The infiltration of inflammatory cells, plasma cells, and lymphocytes was extensive. Epithelial shedding as an effect of the inflammation was also observed (Figures 2(c) and 2(d)). Interestingly, tooth structure components with lamellar structures of cementum were found irregularly at the inner surface of the proximal part of the lesion (Figure 2(c)). The distal part showed severe inflammation without tooth structure components (Figure 2(d)).

3. Discussion

A radicular cyst is the most common odontogenic cyst, accounting for 55% of odontogenic cysts and 52%–68% of all of the cysts of the jaw in humans. Radicular cysts are observed mostly in the third and fourth decades of life, and they have shown male predilection. A "radicular cyst" is defined as a cyst arising from the epithelial residues in the periodontal ligament as a consequence of inflammation following necrosis of the dental pulp. The most common etiology is dental caries with pulp involvement [1, 2]. Radiographically, a radicular cyst presents well-defined unilocular radiolucency located periapical to a tooth with pulp involvement. In our patient's case, the radiographic appearance showed bilocular radiolucency apart from the usual radiolucency. There have been very few reports of a radicular cyst with multilocular radiolucency [2–4].

Before a pathological diagnosis, in addition to the radicular cyst, a differential diagnosis in similar cases should include ameloblastoma, odontogenic keratocyst, enamel epithelium fibroma, odontogenic fibroma, odontogenic myxoma, jawbone central hemangioma, schwannoma, giant cell

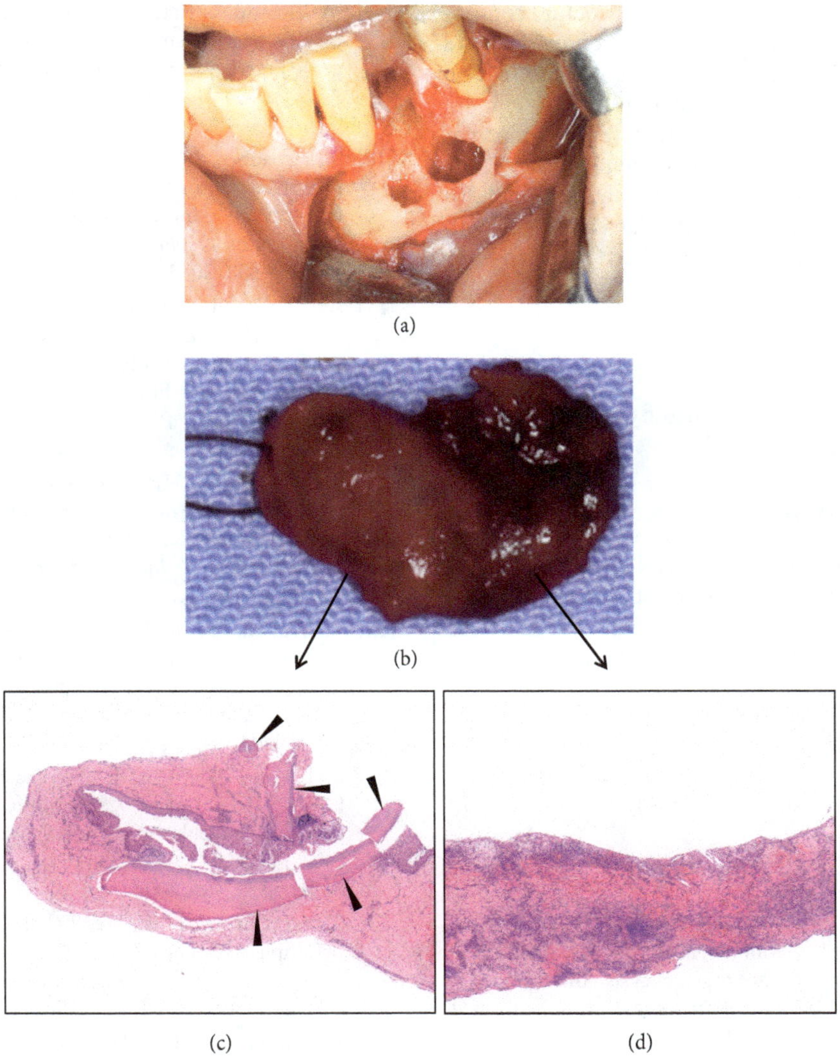

Figure 2: Intraoperative and pathological findings of the bilocular lesion in the mandible. (a) Bicameral bone resorption after resection of the bilocular lesion. After total resection of the bilocular lesion and extraction of the 1st premolar, bicameral alveolar bone resorption was observed. (b) The resected bilocular lesion. The left half is the proximal part of the lesion and the right side is the distal part. The proximal part is in bright red and the distal part is in dark red. (c) Pathological findings of the proximal part of the lesion. The components of hard tissue in the proximal part of the lesion represented lamellar structures of cementum (arrowheads). (d) Pathological findings of the distal part of the lesion, which showed severe inflammation without tooth structure components inside.

granuloma, and pseudocysts (simple bone cyst, aneurysmal bone cyst, and latent bone cyst) [6–9]. We suspected ameloblastoma in the present case because knife-edge root resorption was observed in the 2nd premolar. The possibility of a hybrid lesion (cyst with cyst, cyst with tumor, and tumor with tumor) was also discussed, although such hybrids are uncommon [10–16]. Although dentigerous cysts associated with an adenomatoid odontogenic tumor have been reported in several cases, a radicular cyst associated with other cysts or tumors has not been reported, to the best of our knowledge [15, 16].

In our patient's case, tumors and pseudocysts were denied as the pathological diagnosis because the lesion had an apparent cystic wall. The whole resected tissue showed a stratified squamous epithelial lining. The wall of the lesion consisted of dense fibrous connective tissue, with an inflammatory infiltrate containing lymphocytes mixed with neutrophils, plasma cells, and histiocytes. These findings are in accordance with the pathology of a radicular cyst [17]. There was no clear border between the proximal and distal parts of the lesion. In only the proximal part of the lesion, tooth structure components were found irregularly at the inner surface of the cyst. The lesion was eventually considered a radicular cyst with tooth structure components that showed lamellar structures of cementum.

Although a radicular cyst with tooth structure components has not been reported, it is reasonable to speculate that the cementum-like structure in our patient's case was derived from odontogenic cells present in the wall that, under inflammatory stimulation, started to produce the structure over the years. As another hypothesis, we suspect that the cementum-like structure was derived from tooth fragments by the root canal treatments of the 1st premolar which had been performed several years before. The distal part of the lesion showed severe inflammation without tooth structure components. This suggested that a secondary infection that had occurred in the unilocular lesion caused severe inflammation which led to the formation of a bilocular cyst.

In summary, we experienced a rare case of a bilocular radicular cyst with tooth structure components inside. There are numerous reports about radicular cysts, but the multilocular type is quite uncommon. A radicular cyst with tooth structure components has apparently not been reported prior to this case.

Consent

Written informed consent was obtained from the patient for his data and images to be published.

Authors' Contributions

MA conceived and designed the study. AN and MA collected the clinical data and wrote the manuscript. AS and YO contributed the pathological findings. LZ, TA, and KH reviewed the manuscript. All authors have read and approved the final manuscript.

Acknowledgments

We thank Dr. Mamoru Nakamura for his great clinical effort for the patient.

References

[1] N. R. Johnson, O. M. Gannon, N. W. Savage, and M. D. Batstone, "Frequency of odontogenic cysts and tumors: a systematic review," *Journal of Investigative and Clinical Dentistry*, vol. 5, no. 1, pp. 9–14, 2014.

[2] P. Shivhare, A. Singh, N. Haidry, M. Yadav, and L. Shankarnarayan, "Multilocular radicular cyst – a common pathology with uncommon radiological appearance," *Journal of Clinical and Diagnostic Research*, vol. 10, no. 3, pp. Zd13–Zd15, 2016.

[3] E. C. Armbrecht and W. A. Waterman, "Multilocular radicular cysts of the mandible," *Oral Surgery, Oral Medicine, and Oral Pathology*, vol. 5, no. 8, pp. 827–829, 1952.

[4] V. Krishnamurthy, S. Haridas, M. Garud, S. Vahanwala, C. D. Nayak, and S. S. Pagare, "Radicular cyst masquerading as a multilocular radiolucency," *Quintessence International*, vol. 44, no. 1, pp. 71–73, 2013.

[5] M. P. V. Prabhat, P. Deshpande, S. Gummadapu, S. Babburi, R. L. Chintamaneni, and B. Sujanamulk, "Dual lesions: a diagnostic dilemma," *Case Reports in Dentistry*, vol. 2013, Article ID 539234, 5 pages, 2013.

[6] M. Abe, L. Zong, T. Abe, and K. Hoshi, "A turning point in therapy for ameloblastomas," *Oral Oncology*, vol. 80, pp. 95-96, 2018.

[7] M. Abe, L. Zong, T. Abe et al., "BRAF inhibitor: a novel therapy for ameloblastoma in mandible," *Chinese Journal of Cancer Research*, vol. 30, no. 6, pp. 677-678, 2018.

[8] D. M. Laskin, J. A. Giglio, and L. F. Ferrer-Nuin, "Multilocular lesion in the body of the mandible," *Journal of Oral and Maxillofacial Surgery*, vol. 60, no. 9, pp. 1045–1048, 2002.

[9] M. Minami, T. Kaneda, K. Ozawa et al., "Cystic lesions of the maxillomandibular region: MR imaging distinction of odontogenic keratocysts and ameloblastomas from other cysts," *AJR American Journal of Roentgenology*, vol. 166, no. 4, pp. 943–949, 1996.

[10] S. S. Chaubey, S. S. Mishra, S. S. Degwekar, and S. Chaubey, "A rare presentation of hybrid odontogenic tumor involving calcifying cystic odontogenic tumor and plexiform ameloblastoma," *Contemporary Clinical Dentistry*, vol. 4, no. 3, pp. 406–408, 2013.

[11] A. N. Neuman, L. Montague, D. Cohen, N. Islam, and I. Bhattacharyya, "Report of two cases of combined odontogenic tumors: ameloblastoma with odontogenic keratocyst and ameloblastic fibroma with calcifying odontogenic cyst," *Head and Neck Pathology*, vol. 9, no. 3, pp. 417–420, 2015.

[12] M. D. Phillips, J. J. Closmann, M. R. Baus, K. R. Torske, and S. B. Williams, "Hybrid odontogenic tumor with features of ameloblastic fibro-odontoma, calcifying odontogenic cyst, and adenomatoid odontogenic tumor: a case report and review of the literature," *Journal of Oral and Maxillofacial Surgery*, vol. 68, no. 2, pp. 470–474, 2010.

[13] M. Wakoh, T. Harada, and T. Inoue, "Follicular/desmoplastic hybrid ameloblastoma with radiographic features of concomitant fibro-osseous and solitary cystic lesions," *Oral Surgery, Oral Medicine, Oral Pathology, Oral Radiology, and Endodontics*, vol. 94, no. 6, pp. 774–780, 2002.

[14] J. H. Yoon, H. J. Kim, J. In Yook, I. H. Cha, G. L. Ellis, and J. Kim, "Hybrid odontogenic tumor of calcifying odontogenic cyst and ameloblastic fibroma," *Oral Surgery, Oral Medicine, Oral Pathology, Oral Radiology, and Endodontics*, vol. 98, no. 1, pp. 80–84, 2004.

[15] S. Durga Sreenivas, C. Sree Lalita, G. Harsha, and C. V. Rao, "Multiple pathology in a single lesion: AOT associated with dentigerous cyst," *Journal of Maxillofacial and Oral Surgery*, vol. 14, Supplement 1, pp. 215–221, 2015.

[16] S. Majumdar, D. Uppala, A. K. Rao, S. Talasila, and M. Babu, "Dentigerous cyst associated with adenomatoid odontogenic tumour," *Journal Of Clinical And Diagnostic Research*, vol. 9, no. 5, article Zd01-04, 2015.

[17] K. S. Uloopi, R. U. Shivaji, C. Vinay, S. P. S. Pavitra, and R. Chandrasekhar, "Conservative management of large radicular cysts associated with non-vital primary teeth: a case series and literature review," *Journal of the Indian Society of Pedodontics and Preventive Dentistry*, vol. 33, no. 1, pp. 53–56, 2015.

17

A Case of Drastic Reduction of Membranous Substances in the Pharynx by Interprofessional Cooperative Oral Care

Masahiko Okubo,[1,2] Hideyuki Kamimura,[2] Tsuyoshi Sato,[1] and Shoichiro Kokabu[3]

[1]*Department of Oral and Maxillofacial Surgery, Faculty of Medicine, Saitama Medical University, 38 Morohongo, Moroyama-machi, Iruma-gun, Saitama, Japan 350-0495*
[2]*Kamimura Dental and Orthodontics Clinic, 3-246-1, Sagami-chou, Koshigaya-shi, Saitama, Japan 343-0823*
[3]*Division of Molecular Signaling and Biochemistry, Department of Health Improvement, Kyushu Dental University, 2-6-1 Manazuru, Kokurakita-ku, Kitakyusyu-shi, Japan 803-8580*

Correspondence should be addressed to Shoichiro Kokabu; r14kokabu@fa.kyu-dent.ac.jp

Academic Editor: Rui Amaral Mendes

Membranous substances in the pharynx are occasionally observed in tube feeding patients during the fiberoptic endoscopic evaluation of swallowing. Although the mechanism of the formation of these deposits sometimes causes problems, such as dysphagia, asphyxia, or aspiration pneumonia, a 91-year-old male complained about difficulty of swallowing. He had a history of cerebral infarction and aspiration pneumonitis. There was a large amount of oral desquamated epithelium, dental plaque, and calculus in his mouth. Nurses and care workers administered oral care such as rubbing the tongue and buccal mucosa daily. Dentists and oral hygienists visited and provided special oral care three times per week. At least for 77 days, the patient had no recurrence of pneumonitis. The oral desquamated epithelium and membranous substances in the pharynx decreased drastically. 2 months after the first examination, the patient was able to start rehabilitation with food. Some studies have indicated that pharyngeal deposits are derived from the oral mucosa, and through our case, we realized the importance of daily oral care by interprofessional work to reduce membranous substances in the pharynx.

1. Introduction

Membranous substances in the pharynx are occasionally observed in tube feeding patients during the fiberoptic endoscopic evaluation of swallowing. Although some studies have indicated that pharyngeal deposits are derived from the oral mucosa [1], the mechanism of depositing these membranous substances on the pharynx remains largely unknown. These deposits sometimes cause problems, such as dysphagia, asphyxia, or aspiration pneumonia. Membranous substances are usually removed using tweezers or aspirators. However, this method is associated with a risk of bleeding. In this paper, we report a case in which intensive oral care completely removed the pharyngeal deposits, and the patient could take food intraorally.

2. Case Report

We visited a 91-year-old male with difficulty in swallowing. He had a history of heart failure, type 2 diabetes, bladder cancer, cerebral infarction, and aspiration pneumonitis. A month before the first visit, the patient had aspiration pneumonitis. After his pneumonitis had been treated with antibiotics, he come back to his nursing home. His physician supposed that he had severe dysphagia and then discharged with a gastrostomy feeding tube. However, his ability of swallowing was not thoroughly accessed. Therefore, his physician asked us to assess his dysphagia and provide rehabilitation for it. At the first examination, the Japan Coma Scale score was I-2. Oxygen saturation (SpO2) was 88% (reference range, ≥95%). Fiberoptic endoscopic evaluation of

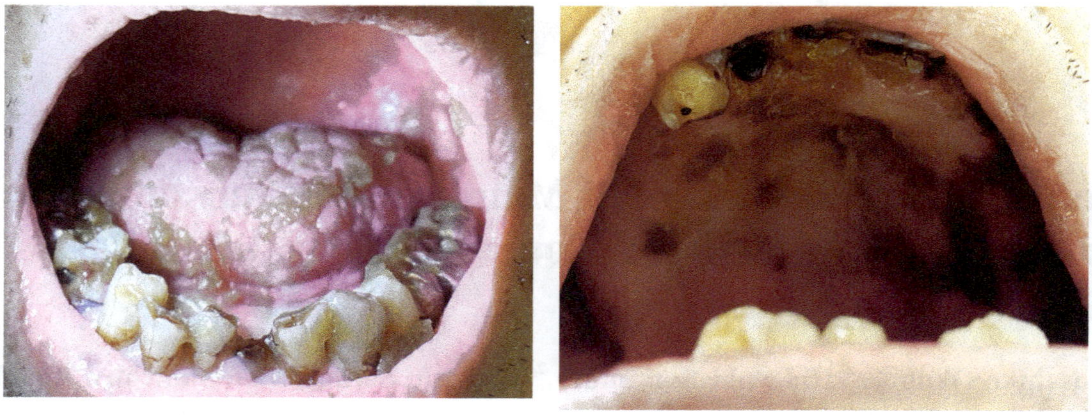

(a) (b)

Figure 1: There was a large amount of oral desquamated epithelium. (a) Lower jaw and (b) upper jaw.

swallowing (FEES) revealed that there was a large amount of oral desquamated epithelium, dental plaque, and calculus in his mouth (Figure 1). We could not examine the pharynx for swallowing evaluation even during fiberoptic endoscopy due to the deposits (Figure 2(a)). The patient was deemed to require oral care, pharyngeal deposit removal, and dysphagia rehabilitation without food before initiating oral food intake. First, we changed the type of moisturizing agent from gel to liquid. Nurses and care workers administered oral care such as rubbing the tongue and buccal mucosa daily. Dentists and oral hygienists visited and provided special oral care three times per week. The patient had no recurrence of pneumonitis at least for 77 days. In addition to daily oral care, we evaluated his dysphagia by FEES on 14 days, 37 days, and 61 days after the first examination. The responsiveness, reflection, and movement of the pharynx were improved day by day. The oral desquamated epithelium and membranous substances in the pharynx also decreased drastically (Figures 2(b)–2(d)), and SpO2 improved (98%). Therefore, 2 months after the first examination, the patient was able to eat the special nonprotein foods for rehabilitation of dysphagia.

3. Discussion

Membranous substances in the pharynx can cause suffocation and decrease the ability to eat and swallow; hence, they are associated with aspiration pneumonia. The SpO_2 in our patient was 88% at the first examination, but after removing the pharyngeal deposits, his SpO_2 increased to 98%. He had no recurrence of pneumonia after the removal of the membranous substances in the pharynx.

The formation of pharyngeal deposits is closely related to membranous substances in the oral cavity. The prevalence of membranous substances in the oral cavity in tube feeding patients is 40% (10/25). Within these 40% patients, 70% (7/10) have membranous substances in the pharynx [1]. Histologically, membranous substances in both the pharynx and oral cavity are composed of cornified squamous epithelium [1–3]. Therefore, the origin of deposits in the pharynx is, at least in part, squamous epithelium, that is, membranous substances in the oral cavity, although the appearance of membranous substances in the pharynx seemed to be crust-like or sputum-like when we observed them by endoscopy [1]. Indeed, in our case, the membranous substances in the pharynx were clearly reduced in the oral cavity by intensive oral care. We speculated oral care reduced the membranous substances in the oral cavity in consequence and also reduced the substances, which had dropped into the pharynx and attached to the surrounding membrane. In addition, other mechanisms may be involved in the reduction of membranous substances in the pharynx by oral care. Because intensive oral care increases the cough reflex sensitivity in the pharynx [4] and stimulates the swallowing reflex [5] through the production of substance, of course, future research is needed to comprehend the relationship between oral care and membrane substances in the pharynx.

As described above, membranous substances in the oral cavity contain stratified squamous epithelium. Therefore, these are regarded as desquamated epithelium from the oral mucosa [1]. Dry conditions are the main risk factor for the formation of desquamated epithelium in the oral cavity [2–8]. Under dry conditions, the surface of the epithelium is denatured, and the epithelium is peeled from the lower layer [9]. Dry conditions also reduce the function of exfoliating enzymes, disturb epidermal turnover, and cause the accumulation of the stratum corneum in the oral mucosa. Therefore, the mucosa is peeled and caked under dry conditions compared to normal conditions [9, 10].

As mentioned above, since the formation of desquamated epithelium is closely related to dry mouth, the use of moisturizing agents is recommended to prevent this process in tube feeding patients [10, 11]. Oral care with moisturizing agents has been shown to prevent membranous substances at the oral membrane in tube feeding patients [3]. However, gel-type moisturizing agents should be used carefully because too much gel may contribute to the formation of membranous substances [11]. In our case, after changing

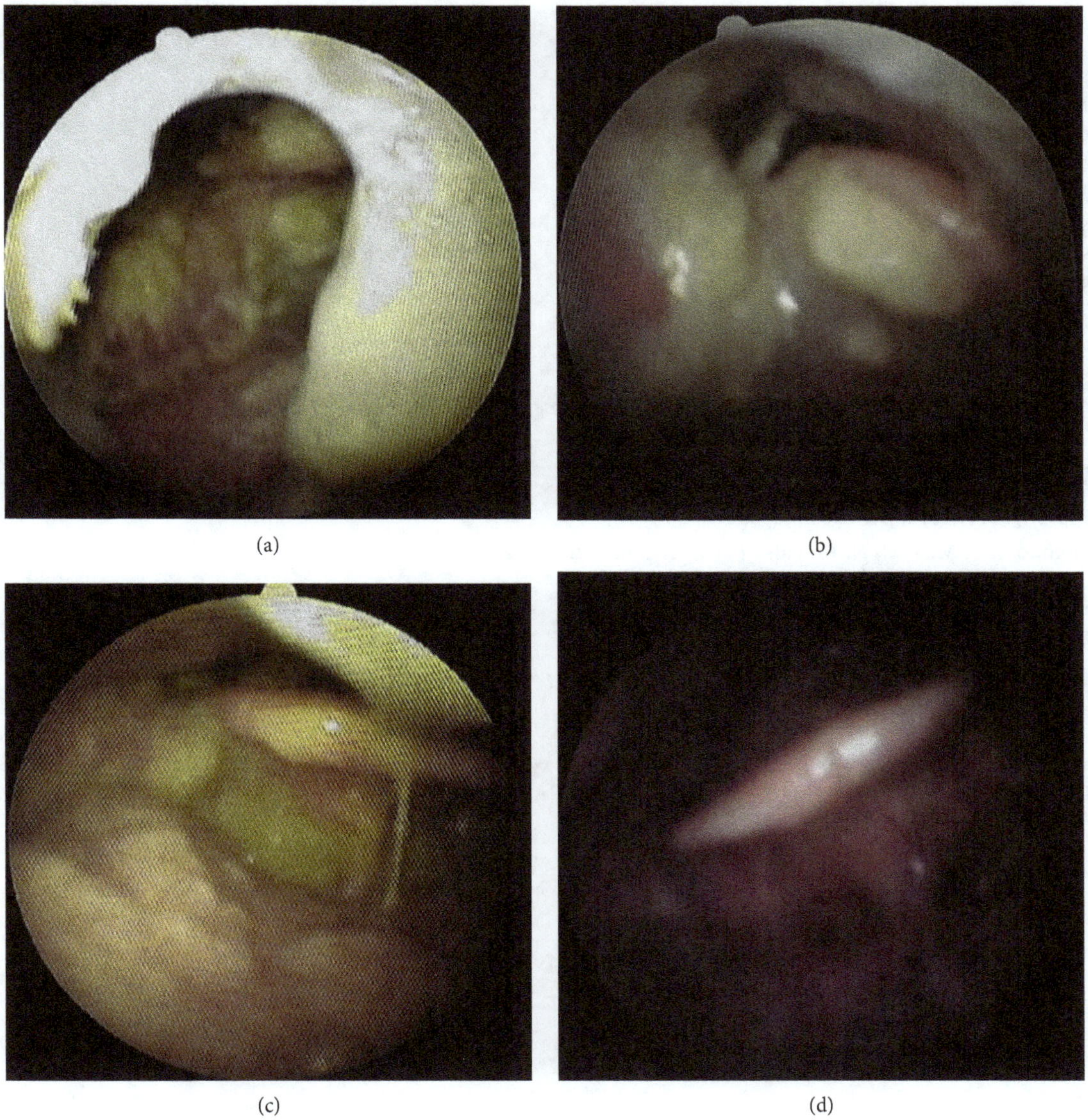

FIGURE 2: The membranous substances in the pharynx decreased gradually. Fiberoptic endoscopic pictures in the pharynx. (a) First examination, (b)14 days, (c) 37 days, and (d) 61 days after the first examination.

the moisturizing agent from gel to liquid, the amount of membranous deposits was drastically reduced.

4. Conclusions

We reported that daily oral care by interprofessional workers, such as dentists, hygienists, nurses, and care workers, drastically reduces membranous substances in the pharynx and improves swallowing functions.

Consent

Consent to publish the case report was not obtained. The report does not contain any personal information that could lead to identifying the patient.

References

[1] K. Shinotsuka, T. Ogasawara, H. Iwasaki et al., "Causative factors of the formation of deposition on the pharyngeal mucosal surface of persons requiring nursing care with tube feeding," *Journal of the Japanese Society for Disability and Oral Health*, vol. 37, pp. 22–27, 2016.

[2] Y. Kawase, T. Ogasawara, S. Kawase et al., "Factors affecting the formation of membranous substances in the palates of elderly persons requiring nursing care," *Gerodontology*, vol. 31, no. 3, pp. 184–193, 2014.

[3] T. Ogasawara, Y. Kawase, K. Isono et al., "Formative factors of membranous substances on dorsum of tongue, teeth, buccal mucosa in elderly persons requiring nursing care," *Japanese Journal of Gerodontology*, vol. 29, pp. 11–20, 2014, [Article in Japanese].

[4] A. Watando, S. Ebihara, T. Ebihara et al., "Daily oral care and cough reflex sensitivity in elderly nursing home patients," *Chest*, vol. 126, no. 4, pp. 1066–1070, 2004.

[5] A. Yoshino, E. Ebihara, S. Ebihara, H. Fujii, and H. Sasaki, "Daily oral care and risk factors for pneumonia among elderly nursing home patients," *JAMA*, vol. 286, no. 18, pp. 2235-2236, 2001.

[6] T. Ogasawara, N. Andou, S. Kawase et al., "Potential factors responsible for dryness of the dorsum of the tongue in elderly requiring care," *Gerodontology*, vol. 25, no. 4, pp. 217–221, 2008.

[7] S. S. Nakamura, "Classification and diagnosis of dry mouth," *Japanese Journal of Oral and Maxillofacial Surgery*, vol. 55, no. 4, pp. 169–176, 2009, [Article in Japanese].

[8] T. Ooka, M. Watanabe, N. Kimura et al., "A study of oral health care and improvement of oral hygiene at an emergency hospital," *The Japanese Society for Disability and Oral Health*, vol. 31, pp. 749–757, 2010, [Article in Japanese].

[9] C. A. Borgoño, I. P. Michael, N. Komatsu et al., "A potential role for multiple tissue kallikrein serine proteases in epidermal desquamation∗," *The Journal of Biological Chemistry*, vol. 282, no. 6, pp. 3640–3652, 2007.

[10] H. Tagami, "Approach to dry skin (xerosis): lessons from the past," *Journal of Japanese Cosmetic Science Society*, vol. 38, pp. 15–21, 2014, [Article in Japanese].

[11] H. Iwasaki, T. Ogasawara, K. Shinotsuka et al., "A study on preventing the formation of membranous substances in the oral cavity by moisturizer," *The Japanese Journal of Dysphagia Rehabilitation*, vol. 20, pp. 86–93, 2016, [Article in Japanese].

18

A Case of Multiple Phleboliths on the Medial Side of the Right Mandible

Shinichi Sato,[1,2] **Masato Takahashi**,[1] **and Tetsu Takahashi**[2]

[1] *Oral and Maxillofacial Surgery, Japan Community Health Care Organization Sendai Hospital, 3-16-1 Tsutsumimachi, Aoba-ku, Sendai 981-8501, Japan*
[2] *Division of Oral and Maxillofacial Surgery, Tohoku University Graduate School of Dentistry, 4-1, Seiryo-machi, Aoba-ku, Sendai 980-8575, Japan*

Correspondence should be addressed to Shinichi Sato; first.sato@gmail.com

Academic Editor: Giuseppe Alessandro Scardina

A 66-year-old female patient was admitted to the orthopedic department due to a left femoral neck fracture. She received perioperative oral management prior to femoral head replacement. Laboratory blood tests indicated an elevated D-dimer level, which suggested the presence of a venous malformation. Computed tomography, magnetic resonance imaging, and short TI inversion recovery indicated the presence of multiple phleboliths medial to the right mandibular ramus. No swelling, redness, or salivary colic pain was observed. Owing to the absence of clinical symptoms, the patient elected to undergo observation of the lesion, as opposed to surgical treatment.

1. Introduction

Calcifications in the soft tissues of the maxillofacial region may present as sialoliths, phleboliths, calcified epitheliomas, or lymph node calcifications. Phleboliths are found in venous malformations and are thought to be caused by the calcification of intravenous thrombi [1, 2]. In this report, we describe a case in which numerous phleboliths were diagnosed in relation to the right mandible.

2. Case Presentation

A 66-year-old woman suffered a fall at home in January 2020 and was admitted to our orthopedic department due to a left femoral neck fracture. She was subsequently referred to our oral surgery department for perioperative oral management prior to femoral head replacement surgery. The patient provided written informed consent prior to treatment. The appropriate institutional review board waived the requirement for ethical approval.

The patient's height and weight were 160 cm and 62.9 kg, respectively, and the only medical history was the removal of a colorectal polyp.

No facial asymmetry, swelling, or redness was observed extraorally (Figure 1). Upon intraoral examination, no redness or swelling was detected in the buccal mucosa (Figure 2). Laboratory blood tests indicated that the platelet count ($31.4 \times 10^4/\mu L$) and fibrinogen level (228 mg/dL) were both within normal ranges; however, the D-dimer level (36.62 μg/mL) was elevated.

Panoramic radiographs showed a dissemination of calcifications in the head and neck region that were suspected to be venous stones (Figure 3). On computed tomography, numerous calcifications of unequal size were observed medial to the right mandible (Figure 4). The short TI inversion recovery (STIR) showed a higher signal in the area of the lesions compared to the surrounding tissues (Figure 5) [3].

A clinical diagnosis of suspected multiple phleboliths within the right mandibular vein was made. There was no swelling, redness, or pain in the right mandible. No aggressive treatment was performed, since the patient preferred to

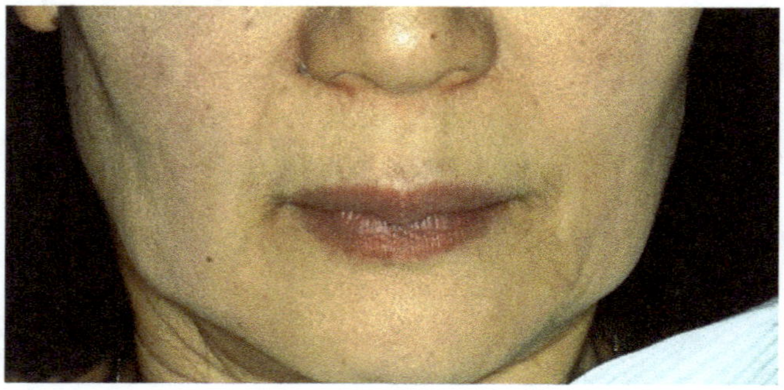

Figure 1: Extraoral photograph showing symmetrical facial features.

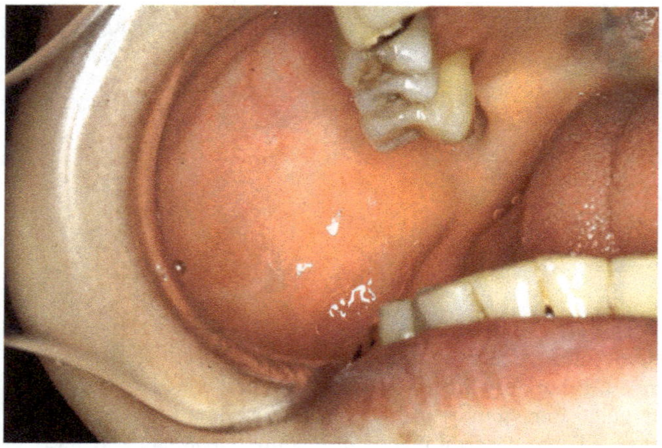

Figure 2: Intraoral photograph showing the absence of swelling or redness.

be reviewed at regular intervals by the doctor. To date, the patient has remained asymptomatic.

She was also examined by our otolaryngology department; as she was, asymptomatic, the follow-up protocol was continued.

3. Discussion

Venous malformations are the most common among all vascular malformations, with a male-to-female ratio ranging from 1 : 1 to 1 : 2. The size and distribution of venous malformations vary, with 40–50% of all hemangiomas occurring in the head and neck region, particularly in the tongue, buccal mucosa, and lips [3]. The incidence of phleboliths in the head and neck region has been reported to range from 5% to 20% [4].

While the association of hemangiomas with phleboliths has been reported in approximately 5% of all oral surgery cases, internal hemangiomas in the mandible are a much rarer occurrence [5]. The submandibular region is considered the most common site for phleboliths. In the present case, the presence of phleboliths was indicated by areas with high absorption on the magnetic resonance T2-weighted image and STIR image; they were observed on the inner side of the right mandible on computed tomography, outside of the submandibular region.

Phleboliths are characterized by a high degree of calcification and are thought to be caused by the dystrophic calcification of intravenous thrombi [6, 7]. When swelling or hard masses occur in the buccal or submandibular region, it is necessary to distinguish phleboliths from sialoliths in the parotid or submandibular glands [8]. The key to this differentiation is that both painful swelling and salivary colic are observed with sialoliths, whereas painless swelling is associated with phleboliths [8, 9].

While hemangiomas and vascular malformations are often referred to as hemangiomas, the International Society for the Study of Vascular Anomalies (ISSVA) has previously proposed that they should be classified as either vascular tumors or vascular malformations, based on the presence or absence of vascular endothelial cell proliferation [4]. The diagnostic criteria and treatment policy proposed by the ISSVA have recently become internationally standardized. According to the ISSVA classification, an autopsy case is considered a venous malformation. D-dimer levels are elevated in approximately 42% of patients with vascular malformations, due to thrombus formation [4]; the patient in this report had an elevated D-dimer level (36.62 μg/mL), suggesting the presence of a venous malformation.

Inflammatory and cystic masses (e.g., lymphadenitis, cystoid cyst, salivary gland inflammation, calcified epithelioma, and sialolith), benign tumors (e.g., schwannoma, lymphangioma, and pleomorphic adenoma), and malignant lesions (e.g., adenoid cystic carcinoma) have been typically considered in the differential diagnosis of deep-seated hemangiomas in the past.

There was an extensive high-intensity signal on the medial aspect of the right side of the face in the STIR image. Computed tomography clearly differentiated the inferior margin of the right mandible from the submandibular gland, and numerous calcifications were observed. Sialoliths were excluded due to the absence of pain associated with the salivary glands. However, a definitive diagnosis of multiple phleboliths could not be made, as they were not removed, and a biopsy was not performed.

Surgical removal, packing, cryosurgery, tissue sclerotherapy, and radiation therapy [10, 11] have been reported as treatment methods for venous malformations. Nevertheless, the choice of treatment should take into consideration the patient's age, as well as the size, site of origin, and characteristics (including its relationship with surrounding tissues and nutrient vessels) of the tumor. In the present case, after explaining the advantages and disadvantages of surgical treatment to the patient, she elected to undergo observation of the lesion only. To date, no swelling, redness, or pain has been observed in the right side of the mandible.

Taken together, we described a case in which multiple phleboliths were diagnosed in the right mandibular region.

Despite the absence of a cardiovascular event, an elevated D-dimer level was evident. Thus, this case illustrates that even in the absence of symptoms or asymptomatic, facial, or orofacial abnormalities, an elevated D-dimer level

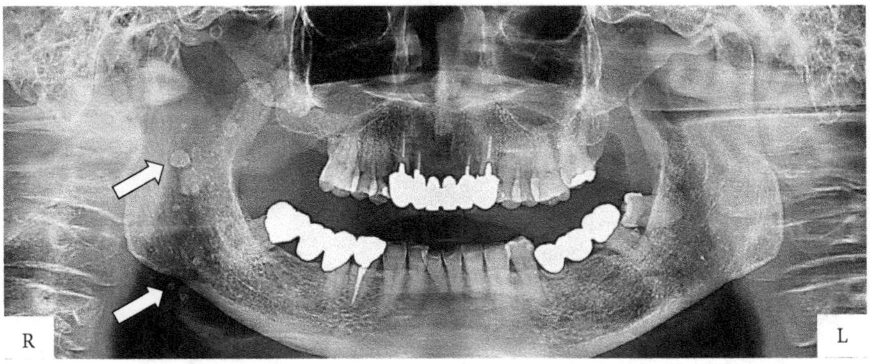

FIGURE 3: A panoramic radiograph during initial examination. Scattered opaque material suspected to be venous stones is noted. A circular opacity is evident (arrow).

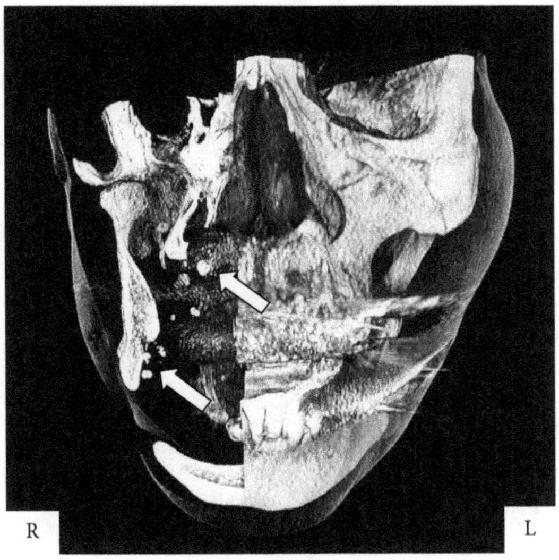

FIGURE 4: Computed tomography image showing numerous calcifications of unequal size in the medial portion of the right mandible. Circular hard tissue is evident (arrow).

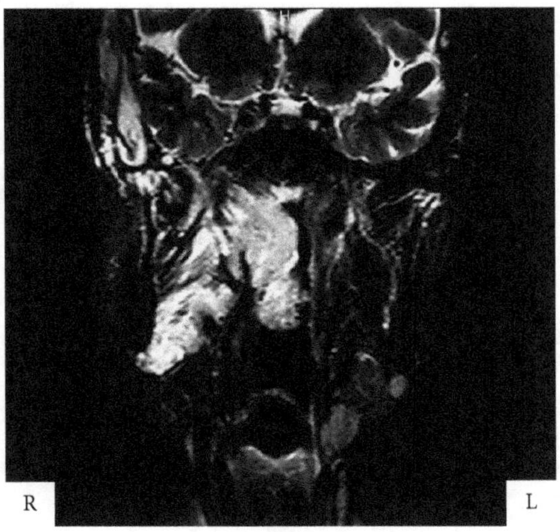

FIGURE 5: Short TI inversion recovery image showing a higher signal in the area of the lesions compared to the surrounding tissues.

may indicate the presence of venous malformations in the head and neck region and the need for further investigations.

Authors' Contributions

SS conceived this report, drafted the article, and critically revised it for important intellectual content. TM and TT helped to draft the manuscript. All authors have read and approved the final manuscript.

Acknowledgments

I would like to thank Dr. Yuri Nomura, Dr. Hiyori Takahashi (Department of Otorhinolaryngology), and Dr. Hideaki Mitsui (of the Department of Radiology), Sendai Hospital, Japan Agency for the Promotion of Regional Medical Care, for their advice on the preparation of this manuscript. We would like to thank Editage (http://www.editage.com) for English language editing.

References

[1] C. C. Chuang, H. C. Lin, and C. W. Huang, "Submandibular cavernous hemangiomas with multiple phleboliths masquerading as sialolithiasis," *Journal of the Chinese Medical Association*, vol. 68, no. 9, pp. 441–443, 2005.

[2] M. M. Suarez-Cunqueiro, J. Dueker, J. Seoane-Leston, and R. Schmelzeisen, "Tonsilloliths associated with sialolithiasis in the submandibular gland," *Journal of Oral and Maxillofacial Surgery*, vol. 66, no. 2, pp. 370–373, 2008.

[3] A. Tekes, J. Koshy, T. O. Kalayci et al., "S.E. Mitchell Vascular Anomalies Flow Chart (SEMVAFC): a visual pathway combining clinical and imaging findings for classification of soft-tissue vascular anomalies," *Clinical Radiology*, vol. 69, no. 5, pp. 443–457, 2014.

[4] F. Marchal and P. Dulguerov, "Sialolithiasis management," *Archives of Otolaryngology— Head & Neck Surgery*, vol. 129, no. 9, pp. 951–956, 2003.

[5] K. Sano, A. Ogawa, T. Inokuchi, H. Takahashi, and K. Hisatsune, "Buccal hemangioma with phleboliths: report of two cases," *Oral Surgery, Oral Medicine, and Oral Pathology*, vol. 65, no. 2, pp. 151–156, 1988.

[6] S. Okura, C. Igarashi, S. Wakae-Morita et al., "A case of venous malformation of the mandible," *Oral Radiology*, vol. 35, no. 2, pp. 194–197, 2019.

[7] T. C. Huang, J. B. Dalton, F. N. Monsour, and N. W. Savage, "Multiple, large sialoliths of the submandibular gland duct: a case report," *Australian Dental Journal*, vol. 54, no. 1, pp. 61–65, 2009.

[8] M. McMenamin, A. Quinn, H. Barry, D. Sleeman, G. Wilson, and M. Toner, "Cavernous hemangioma in the submandibular gland masquerading as sialadenitis: case report," *Oral Surgery, Oral Medicine, Oral Pathology, Oral Radiology, and Endodontics*, vol. 84, no. 2, pp. 146–148, 1997.

[9] D. M. Levy, W. H. Remine, and K. D. Devine, "Salivary gland Calculi," *Journal of the American Medical Association*, vol. 181, no. 13, pp. 1115–1119, 1962.

[10] O. Enjolras, M. Wassef, and R. Chapot, *Color atlas of vascular tumors and vascular malformations*, Cambridge University Press, New York, 2007.

[11] J. Lustmann, E. Regev, and Y. Melamed, "Sialolithiasis: A survey on 245 patients and a review of the literature," *International Journal of Oral and Maxillofacial Surgery*, vol. 19, no. 3, pp. 135–138, 1990.

19

Augmentation of the Atrophic Mandible with a Block Corticomedullary Graft

Layla Louise de Amorim Rocha,[1] **Matheus Francisco Barros Rodrigues**,[1] **Rodrigo da Franca Acioly**,[2] **Daniel do Carmo Carvalho**,[2] **and Cristofe Coelho Lopes da Rocha**[3]

[1]*Dentistry Course, Faculdade Cathedral, Boa Vista 69307-053, Brazil*
[2]*Department of Oral and Maxillofacial Surgery and Traumatology, Hospital Geral, Boa Vista 69305-455, Brazil*
[3]*Department of Infrastructure, Federal Institute, Boa Vista 69303-340, Brazil*

Correspondence should be addressed to Layla Louise de Amorim Rocha; layla2rocha@gmail.com

Academic Editor: Daniel Torres-Lagares

The gradual loss of the dental alveolus leads to bone resorption, which may cause atrophy of the maxilla and mandible. One of the most complex procedures in reconstructive surgery is the rehabilitation of patients with atrophic mandibles. Herein, we present a clinical case study of atrophic mandible augmentation with grafts obtained from the iliac crest. The use of reconstruction plates may represent a feasible mechanism for treatment as well as fracture prevention. Mandible augmentation performed by grafting the donor site of the iliac crest showed satisfactory results and resolution of the aesthetic and functional impairments.

1. Introduction

Edentulism is a condition that affects a large number of individuals worldwide, especially elderly people [1–3]. The gradual loss of the dental alveolus leads to bone resorption, which may cause atrophy of the maxillae [4]. This atrophy makes the bone fragile and vulnerable to fractures, since the bone mass is reduced [5].

One of the most complex procedures in reconstructive surgeries is the rehabilitation of patients with an atrophic mandible [6]. Factors related to bone quantity and quality, reduced contact area between fractured segments, and inadequate blood supply increase the complexity of this treatment procedure [1]. Several treatment options for these procedures have been reported in the literature, including short implants, bone grafting, and repositioning of the inferior alveolar neurovascular bundle [2].

Techniques for increasing the alveolar dimensions are recommended according to the level of existing bone loss [7]. Monocortical grafts or guided bone grafts are useful for small augmentations, and the interposition graft better suits moderate defects [7]. For defects that are more extensive, osteogenic distraction or reconstruction with grafts from the iliac bone is applied; however, before using these techniques, it is necessary to determine if there is enough bone for distraction [7].

Various types of grafts, including allografts, xenografts, and autografts, are used in the field of dentistry [8]. The autologous bone is considered to be the "gold standard" and the most effective material in bone regeneration procedures owing to its favorable properties and the absence of immunological reactions, showing an optimal combination of osteoconductive, osteoinductive, and osteogenic characteristics when compared to different types of grafts [9, 10]. It may be obtained through donor intraoral areas, such as the maxillary tuberosity, mandibular symphysis, mandibular body, ascending ramus, and zygomatic bone, and through extraoral areas by using the skull bone and the iliac crest [8]. The iliac crest stands out in grafting procedures in cases of atrophy of the jaws due to its high bone volume, relative ease of operation, and low prevalence of morbidity and complications [11]. Graft placement may be performed

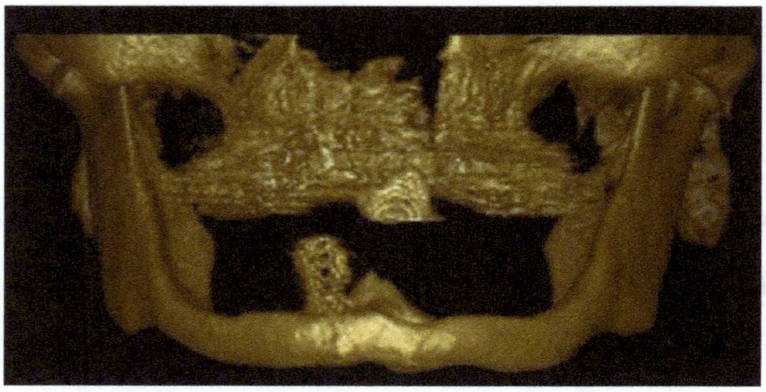

Figure 1: Three-dimensional computed tomography revealing severe mandibular atrophy with perforations at the implant sites.

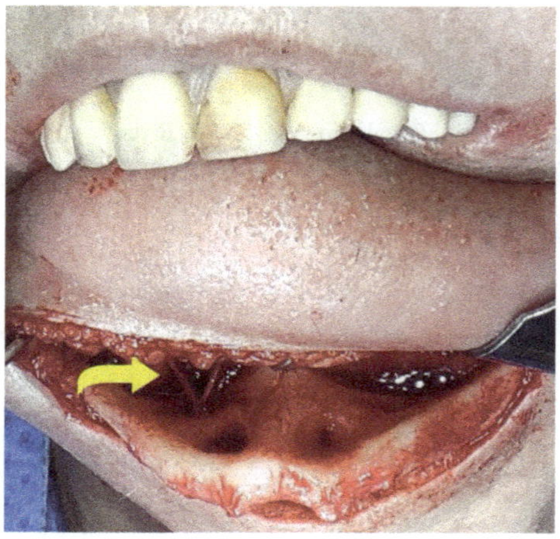

Figure 2: Mandible with severe bone resorption and exposure of the inferior alveolar nerve (yellow arrow).

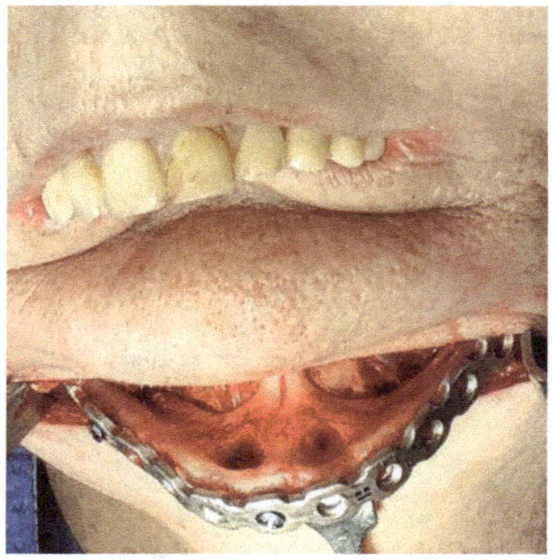

Figure 3: Fixation of the reconstruction plate.

through intraoral or extraoral access at the discretion of each surgeon [7].

The objective of this study is to present a clinical case involving atrophic mandible augmentation with a graft obtained from the iliac crest, with discussion of the clinical, surgical, and radiographic aspects in addition to a review of the main concepts involved. Considering the possibility of jaw fractures due to severe bone loss, adoption of a grafting procedure can facilitate the patient's functional and aesthetic rehabilitation and fracture prevention.

2. Case Presentation

A 72-year-old female patient presented to the dental office with complaints including chewing difficulty and aesthetic dissatisfaction owing to the absence of dental elements. The anamnesis revealed a frustrated rehabilitation attempt approximately 10 years previously, with an overdenture prosthesis in the O-ring on the bottom part under two implants. As time went by, bone resorption occurred.

The patient underwent a computed tomography scan with 3D reconstruction and orthopantomography. Clinical and radiographic examinations revealed severe mandibular atrophy with bilateral exposure of the lower alveolar nerve, perforations at the implant sites (Figure 1), and a bone height of 7 mm (Class VI, Cawood and Howell). In order to obtain assistance during the surgical procedure and to optimize the preoperative planning, a mandibular biomodel was made, which enabled manipulation of the reconstruction plate before the surgical procedure.

Rehabilitative surgical treatment was planned using bone blocks obtained in the iliac crest region to be positioned in the mandible in order to achieve bone height and avoid mandibular fracture [7].

The patient received general anesthesia and was administered corticosteroids (dexamethasone 8 mg intravenously) and anti-inflammatory (tenoxicam 40 mg endovenous) and analgesic (dipyrone sodium 1 g endovenous) drugs after anesthetic induction. For the operation, extraoral access was chosen, with a submental incision followed by divulsion and detachment, exposing the mandible and visualizing the areas of exposure of the alveolar nerve. The nerves were disinserted with the aid of a piezoelectric device, after which the reconstruction plate with 16 holes was fixed using seven fixed screws, three in the region of the genial spines and two on the angles of the mandible intended to prevent fractures and reinforce the mandible to make it functional (Figures 2 and 3). The presence of perforations corresponding to the site of the implants was observed (Figure 2).

The graft removed from the iliac crest was decorticalized, and its bed was perforated in order to expose the medullary part to facilitate neovascularization. Then, grafting of the three blocks from the iliac crest was performed with one screw in each block (Figure 4).

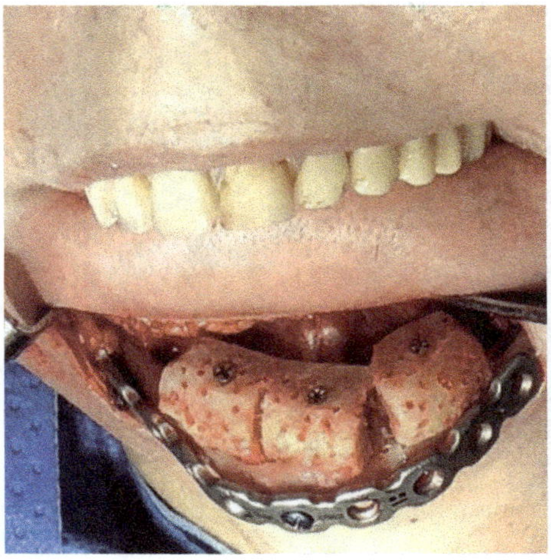

Figure 4: Fixation of the graft.

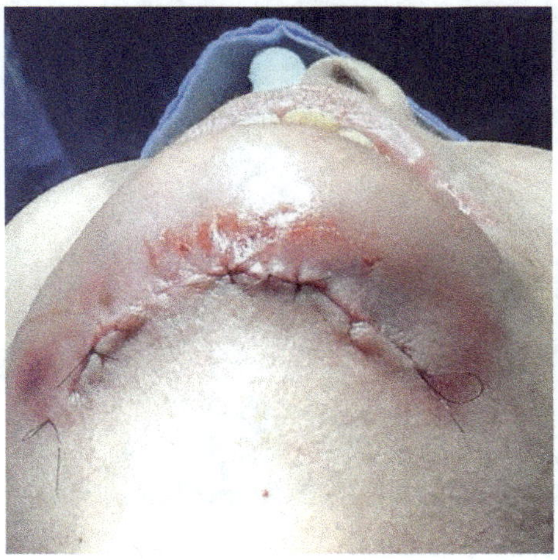

Figure 5: Tissue repositioning with a synthesis operation on the suprahyoid muscles.

For osteoconduction, bioactive NovaBone putty was applied to the bone cement blocks in order to protect the graft and fill the spaces between the bone blocks. Finally, tissue repositioning was performed with a synthesis operation on the suprahyoid muscles by using simple stitches interrupted with Monocryl 4.0 thread and skin and intradermal sutures with 5.0 nylon thread and interrupted simple reinforcement stitches (Figure 5).

The patient remained hospitalized for 2 days, and the postoperative medication protocol consisted of antibiotics (amoxicillin 500 mg every 8 hours for 7 days), corticosteroids (dexamethasone 4 mg every 12 hours for 3 days), anti-inflammatory (tenoxicam 20 mg every 12 hours for 5 days), and an analgesic (dipyrone sodium 500 mg every 6 hours for 3 days) in case of pain or discomfort. To assist in the treatment of neuralgia, Citoneurin was prescribed. During the postoperative period, the patient reported mild-to-moderate pain and mild paresthesia for the first few days, with no progression of the condition, besides presenting with edema and ecchymosis, which are clinical signs eventually observed in these cases. On the seventh postoperative day, the sutures were removed.

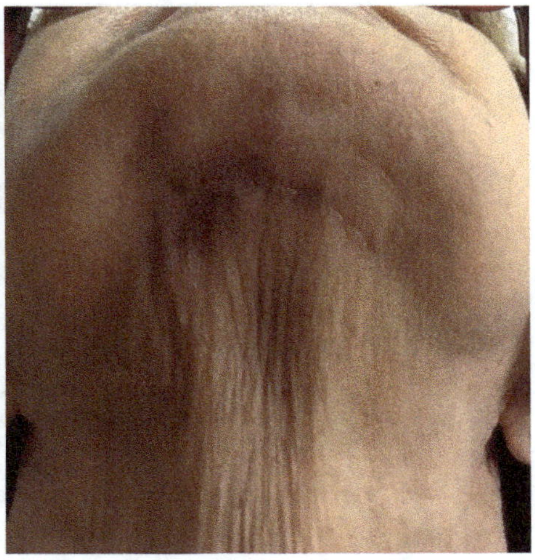

Figure 6: Postoperative healing of the extraoral access site (2 months).

After waiting 20 days in order to restore masticatory function, the old prosthesis was repackaged and adapted for the patient to use while waiting for placement of the implants. The extraoral access site showed satisfactory healing and no sequelae (Figure 6).

After four months, the patient returned complaining of pain as a result of the side screws. These were removed to avoid graft exposure and provide comfort. The patient was followed for 6 months, at which point imaging studies revealed successful grafting, and an increase of 9 mm was seen in the jawbone height, which indicated favorable conditions for beginning the dental implant process (Figures 7 and 8).

3. Discussion

There are several reports in the literature describing the occurrence of fractures in patients with mandibles showing severe bone resorption [3]. This condition makes the bone fragile and vulnerable to fractures since the bone mass is reduced [5]. Therefore, the surgeon must employ techniques that help prevent fractures in addition to reinforcing the mandible to ensure its functionality.

The therapeutic choice must be based on the patient's age, the severity of the case, and the condition of the bone involved [12]. Although the surgical procedure for insertion of reconstruction plates requires more time, it represents a viable approach both for treatment and fracture prevention [12].

Moreover, the time required for the procedure can be optimized by making a biomodel [13], which, in addition to reducing the incision length, allows visualization and a better understanding of the anatomical region of interest [14] and allows the plate to be molded preoperatively. Thus, during the surgery, the patient's mandible is easily adapted.

Regarding the surgical access point, there is no evidence favoring one over the other [5]. Intraoral access has some disadvantages, such as the presence of the mental nerve on the upper part of the jawbone, which could be injured upon incision and dissection, causing hemilabial hypoesthesia,

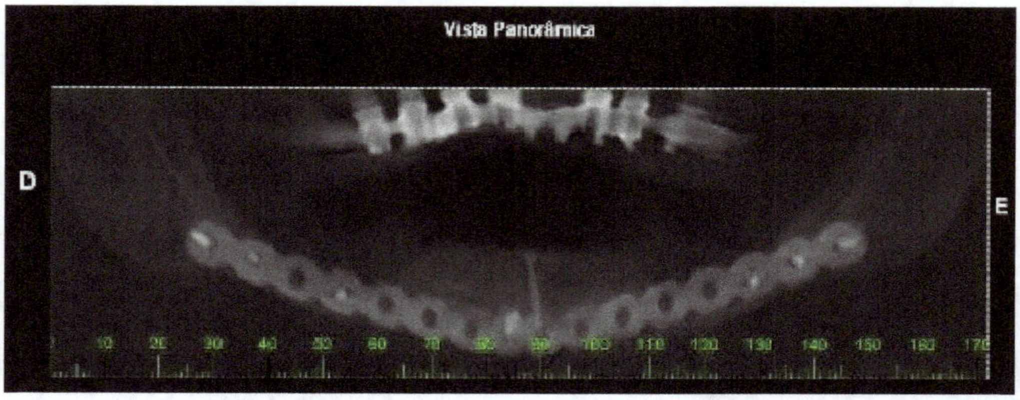

Figure 7: Postoperative panoramic radiography (6 months) demonstrating increased bone height.

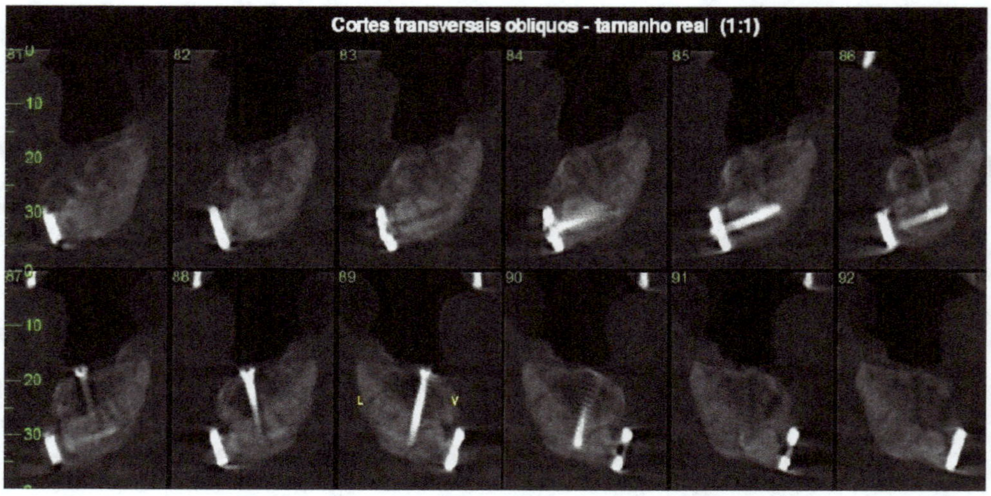

Figure 8: Postoperative computed tomography (6 months).

and possible contamination of the fracture by the oral bacterial fauna, increasing the risk of infection during and after surgery [5]. In turn, extraoral access, despite the possibility of injury to the facial nerve or other anatomic structures, provides the surgeon with a direct view of the fracture, reducing the procedure's complexity compared to intraoral access [5, 15].

Lateralization of the lower alveolar nerve is one of the options for prosthetic-based rehabilitation of patients with moderate-to-severe alveolar reabsorption in the posterior region of the jaw [3]. However, there may be postsurgical consequences resulting from this technique such as neurosensory disorders (neurapraxia, axonotmesis, and neurotmesis) [3]. A high degree of mandibular reabsorption implies a risk of fracture, and this approach is, therefore, not recommended in such cases [3].

4. Conclusions

The various risks surrounding mandible atrophy necessitate procedures to prevent further damage and ensure effective treatment depending on the bone loss observed. Jawbone augmentation with an iliac crest graft provided satisfactory results in our patient. Extraoral access allowed for a reduction in case complexity and demonstrated satisfactory scarring without aesthetic problems for the patient. Six months after surgery, an increase of 9 mm was found in the jawbone height, which indicated favorable conditions for beginning the dental implant process.

References

[1] M. Brucoli, P. Boffano, I. Romeo et al., "Surgical management of unilateral body fractures of the edentulous atrophic mandible," *Oral and Maxillofacial Surgery*, vol. 24, no. 1, pp. 65–71, 2020.

[2] M. Nasser, Z. Fedorowicz, and A. Ebadifar, "Management of the fractured edentulous atrophic mandible," *Cochrane Database of Systematic Reviews*, no. 1, 2007.

[3] R. L. Alvarenga, E. Akaki, A. C. R. A. de Souza, and L. N. de Souza, "Rehabilitation atrophic mandible with short dental implants and titanium plate: a case report," *Revista Portuguesa de Estomatologia, Medicina Dentária e Cirurgia Maxilofacial*, vol. 54, no. 4, pp. 217–221, 2013.

[4] C. F. Nóia, H. D. de Miranda Chaves Netto, R. O. Lopes, J. Rodríguez-Chessa, and R. Mazzonetto, "Uso de Enxerto Ósseo Autogeno nas Reconstruçoes da Cavidade Bucal. Analise Retrospectiva de 07 Anos," *Revista Portuguesa de Estomatologia, Medicina Dentária e Cirurgia Maxilofacial*, vol. 50, no. 4, pp. 221–225, 2009.

[5] M. Marcelo Mardones, G. Eduardo Navia, A. Rodrigo Bravo, and O. Cristopher Mayer, "Tratamiento de fracturas en mandíbulas atróficas: presentación de dos casos clínicos," *International Journal of Odontostomatology*, vol. 5, no. 2, pp. 126–132, 2011.

[6] R. D. S. Pereira, J. P. Bonardi, J. R. da Silva, C. F. d. A. B. Mourão, P. R. Barbosa Júnior, and L. F. Magacho, "Tratamento cirúrgico da fratura de mandibula atrófica pela técnica AO: relato de caso," *Archives of Health Investigation*, vol. 6, no. 3, 2017.

[7] M. Miloro et al., *Princípios de Cirurgia Bucomaxilofacial de Peterson*, Santos Editora, São Paulo, 2 edition, 2010.

[8] A. C. Fardin, E. C. G. Jardim, F. C. Pereira, M. H. Guskuma, A. M. Aranega, and I. R. G. Júnior, "Enxerto ósseo em odontologia: revisão de literatura," *Innovations Implant Journal*, vol. 5, no. 3, pp. 48–52, 2010.

[9] A. Sakkas, F. Wilde, M. Heufelder, K. Winter, and A. Schramm, "Autogenous bone grafts in oral implantology—is it still a "gold standard"? A consecutive review of 279 patients with 456 clinical procedures," *International Journal of Implant Dentistry*, vol. 3, no. 1, p. 23, 2017.

[10] M. A. Talmaç, M. A. Görgel, M. Kanar, S. Erinç, A. H. Olçar, and H. M. Özdemir, "Anterior and posterior iliac crest bone graft donor site morbidities: a comparing retrospective study," *Medical Journal of Bakirkoy*, vol. 15, no. 3, pp. 244–249, 2019.

[11] E. Cansiz, D. Karabulut, S. C. Dogru, N. E. Akalan, Y. Temelli, and Y. Z. Arslan, "Gait analysis of patients subjected to the atrophic mandible augmentation with iliac bone graft," *Applied Bionics and Biomechanics*, vol. 2019, Article ID 8203597, 9 pages, 2019.

[12] L. B. Lima, M. T. F. Oliveira, J. D. Batista, F. S. Rocha, M. C. P. da Silva, and C. J. Silva, "Tratamento cirúrgico de fratura em mandíbula atrófica," *Revista Odontológica do Brasil Central*, vol. 23, no. 67, 2014.

[13] L. C. Safira, A. D. S. Maciel, J. C. C. Souto-Maior et al., "Aplicação dos biomodelos de prototipagem rápida na Odontologia, confeccionados pela técnica da impressão tridimensional," *Revista de Ciências Médicas e Biológicas*, vol. 9, no. 3, pp. 240–246, 2011.

[14] E. G. Ferraz, *Efeito do processamento de reconstruções tridimensionais virtuais para confecção de biomodelos de prototipagem rápida: estudo experimental em mandíbulas secas humanas*, 2009.

[15] H. C. Lima e Silva, L. R. Knoll, S. L. de Miranda, and R. Moreno, "Fratura em mandíbula atrófica: relato de caso," *Archives of Health Investigation*, vol. 6.1, 2017.

20

Microscopic Polyangiitis Initially Presumed to be Endocarditis

Takahiro Kaneko, Shunsuke Hino, Yosuke Iijima, and Norio Horie

Department of Oral and Maxillofacial Surgery, Saitama Medical Center, Saitama Medical University, Saitama, Japan

Correspondence should be addressed to Takahiro Kaneko; t_kaneko@saitama-med.ac.jp

Academic Editor: Ronald S. Brown

The antineutrophil cytoplasmic antibody- (ANCA-) associated vasculitides (AAVs), which include fever of unknown origin (FUO), are rare diseases characterized by necrotizing inflammation of small blood vessels and the presence of ANCAs. Microscopic polyangiitis (MPA) is a subtype of the AAVs. Although the prevalence of AAVs has generally increased over the last 20 years, there have been rare reports from the dental and oral surgery field. In this article, we present a case of MPA suspected to be infective endocarditis (IE) following tooth extraction.

1. Introduction

Fever of unknown origin (FUO) can be caused by a wide group of diseases including infections, noninfectious inflammatory diseases, malignancies, and miscellaneous diseases [1]. However, diagnosing certain causes of FUO has remained difficult. The antineutrophil cytoplasmic antibody- (ANCA-) associated vasculitides (AAVs) are rare diseases included in FUO characterized by necrotizing inflammation of small blood vessels and the presence of ANCAs [2]. AAVs can be classified into three phenotypically distinct processes: microscopic polyangiitis (MPA), granulomatosis with polyangiitis (GPA), and eosinophilic granulomatosis with polyangiitis (EGPA). Two main types of ANCA can be detected in patients with AAV: leukocyte proteinase 3 (PR3) and myeloperoxidase (MPO) [2]. Patients with GPA are predominantly PR3-ANCA-positive, whereas those with MPA or EGPA are predominantly MPO-ANCA-positive [2]. These antibodies are checked not only at diagnosis but also in follow-up as disease activity markers [3].

The prevalence of AAV is estimated to be 46–184/million people, and the numbers of patients with AAV have generally increased [4]. There is a relatively high prevalence of AAV among middle-aged and elderly persons [5], affecting both sexes equally (quite unlike most systemic autoimmune diseases) [5]. There is a geographic difference in the occurrence of AAVs.

Recently considered risk factors for AAVs include ultraviolet radiation and silica, which is commonly inhaled [4]. Although there have been studies that suggested infection as a risk factor, the long-held view that there is an infectious trigger has not been borne out [4].

The clinical presentation of AAVs begins with fever and weight loss, followed by systemic vasculitis characterized by renal and respiratory dysfunction [6]. In cases of MPA, necrotizing glomerulonephritis occurs rapidly, and it frequently progresses to renal failure [6]. Laboratory tests show increased C-reactive protein (CRP) and serum creatinine levels with increased MPO-ANCA [7]. In GPA, hemorrhages of the lung and upper respiratory tract and destructive lesions of the ear, nose, and throat are prominent [8]. EGPA patients typically have a long-standing history of asthma and allergic rhinitis [9].

Induction therapy for AAVs includes treatment with high-dose glucocorticoids (GCs) in combination with another immunosuppressive agent such as cyclophosphamide (CYC) or rituximab (RTX) [3]. RTX is more effective than CYC in refractory AAVs [3]. Patients with AAVs presenting with severe renal failure may be treated with pulsed CYC and GCs, with adjuvant plasma exchange [3].

Patients with FUO may visit dental or oral surgery clinics following recent dental treatment or have discomfort in the oral cavity. In this article, a rare case of MPA that was first referred to an oral surgery clinic for postextraction fever with dysgeusia and numbness of the tongue was presented. Initially, the authors suspected that the patient had infective endocarditis (IE) and thus consulted with specialists in cardiac medicine. However, IE was ruled out, with further detailed evaluations determining the presence of MPA.

2. Case Report

A 75-year-old woman was referred to the oral surgery clinic for a suspected dental infection. Her medical history included tuberculosis, hypertension, hyperlipidemia, and neurogenic bladder. Her surgical history included hip joint surgery at the ages of 11, 27, and 68 years. Four weeks earlier, the patient visited an otolaryngologist for otorrhea of the right ear and was diagnosed with otitis media and treated with antibiotics. On the same day, the patient underwent extraction of the right mandibular canine and lateral incisor by the patient's family dentist. Two weeks earlier, the patient had visited the primary care doctor for regular follow-up and complained of fatigue, fever, dysgeusia, swelling and numbness of the neck, and backache, which continued after the extraction. On laboratory examination, C-reactive protein (CRP) was 11.46 mg/dL, and the white blood cell count was 11,000/μL. Subsequently, chest X-ray and computed tomography (CT) showed no abnormal findings, and she tested negative for influenza virus. The patient then developed trismus and pain at the apex of the tongue and was referred to the oral surgery clinic.

On examination, the patient complained of fever and discomfort of the tongue with dysgeusia. Although usually both the maxilla and mandible cause dentures to wear, this does not occur when the teeth have been extracted. Salivary function was relatively good, and there was no xerostomia observed. No trismus was found; the teeth extraction sockets had healed well. None of the other residual teeth exhibited any prominent caries or periodontal disease. There were no abnormal findings in the orofacial region except for the dysgeusia and redness and numbness at the apex of the tongue (Figure 1). Orthopantomography revealed no abnormal findings, including maxillary sinuses and temporomandibular joints (Figure 2). On physical examination, the patient's temperature was 38.5°C, and blood pressure was 125/75 mmHg. The serum CRP concentration was 19.4 mg/dL, and the WBC count was 14,700/μL (Table 1). Given the history of tooth extraction, the patient was immediately referred to the division of cardiology for suspected IE.

The cardiologist took blood cultures, which were negative for bacteria, and an ultrasound cardiogram and transesophageal echocardiography showed neither clear vegetations nor regurgitation. For the remittent fever of more than 38.0°C, the patient was admitted to the cardiology clinic three days after the first visit and underwent a complete examination. Serum examination showed the following: PR3-ANCA < 1 IU/mL, MPO-ANCA 124.0 IU/mL, cytomegalovirus complement fixation test 8, ferritin 471 ng/mL, and CH50 60.0 U/mL. Sputum cultures, acid-fast bacterial cultures, and fecal cultures were negative. CT imaging showed no abnormal findings causing fever, and deep vein thrombosis was not found on ultrasonography of the veins of the lower extremities. There were no active symptoms related to the right otitis media other than depression of the eardrum on otolaryngological examination.

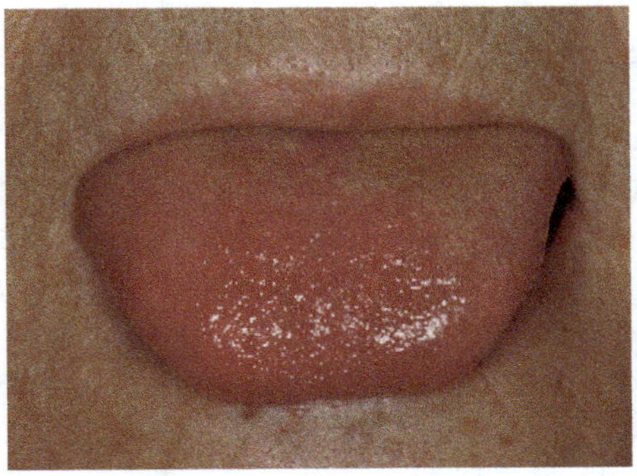

FIGURE 1: The apex of the tongue showing slight redness.

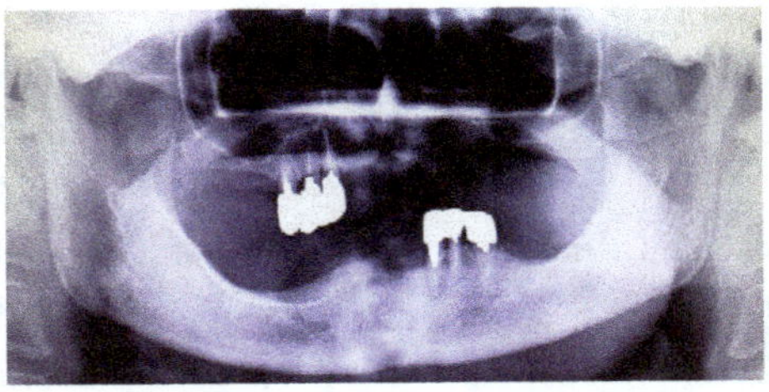

FIGURE 2: Orthopantomography at the first examination showing the sockets of the right mandibular canine and lateral incisor.

Fourteen days after the first visit, the patient was transferred to the Department of Rheumatology and Clinical Immunology because of the high suspicion of AAV, although renal dysfunction and findings of interstitial pneumonia were not evident. Twenty-seven days after the first visit, a renal biopsy was planned, but it was postponed due to influenza A infection. After the renal biopsy, which showed the findings of necrotizing glomerulonephritis, the patient was finally diagnosed with MPA (fever, MPO-ANCA-positive, CRP elevation, proteinuria, and histopathological findings of renal biopsy) 40 days after the first visit. Steroid therapy was then started with 30 mg prednisolone/day without immunosuppressive agents, and four days later, the patient was discharged. The inflammatory symptoms improved well, and the dysgeusia and numbness at the apex of the tongue disappeared four weeks later. At 20-week follow-up, prednisolone was tapered to 10 mg/day, and she was MPO-ANCA-negative.

The protocol of the report has been approved by the ethical review board of the university.

3. Discussion

To finally diagnose cases of FUO, detailed medical examination with various investigations and a longer time is needed. Dentists and oral surgeons should refer patients with fever to a physician immediately when the odontogenic diseases do not appear related to the cause of the fever. In addition, other

TABLE 1: Laboratory data of the first examination.

		Normal range			Normal range
Complete blood cell count					
WBC ($\times 10^3/\mu$L)	14.7	3.25–8.59	Neutrophils (%)	91.7	40.30-71.70
RBC ($\times 10^6/\mu$L)	4.29	3.58-4.90	Hemoglobin (g/dL)	12.7	11.10–15.50
Platelets ($\times 10^4/\mu$L)	530	148.00–336.00			
Blood chemistry					
TP (g/dL)	6.5	6.50-8.00	ALB (g/dL)	2.6	3.70–5.00
CPK (U/L)	29	0.00-140.00	AST (U/L)	61	8.00–38.00
ALT (U/L)	53	4.00–43.00	LDH (U/L)	255	115-280
ALP	426	115.00-340.00	γ GTP (U/L)	44	10.00-47.00
Creatinine (mg/dL)	0.70	0.30–1.00	BUN (mg/dL)	8	5.00–22.00
UA mg/dL	1.4	2.00–6.20	eGFRcreat	61.3	90.00–999.90
Na (mEq/L)	138	136.00–145.00	Cl (mEq/L)	99	98-109
K (mEq/L)	3.6	3.30–5.00	Ca (mg/dL)	8.2	8.30–10.20
Zn (μg/dL)	57	65.00-110.00	T-Bil (mg/dL)	0.5	0.20–1.00
CH50	60	31.60–57.60	CRP (mg/dL)	19.4	0.00–0.30
Procalcitonin (ng/mL)	0.1	0.00–0.40	cTnI (ng/mL)	0.00	0.00-0.09
Ferritin (ng/mL)*	471	8.00–120.00	ASO* (IU/mL)	18	0.00–140.00
RF (IU/mL)*	<11	0.00–15.00			
Immune tests					
β-D-Glucan (pg/mL)	≤5.0	0.00–10.90	ANA	80	0.00–80.00
Cryoglobulin	(-)	(-)	PR3-ANCA (U/mL)*	<1	0.00–3.40
MPO-ANCA (U/mL)*	124.0	0.00–3.40			
Viral tests					
CMV-CF	8	0.00–3.00	EB Anti-VCA/IgM-FA	<10	0.00-9.00
Tumor markers					
CEA-FEIA (ng/mL)*	2.3	0.00–6.70	CA19-9 (U/mL)*	10	0.00-37.00

These data include results of both examinations performed at the Oral and Maxillofacial Clinic and the Internal Medicine Clinic. *Data obtained later (day six to day ten after the first visit). WBC: white blood cell (count); RBC: red blood cell (count); TP: total protein; ALB: albumen; CPK: creatine phosphokinase; AST: aspartate aminotransferase; ALT: alanine aminotransferase; LDH: lactate dehydrogenase; ALP: alkaline phosphatase; γ GTP: γ glutamyl transpeptidase; BUN: blood urea nitrogen; UA: uric acid; eGFRcreat: estimated glomerular filtration rate based on serum creatinine; T-Bil: total bilirubin; CH50: 50% hemolytic complement activity; CRP: C-reactive protein; cTnI: cardiac troponin I; ASO: anti-streptolysin O antibody; RF: rheumatoid factor; ANA: antinuclear antibody; PR3-ANCA: proteinase 3-antineutrophil cytoplasmic antibody; MPO-ANCA: myeloperoxidase-antineutrophil cytoplasmic antibody; CMV-CF: cytomegalovirus complement fixation test; EB Anti-VCA/IgM-FA: Epstein-Barr antiviral capsid antigens/IgM fluorescence assay; CEA-FEIA: carcinoembryonic antigen fluorometric enzyme immunoassay; CA19-9: carbohydrate antigen 19-9.

differential diagnoses with FUO that may be initially encountered include Castleman's disease and adult-onset Still's disease [10].

In the present study, it seemed appropriate to initially diagnose the patient with suspected IE, because dentists are extremely well aware of the association between tooth extraction and IE. IE is defined as an infection of a native or prosthetic heart valve, the endocardial surface, or of an indwelling cardiac device. In this case, it was obviously important to refer the patient to a physician for meticulous examination. However, it is of note that there were oral symptoms that were overlooked and might suggest the occurrence of an AAV. The patient showed dysgeusia that had lasted for four weeks. AAVs frequently affect the peripheral and central nervous systems [11], and there was a case report of MPA that described multiple cranial neuropathies including dysgeusia [12]. As a matter of fact, diseases with both continuous fever and dysgeusia are few [13]. The patient felt numbness at the apex of the tongue. Numbness of the extremities and face has been reported in AAVs [14]. The numbness of the tongue may also be a sensory symptom caused by AAVs. In the present case, the dysgeusia and numbness of the tongue improved with the steroid therapy for MPA.

The patient had developed otitis media just before the tooth extractions. There are cases of AAVs that are complicated with otitis media, and the concept of otitis media with ANCA-associated vasculitis (OMAAV) has been proposed [15]. The criteria of OMAAV include otitis media with effusion or granulation resistant to antibiotics and insertion of tympanic ventilation tubes. It is unclear whether the otitis media in the present case could be considered OMAAV, because it improved before steroid therapy.

GPA, which was formerly known as Wegener's granulomatosis, has characteristic oral lesions of gingival swellings and nonspecific ulcerations, which are identified in 6-13% of cases [16]. However, there has been no report describing the other characteristics of AAV in the oral cavity. The dysgeusia and numbness of the tongue in the present case might be manifestations of AAVs that can be found in the oral cavity.

The patient's medical history revealed there were several previous issues, including tuberculosis, hypertension, hyperlipidemia, and neurogenic bladder. However, there was no indication of any association between these diseases and the AAVs.

4. Conclusion

The prevalence of AAVs has generally increased over the last 20 years, and AAVs are associated with high morbidity or mortality, especially if not immediately diagnosed and treated [4, 17]. Therefore, dentists and oral surgeons should keep AAVs in mind. At the same time, there may be hidden oral signs, such as the dysgeusia and numbness of the tongue in the present case, that may help make the diagnosis.

Consent

Informed consent was obtained from an individual participant included in the study.

References

[1] B. A. Cunha, "Fever of unknown origin: focused diagnostic approach based on clinical clues from the history, physical examination, and laboratory tests," *Infectious Disease Clinics of North America*, vol. 21, no. 4, pp. 1137–87, xi, 2007.

[2] D. Cornec, E. Cornec-Le Gall, F. C. Fervenza, and U. Specks, "ANCA-associated vasculitis - clinical utility of using ANCA specificity to classify patients," *Nature Reviews Rheumatology*, vol. 12, no. 10, pp. 570–579, 2016.

[3] E. Ntatsaki, D. Carruthers, K. Chakravarty et al., "BSR and BHPR guideline for the management of adults with ANCA-associated vasculitis," *Rheumatology*, vol. 53, no. 12, pp. 2306–2309, 2014.

[4] R. A. Watts, A. Mahr, A. J. Mohammad, P. Gatenby, N. Basu, and L. F. Flores-Suárez, "Classification, epidemiology and clinical subgrouping of antineutrophil cytoplasmic antibody (ANCA)-associated vasculitis," *Nephrology, Dialysis, Transplantation*, vol. 30, supplement_1, pp. i14–i22, 2015.

[5] A. Mahr, L. Guillevin, M. Poissonnet, and S. Aymé, "Prevalences of polyarteritis nodosa, microscopic polyangiitis, Wegener's granulomatosis, and Churg-Strauss syndrome in a French urban multiethnic population in 2000: a capture-recapture estimate," *Arthritis Care & Research*, vol. 51, no. 1, pp. 92–99, 2004.

[6] J. C. Jannette and R. J. Falk, "Small-vessel vasculitis," *The New England Journal of Medicine*, vol. 337, no. 21, pp. 1512–1523, 1997.

[7] M. A. Hamidou, A. Moreau, C. Toquet, D. Kouri, P. de Faucal, and J. Y. Grolleau, "Temporal arteritis associated with systemic necrotizing vasculitis," *The Journal of Rheumatology*, vol. 30, no. 10, pp. 2165–2169, 2003.

[8] S. Lionaki, E. R. Blyth, S. L. Hogan et al., "Classification of antineutrophil cytoplasmic autoantibody vasculitides: the role of antineutrophil cytoplasmic autoantibody specificity for myeloperoxidase or proteinase 3 in disease recognition and prognosis," *Arthritis and Rheumatism*, vol. 64, no. 10, pp. 3452–3462, 2012.

[9] C. Comarmond, C. Pagnoux, M. Khellaf et al., "Eosinophilic granulomatosis with polyangiitis (Churg-Strauss): clinical characteristics and long-term followup of the 383 patients enrolled in the French Vasculitis Study Group cohort," *Arthritis and Rheumatism*, vol. 65, no. 1, pp. 270–281, 2013.

[10] S. Hino, A. Nakamura, T. Kaneko, N. Horie, and T. Shimoyama, "Adult-onset Still's disease initially thought to be an odontogenic infection: a case report," *Gerodontology*, vol. 35, no. 2, pp. 139–142, 2018.

[11] J. H. Schirmer, M. N. Wright, R. Vonthein et al., "Clinical presentation and long-term outcome of 144 patients with microscopic polyangiitis in a monocentric German cohort," *Rheumatology*, vol. 55, no. 1, pp. 71–79, 2016.

[12] A. Morinaga, K. Ono, K. Komai, and M. Yamada, "Microscopic polyangitis presenting with temporal arteritis and multiple cranial neuropathies," *Journal of the Neurological Sciences*, vol. 256, no. 1-2, pp. 81–83, 2007.

[13] E. Nwokolo, C. Ujuju, J. Anyanti et al., "Misuse of artemisinin combination therapies by clients of medicine retailers suspected to have malaria without prior parasitological confirmation in Nigeria," *International Journal of Health Policy and Management*, vol. 7, no. 6, pp. 542–548, 2018.

[14] T. Kanda, H. Tanio, C. Wu, H. Nishihara, F. Nogaki, and T. Ono, "Churg-Strauss syndrome with severe granulomatous angiitis and crescentic glomerulonephritis, which developed during therapy with a leukotriene receptor antagonist," *Clinical and Experimental Nephrology*, vol. 14, no. 6, pp. 602–607, 2010.

[15] Y. Hisata, E. Sasaki, K. Ishimaru et al., "Do you know otitis media with ANCA-associated vasculitis (OMAAV)?," *Journal of General and Family Medicine*, vol. 18, no. 6, pp. 428–431, 2017.

[16] F. P. Fonseca, B. M. Benites, A. Ferrari et al., "Gingival granulomatosis with polyangiitis (Wegener's granulomatosis) as a primary manifestation of the disease," *Australian Dental Journal*, vol. 62, no. 1, pp. 102–106, 2017.

[17] D. Geetha, Q. Jin, J. Scott et al., "Comparisons of guidelines and recommendations on managing antineutrophil cytoplasmic antibody-associated vasculitis," *Kidney International Reports*, vol. 3, no. 5, pp. 1039–1049, 2018.

21

Anatomical Variant of Spinal Accessory Nerve Passing through Fenestrated Internal Jugular Vein

Shohei Takaoka,[1] Kenji Yamagata,[2] Makiko Okubo-Sato,[1] Satoshi Fukuzawa,[1] Fumihiko Uchida,[2] Naomi Ishibashi-Kanno,[2] and Hiroki Bukawa[2]

[1]*Department of Oral and Maxillofacial Surgery, University of Tsukuba Hospital, Tsukuba, Ibaraki 305-8576, Japan*
[2]*Department of Oral and Maxillofacial Surgery, Institute of Clinical Medicine, Faculty of Medicine, University of Tsukuba, Tsukuba, Ibaraki 305-8575, Japan*

Correspondence should be addressed to Kenji Yamagata; y-kenji@md.tsukuba.ac.jp

Academic Editor: Leandro Napier de Souza

Neck dissection (ND) is a major surgery for head and neck cancer. Currently, some or all of the spinal accessory nerve (SAN), sternocleidomastoid muscle, and internal jugular vein (IJV) are aggressively preserved during ND to reduce postoperative complications. Since the anatomical relationship between the SAN and IJV has several variations, knowledge of these variations is necessary to avoid iatrogenic damage. In the present case, the SAN was observed to pass through the fenestrated IJV at the level of the posterior belly of the digastric muscle during ND in a patient with squamous cell carcinoma of the mandible. Although the anatomical structure of the SAN and IJV is rare, surgeons must be aware of this anatomical variation.

1. Introduction

Neck dissection (ND) is the principal technique for the treatment, prevention, and diagnosis of cervical lymph node metastasis in head and neck cancer. In the early 1900s, radical neck dissection (RND) was reported to remove all lymph nodes belonging to levels I to V, as well as the spinal accessory nerve (SAN), sternocleidomastoid muscle (SCM), internal jugular vein (IJV), and other surrounding tissues [1]. However, this surgery is highly invasive and results in a significant functional loss. In order to prevent postoperative deformity and loss of function, in the 1960s, the concept of functional ND was introduced [2, 3]. The aim of this surgery is to aggressively preserve the SAN, SCM, and IJV. Currently, modified radical neck dissection (mRND) is widely performed based on the principle of functional ND [4]. Mills et al. reported four anatomical relationships between the SAN and IJV [5]. Although the most common variant is the SAN passing laterally to the IJV, the SAN rarely passes through the fenestrated IJV in 0.9%-2.8% of cases [6–10]. Severing or damaging the SAN during ND results in motor deficits such as neck rotation and upper arm elevation. To increase awareness and reduce morbidity associated with iatrogenic SAN injury, surgeons must be aware of these anatomical variations and anticipate them when following the course of the SAN.

In this report, we present a rare case of the SAN passing through the window between the branches of the IJV and also review previous reports regarding this anomaly.

2. Case Presentation

A 62-year-old woman presented with a T4bN2bMo squamous cell carcinoma of the left mandibular gingiva. mRND was performed prior to segmental mandibulectomy and mandible reconstruction with a free fibula flap, using the facial artery and IJV as recipient vessels. At the level of the posterior belly of the digastric muscle (DM), the IJV branched off, with the subsequent rejoining of the branched blood vessels. Fenestration of the IJV was encountered approximately 10 mm above the bifurcation of the common carotid artery. The SAN passed through the window of the

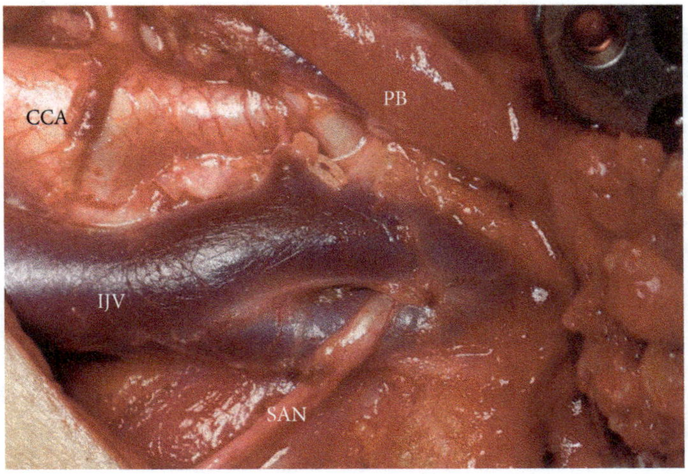

Figure 1: Intraoperative photograph, SAN passes through fenestrated IJV. SAN: spinal accessory nerve; IJV: internal jugular vein; CCA: common carotid artery; PBDM: posterior belly of the digastric muscle.

IJV and coursed medially to the anterior part and laterally to the posterior part of the window (Figure 1). The operative time was 11 h and 20 mins, and the bleeding volume was 277 mL. The postoperative course was uneventful, and there was no functional disorder of the shoulder. The patient is alive with no primary or regional recurrence as confirmed at the two-year postoperative follow-up.

3. Discussion

ND was first performed approximately 100 years ago, and preservation of the SAN, SCM, and IJV has become a basic concept to reduce postoperative complications. Therefore, it is imperative for surgeons to possess knowledge of their anatomical variations to reduce the risk of injury. Mills et al. reported four anatomical relationships of the SAN and IJV at the level of the posterior belly of the DM [5]. The SAN crosses (1) laterally, (2) medially to the IJV, (3) passes through the fenestrated IJV, or (4) goes around the IJV. The most common anatomical variant of the SAN and IJV is the SAN passing laterally to the IJV and is observed in 71.7%-96.6% cases [6–8, 11], while SAN is reported to pass medially to the IJV in 2.6%-28.3% cases [6–8, 11]. The incidence of SAN passing through the fenestrated IJV is 0.9%-2.8% [6–10]. Furthermore, Johal et al. reported that the SAN divided and coursed both laterally and medially around the IJV in 0.5% cases [12].

The SAN has two origins, the brainstem and the spinal cord. The brainstem-derived nerve innervates the pharyngeal and other muscles along with the vagus nerve, and the spinal roots of the SAN innervate the SCM and trapezius muscles [12]. The SAN passes through the jugular foramen and crosses lateral or medial to the IJV. SAN is the commonly used landmark for ND. The posterior belly of the DM was encountered after the resection of the inferior border of the parotid gland. The IJV and SAN were observed at the level of the posterior belly of the DM.

The reason for the passage of SAN through the fenestrated IJV is still unclear. The vascular embryological theory, which is the most acceptable theory for this variation, states that the fenestrated IJV may be caused by inadequate condensation of the embryonic capillary plexus [13]. If part of the venous ring remains at the time of IJV formation, the formation of a window of the IJV around these veins could occur, and this anatomical structure is completed when the SAN enters the window [13]. Few study reports have identified the IJV fenestration; however, the SAN crossed the central part of the IJV and did not pass through the window [14, 15]. Moreover, these cases cannot be explained by vascular embryological theory alone. Thus, further embryological research on both SAN and IJV is needed.

Preoperative diagnosis is crucial for identifying structures with anatomical variations. Abakay et al. reported the importance of ultrasonographic investigation, as they were able to detect fenestration of the IJV using ultrasonography [16]. Hashimoto et al. and Towbin et al. reported that IJV fenestrations were able to observe on contrast-enhanced CT imaging [10, 17]. However, Hashimoto et al. reported that it is very difficult to detect small-fenestration IJV with CT or MRI [10]. To prevent surgical complications, further trials on preoperative examinations to understand the anatomical structures of the SAN and IJV are needed.

4. Conclusion

SAN may penetrate the fenestrated IJV at the level of the posterior belly of the DM. Surgeons must be made aware of this rare anatomical anomaly, perform preoperative diagnosis, and identify the SAN and IJV with attention to its anatomical variation during ND.

References

[1] P. Wistermayer and K. G. Anderson, *Radical Neck Dissection. 2021 Oct 9. In: StatPearls [Internet]*, StatPearls Publishing, Treasure Island (FL), 2021.

[2] E. Bocca, O. Pignataro, and C. T. Sasaki, "Functional neck dissection: a description of operative technique," *Archives of Otolaryngology*, vol. 106, no. 9, pp. 524–527, 1980.

[3] E. Bocca, O. Pignataro, C. Oldini, and C. Cappa, "Functional neck dissection: an evaluation and review of 843 cases," *The Laryngoscope*, vol. 94, no. 7, pp. 942–945, 1984.

[4] S. C. Sheppard, L. Frech, R. Giger, and L. Nisa, "Lymph node yield and ratio in selective and modified radical neck dissection in head and neck cancer-impact on oncological outcome," *Cancers (Basel)*, vol. 13, no. 9, p. 2205, 2021.

[5] S. Mills, C. Aristotelous, L. L. Touil, and R. C. W. James, "Rare anatomical variant of the spinal accessory nerve: case report and comprehensive review," *International Journal of Oral and Maxillofacial Surgery*, vol. 51, no. 21, pp. 467–472, 2021.

[6] C. B. Taylor, J. L. Boone, C. E. Schmalbach, and F. R. Miller, "Intraoperative relationship of the spinal accessory nerve to the internal jugular vein: variation from cadaver studies," *American Journal of Otolaryngology*, vol. 34, no. 5, pp. 527–529, 2013.

[7] M. Saman, P. Etebari, M. N. Pakdaman, and M. L. Urken, "Anatomic relationship between the spinal accessory nerve and the jugular vein: a cadaveric study," *Surgical and Radiologic Anatomy*, vol. 33, no. 2, pp. 175–179, 2011.

[8] M. L. Hinsley and G. K. Hartig, "Anatomic relationship between the spinal accessory nerve and internal jugular vein in the upper neck," *Otolaryngology and Head and Neck Surgery*, vol. 143, no. 2, pp. 239–241, 2010.

[9] S. H. Lee, J. K. Lee, S. M. Jin et al., "Anatomical variations of the spinal accessory nerve and its relevance to level IIb lymph nodes," *Otolaryngology and Head and Neck Surgery*, vol. 141, no. 5, pp. 639–644, 2009.

[10] Y. Hashimoto, N. Otsuki, K. Morimoto, M. Saito, and K. Nibu, "Four cases of spinal accessory nerve passing through the fenestrated internal jugular vein," *Surgical and Radiologic Anatomy*, vol. 34, no. 4, pp. 373–375, 2012.

[11] C. A. F. Freitas, L. R. M. D. Santos, A. N. Santos, A. B. D. Amaral Neto, and L. G. Brandão, "Estudo anatomico do forame jugular no pescoço," *Brazilian Journal of Otorhinolaryngology*, vol. 86, no. 1, pp. 44–48, 2020.

[12] J. Johal, J. Iwanaga, K. Tubbs, M. Loukas, R. J. Oskouian, and R. S. Tubbs, "The accessory nerve: a comprehensive review of its anatomy, development, variations, landmarks and clinical considerations," *Landmarks and Clinical Considerations. Anat Rec (Hoboken)*, vol. 302, no. 4, pp. 620–629, 2019.

[13] J. M. Prades, A. Timoshenko, J. M. Dumollard, M. Durand, N. Merzougui, and C. Martin, "High duplication of the internal jugular vein: clinical incidence in the adult and surgical consequences, a report of three clinical cases," *Surgical and Radiologic Anatomy*, vol. 24, no. 2, pp. 129–132, 2002.

[14] A. Pegot, B. Guichard, J. M. Peron, and O. Trost, "Empty fenestration of the internal jugular vein: a rare phenomenon," *The British Journal of Oral & Maxillofacial Surgery*, vol. 53, no. 1, pp. 78–80, 2015.

[15] E. Cvetko, "Unilateral fenestration of the internal jugular vein: a case report," *Surgical and Radiologic Anatomy*, vol. 37, no. 7, pp. 875–877, 2015.

[16] M. A. Abakay, B. M. Şimşek, B. Olgun, R. Türkay, and S. Güneş, "Ultrasonic identification of internal jugular vein fenestration," *Surgical and Radiologic Anatomy*, vol. 41, no. 9, pp. 1079–1081, 2019.

[17] A. J. Towbin and E. Kanal, "A review of two cases of fenestrated internal jugular veins as seen by CT angiography," *AJNR. American Journal of Neuroradiology*, vol. 25, no. 8, pp. 1433-1434, 2004.

22

Safe and Ultraconservative Rehabilitation of Worn Teeth Patients: How Sectional Clear Aligners May Enhance the Prosthetic Treatment Plan

Camillo D'Arcangelo, Mirco Vadini, Matteo Buonvivere, and Francesco De Angelis

Unit of Restorative Dentistry and Endodontics, Department of Medical, Oral and Biotechnological Science, School of Dentistry, "G. D'Annunzio" University of Chieti, Chieti, Italy

Correspondence should be addressed to Francesco De Angelis; fda580@gmail.com

Academic Editor: Leandro Napier de Souza

This study describes the clinical workflow for occlusal vertical dimension (OVD) increase in patients showing extensive tooth wear and mild teeth misalignment/crowding. A patient affected by dental erosion and occlusal abnormalities was treated to improve her situation. After ascertaining sound condyle and temporomandibular joint (TMJ) conditions, an OVD increase was sought to provide enough inter-occlusal space for the restorations. The use of TMJ three-dimensional imaging throughout the clinical procedures allowed to objectively track the condyle and disk position and confirm a steady condyle–glenoid cavity relationship before definitive restorations placement. Sectional clear aligner therapy prior to totally additive prosthetic rehabilitation allowed obtaining slight derotation and movements of anterior teeth, thus maximizing sound tissue preservation. Adhesively luted restorations were finally delivered on both anterior and posterior sectors. At the end of the treatment, the pre-operative TMJ balance appeared successfully preserved, and the patient was satisfied with the aesthetic and function achieved.

1. Introduction

Aesthetic concerns are nowadays part and parcel of every restorative and prosthetic rehabilitation: a satisfactory aesthetic result is as considerable as a proper functional outcome or a minimally invasive approach.

Simple cases involving frontal teeth aesthetics in the presence of balanced occlusion and proper inter-occlusal space are part of routine clinical practice [1, 2]. Situations involving generalized tooth wear require instead a more comprehensive approach: occlusal vertical dimension (OVD) increase is, in fact, frequently needed to obtain aesthetic improvement in such cases [3–6]. However, the debate regarding the most suitable method to safely increase OVD is still ongoing in the literature [7–20]. Over the last years, the introduction of accurate three-dimensional imaging exams, such as magnetic resonance imaging (MRI) or cone beam computed tomography (CBCT), gave to the clinician an objective tool to take under control the position of the temporomandibular joint (TMJ) during OVD increase.

Additive adhesive dentistry allows to get the most out of OVD increase. Without the need to seek mechanical retention with traditional preparation designs, in fact, sound cervical tooth structure can be saved [1, 2, 21], thus completely preserving the already worn teeth. When tooth wear is coupled with teeth crowding/misalignment, however, an orthodontic treatment with braces or aligners should be performed prior to the prosthetic phase aiming at straightening the teeth, thus providing spaces for minimally invasive intervention. In case of slight misalignment confined to the anterior sector and when posterior teeth do not need to be subjected to any movement, a sectional clear aligner (SCA) therapy might be indicated [22].

In the present clinical case, a safe clinical workflow optimized to aesthetically restore the smile of an asymptomatic patient affected by tooth wear and mild teeth misalignment is described. Adhesive and totally additive lithium disilicate indirect restorations were used in combination with SCAs, to preserve all residual sound tissues and to be as much conservative as possible. An MRI-based diagnostic approach was employed to evaluate the condyle–fossa relationship and keep it unchanged throughout the whole treatment.

2. Case Report

A 65-year-old woman with unremarkable medical history was referred with a chief complaint concerning the unsatisfactory aesthetic of her smile. The intra-oral examination revealed extensive tooth wear involving anterior and posterior teeth on both upper and lower arches, signs of cervical abrasion/erosion, slight misalignment in the upper anterior, and mild crowding in the lower-anterior areas (Figures 1(a) and 1(b)). As showed by the pre-operative panoramic X-ray image, teeth 1.7, 2.5, 2.7, 3.4, and 4.4 were missing, while teeth 1.5 and 1.6 had been previously replaced by implant-supported fixed dental prostheses (Figure 1(c)). Apart from teeth 3.6 and 4.6, which showed small amalgam and composite fillings, all the other elements did not display pre-existing restorations. All teeth were vital. The patient did not report symptoms of temporomandibular disorders (TMDs), and the clinical examination confirmed the absence of any dysfunctions affecting TMJ, masticatory muscles, and the associated structures. The proposed treatment plan consisted of a full mouth adhesive and additive rehabilitation in combination with the use of SCAs, aiming to improve the aesthetics with no tooth preparation, after having established a new and increased OVD.

The presence of physiological and healthy pre-operative TMJ conditions was objectified by MRI sequences taken in maximum intercuspidation using a 3 Tesla MRI system (Philips Ingenia 3.0 T, Philips Medical Systems, Best, The Netherlands) with 6-channel dS Flex M surface coil. *T*1-weighted sagittal sequences with a 2 mm slice thickness were obtained for each TMJ [6]. Both condyles appeared well centered within the glenoid cavities, in an anterior–superior position against the slope of the articular eminences (Figure 1(d)). On the basis of objective MRI analysis and due to the lack of TMD signs/symptoms or muscular contractions, the present preoperative condyle–fossa relationship was presumed to be sound. Thus, care was taken to keep the above-mentioned relationship unchanged throughout the treatment.

After placing a standard cheek/lip retractor, the patient was asked to perform a slight and slow mouth opening, starting from the maximum intercuspidation, up to a degree of tooth separation sufficient to assure enough inter-occlusal clearance for the restorative needs, trying to limit the OVD increase within the boundaries of pure condylar rotation. Any kind of operator-guided manipulation and/or bite registration medium in between the arches were avoided during this step of the procedure. Based on this, an OVD increase of 5 mm interincisally was supposed as appropriate. An indelible marker was used to mark the upper and lower canines and central incisors as references, so as to make the mandible positioning easily repeatable. After pushing two softened three-layer wax wafers (3 mm each) against the occlusal surfaces of left and right mandibular posterior teeth, the patient was asked to close while the operator guided the mandible in the new position, using the previously described marker signs on incisors and canines to prevent unsought excursive movements. The wax wafers were removed, cooled down, and placed back on the teeth to verify accuracy, stability, and fit.

The next step was aimed at objectively verifying that the new mandibular position, in the empirically proposed OVD, was truly within the limit of condylar pure rotation. For this purpose, self-curing low shrinkage acrylic pattern resin (Temp Red; Micerium S.p.A., Avegno, Italy) in dough stage was placed onto the upper anterior teeth before asking the patient to bite with the posterior wax wafers in place, thus obtaining an anterior jig. Following a facebow transfer, the jig, together with the wax wafers, served as inter-occlusal record to mount pre-operative casts on a semi-adjustable articulator (SAM 2P; SAM Präzisionstechnik GmbH, Gauting, Germany). On these casts, temporary and additive posterior splints extending from the second lower premolar to the second lower molar were manufactured with orthodontic acrylic resin (Orthocryl; Dentaurum) through salt-and-pepper technique. The splints extended bilaterally from the second lower premolar to the second lower molar and were fixed intra-orally on the unprepared teeth using a glass-ionomer cement (Ketac Cem; 3M ESPE). The patient was, then, subjected to a second TMJ MRI evaluation while dressing the posterior fixed splints, using the same parameters and the same corrected cross-sections described for the pre-operative exam. Comparing the two MRIs, the condylar position appeared substantially unchanged in respect to the articular fossa (Figure 1(e)), which confirmed that the proposed OVD increase could be safely considered within the limits of a pure rotation.

The posterior splints allowed for an additional diagnostic step, planned to clinically verify in a totally reversible way the real patient adaptation. After having dressed the fixed splints for two months, the patient reported a reassuring subjective adaptation to the new mandibular position, in the absence of TMD and muscle tenderness, which represented the required validation for the new proposed mandible position.

The prosthetic finalization was performed adopting the splint-induced occlusal position as inter-maxillary relationship and took place starting from the left posterior sector. Left-side fixed splint was removed, providing access for restoring both upper and lower left premolars and molars. Sound posterior teeth were left unprepared. Old fillings were removed and replaced with direct composite (Enamel Plus BioFunction; Micerium S.p.A.) build-ups, and the residual sound tissues were not prepared. Polyvinylsiloxane impressions of the upper and lower arches were taken, holding the right-side fixed splint in place. Lithium disilicate (IPS e.max Press HT; Ivoclar Vivadent, Amherst, NY, USA) indirect overlays were manufactured using standard laboratory procedures, etched with 5% hydrofluoric acid, silanized, and adhesively luted: Enabond (Micerium S.p.A.) and warm Enamel Plus BioFunction composite were, respectively, used as adhesive and cement. Once stable and definite occlusal

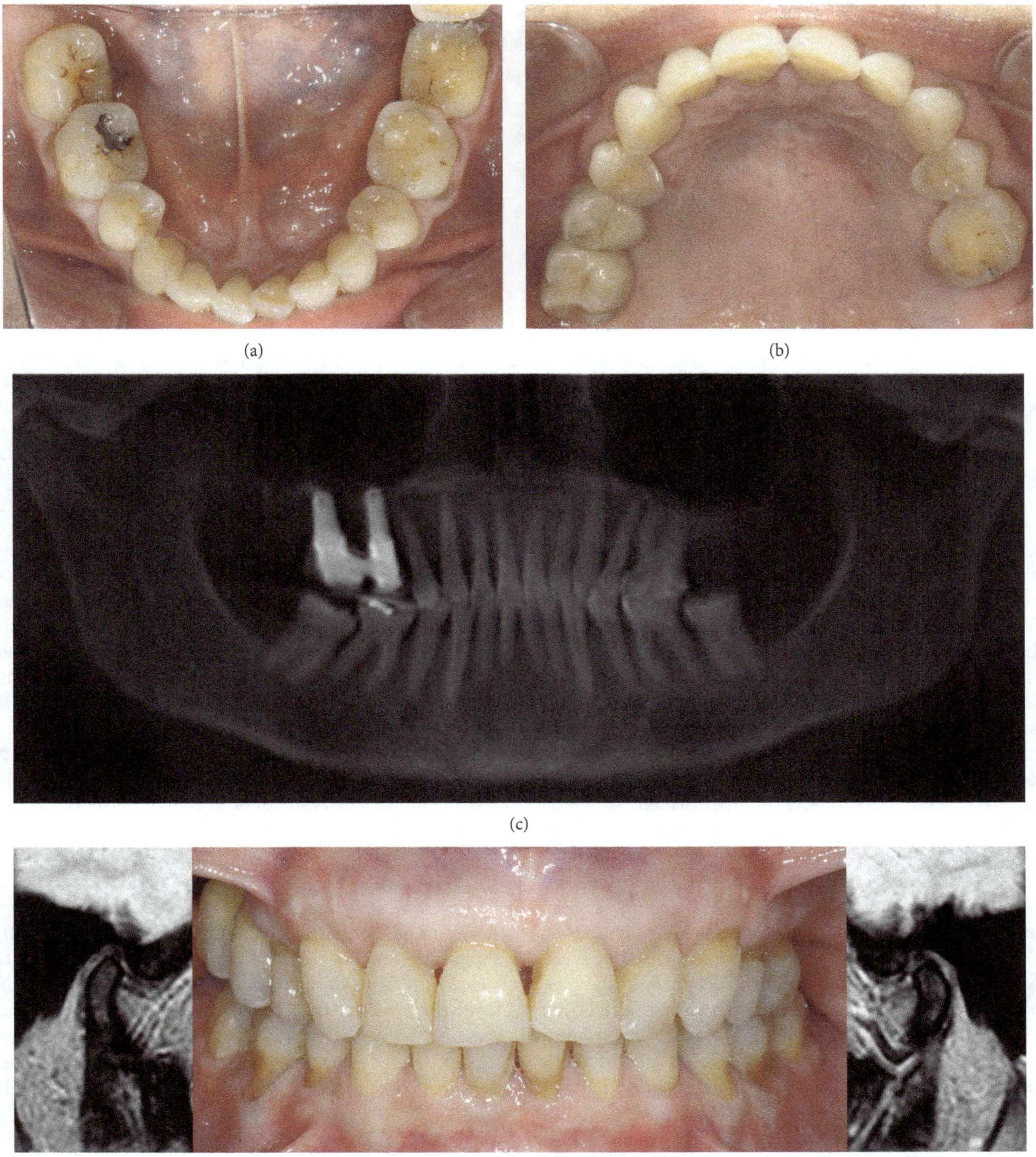

(a) (b) (c) (d)

Figure 1: Continued.

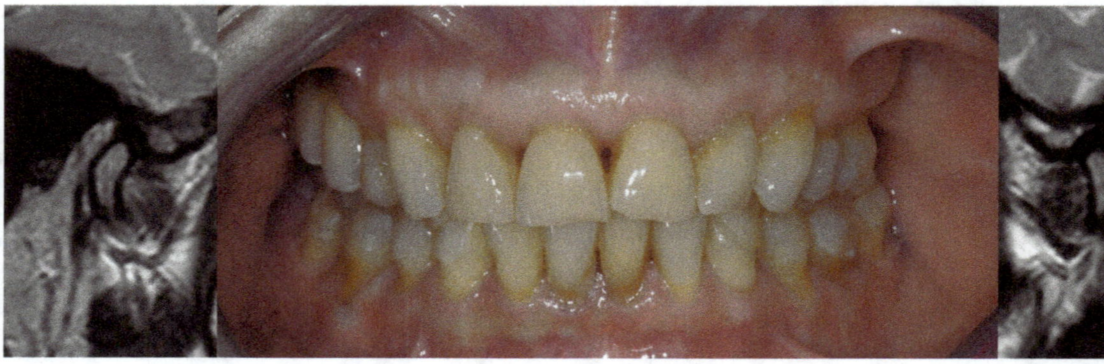

(e)

Figure 1: Clinical workflow for an occlusal vertical dimension increase in a patient showing worn dentition. ((a) and (b)) Pre-operative intra-oral occlusal photographs showing signs of cervical abrasion/erosion, slight misalignment in the upper anterior, and mild crowding in the lower-anterior areas: aesthetics appears negatively affected. (c) Panoramic X-ray image showing the pre-operative initial condition. (d) A pre-operative temporomandibular joint (TMJ MRI) scan was taken, with the patient in maximum intercuspation, showing healthy and balanced condyle–disc–fossa relationship both on the left and right side. (e) A second TMJ MRI scan was taken with patient dressing resin posterior fixed splints in order to check the TMJ status in the new mandibular position.

contacts were established on the left sector, the right-side fixed splint was removed, and both upper and lower right premolars and molars were restored as just described for the left side. Since the patient wanted to keep her pre-existing implant-supported fixed dental prostheses, lithium disilicate overlays were adhesively luted even on the old implant-supported ceramic crowns (teeth 1.5 and 1.6). At this stage, in order to close the residual open bite between upper and lower frontal teeth following the OVD incrementation, SCA therapy in both arches (Invisalign GO, Align Technology, Tempe, AZ, USA) was performed. A digital impression was acquired by means of an intra-oral scanner (iTero, Align Technology) and sent to the manufacturer for the 3D alignment simulation through the ClinCheck software (Align Technology; Figure 2(a)). After the approval, aligners were received, and attachments were bonded on teeth 1.1, 1.3, 1.4, 2.1, 2.2, 2.3, 2.4, and 4.3, respectively. Inter-proximal reduction was performed following the producer's recommendations: 0.2 mm of enamel was removed from both the mesial and distal sides of tooth 1.3; 0.2 mm from the mesial and 0.3 mm from the distal side of tooth 2.3; 0.2 mm from the distal side of tooth 2.4; and 0.2 mm from the mesial side of tooth 2.6. The therapy consisted of 15 aligners: the patient was instructed to wear them at least 22 hours a day and to change them weekly; clinical control was repeated every 4 weeks throughout the treatment. At the end of the treatment, a derotation of teeth 1.1, 1.3, 1.4, 2.2, 2.3, and 4.3 was obtained, as well as a slight increase in tipping of tooth 2.1 and in torque of tooth 2.2. After the SCA therapy, the anterior teeth misalignment was corrected, and an anterior occlusal contact was re-established on natural enamel, leaving an appropriate overjet to safely restore the upper anterior teeth. Moreover, teeth position was optimized for the subsequent prosthetic phase. The six maxillary anterior teeth were restored using an indirect additive solution. New polyvinyl-siloxane impressions were taken, and the poured casts were placed on to the articulator to fabricate six no-prep lithium disilicate (IPS e.max Press HT; Ivoclar Vivadent) veneers. The veneers were etched using 5% hydrofluoric acid and silanized. Subsequently, they were adhesively luted, using Enabond (Micerium S.p.A.) as adhesive and pre-warmed with composite heating conditioner (Ena Heat; Micerium S.p.A.) Enamel Plus BioFunction (Micerium S.p.A.) as cement. A life-long retention protocol (Vivera Retainer, Align Technology) was prescribed to stabilize teeth position achieved after SCA therapy.

After one week, the patient was recalled to collect post-operative clinical photographs (Figures 2(b), 2(c), and 2(d)). The patient aesthetic and functional needs appeared to be successfully satisfied.

3. Discussion

A full-mouth adhesive rehabilitation of a patient with no signs/symptoms of TMD, while showing generalized tooth wear and signs of malocclusion, was performed using a three-dimensional imaging to keep under control the TMJ conditions throughout the treatment. Totally additive prosthodontic procedures in combination with SCAs represented the ideal clinical choice to preserve all residual enamel and dentine structures.

The absence of pre-operative symptoms confirms that an OVD loss or a malocclusion is not always associated with a clinical TMJ impairment. When, in similar situations, a full-mouth rehabilitation is required for aesthetic purposes, it could be wise to limit the introduction of additional occlusal changes since they could become detrimental if the TMJ was just precariously balanced [23–27].

With the support of a solid MRI or CBCT validation of the proposed OVD increase, the use of temporary and additive fixed splints for two months provides a supplementary non-invasive diagnostic phase to rule out any risk of irremediable TMJ damage due to the abrupt occlusal change [23, 24, 27]. In this way, if any TMJ alteration or muscular abnormal response was identified during this reversible two-month-lasting step, the original occlusal conditions

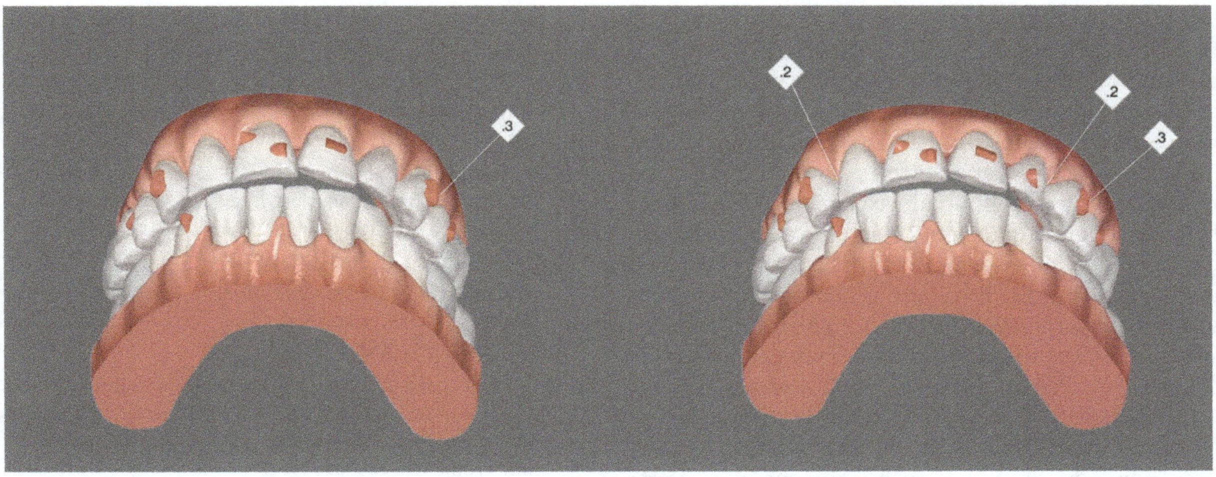

(a)

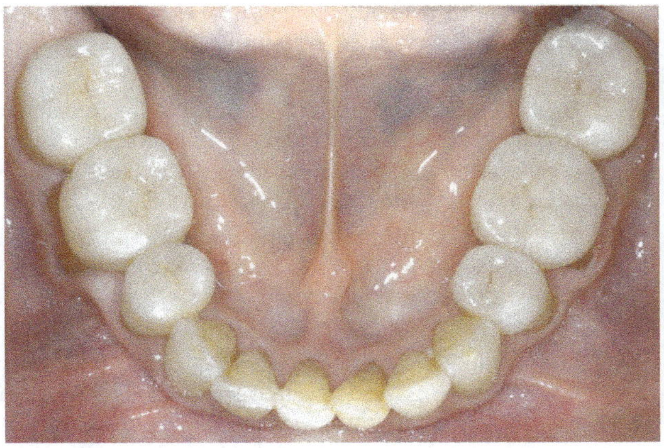

(b)

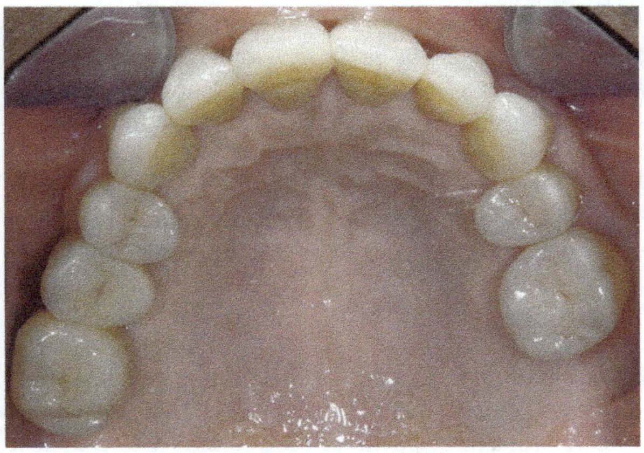

(c)

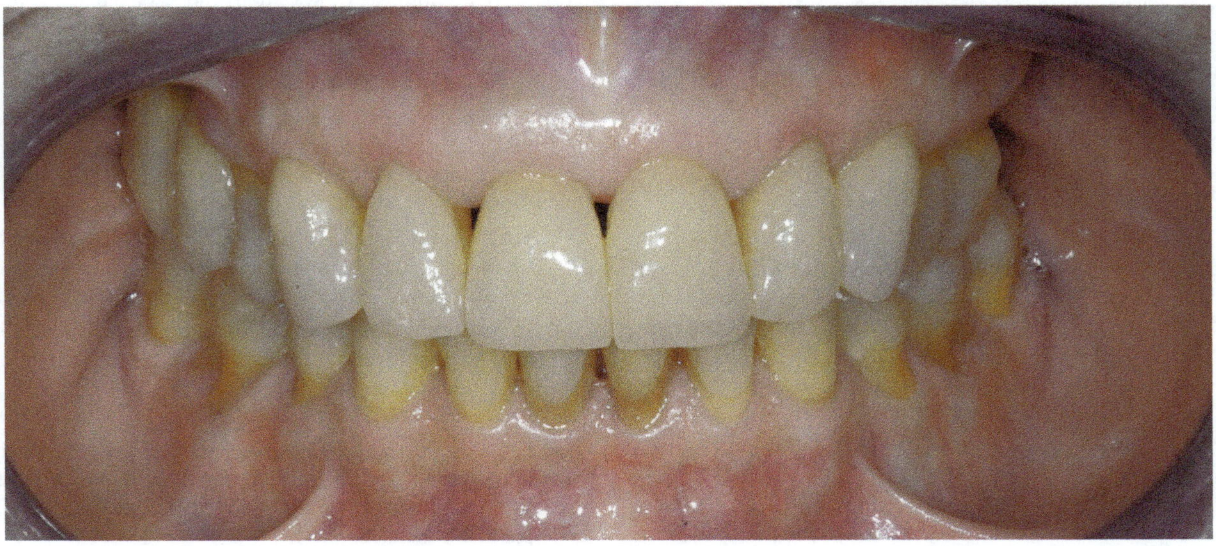

(d)

FIGURE 2: Sectional clear aligner therapy and final restorations. (a) 3D alignment simulation through ClinCheck software showing attachments bonded on teeth 1.1, 1.3, 1.4, 2.1, 2.2, 2.3, 2.4, and 4.3 and interproximal enamel reduction required on teeth 1.3, 2.3, 2.4, and 2.6. ((b)–(d)) Post-operative occlusal and frontal views. The main movements achieved after the clear aligner therapy were: derotation on teeth 1.1, 1.3, 1.4, 2.2, 2.3, and 4.3; tipping increase on tooth 2.1; torque increase on tooth 2.2.

could be readily reestablished through the simple removal of the fixed splints. Among the multiple benefits offered by this clinical workflow, the prompt evidence of a potential condyle misplacement and the objective knowledge of the real jaw/condyle/disc positions prior to any permanent therapy seem to be of particular importance.

When dealing with full mouth rehabilitation cases, pre-prosthetic orthodontic treatment could represent a valid aid to achieve the desired aesthetical and functional outcomes. Correcting misalignment and crowding and closing open bite before the prosthetic phase, in fact, allow to perform less invasive procedures, thus maximizing the preservation of tooth sound tissues. Nowadays, however, adult patients tend to reject the unaesthetic conventional labial fixed appliances. Lingual orthodontics could be an adequate alternative, but still shows some disadvantages, such as tongue discomfort, speech problems, and masticatory difficulties [28]. Moreover, both labial and lingual appliances require a well-trained orthodontist. In this light, newly developed SCAs [22] could constitute a valuable option to combine patient's demands with dentist's needs. Being limited to the aesthetic sectors, SCA therapy is perceived as quick and comfortable by the patients, while representing a valid tool for restorative dentists aiming at simplifying their prosthodontic procedures by treating cases with inter-disciplinary mindset [22].

4. Conclusion

Totally additive restorations in combination with SCAs appear to be the best solution in patients showing extensive tooth wear, with a large portion of sound tissues already lost. An OVD increase, adequately supported by TMJ three-dimensional imaging (MRI or CBCT), is always necessary to re-establish good aesthetics in these patients.

Paired with adhesively luted restorations, SCA therapy may represent an additional tool to approach these complex clinical cases in the least invasive way possible.

References

[1] C. D'Arcangelo, M. Vadini, M. D'Amario, Z. Chiavaroli, and F. De Angelis, "Protocol for a new concept of no-prep ultrathin ceramic veneers," *Journal of Esthetic and Restorative Dentistry*, vol. 30, no. 3, pp. 173–179, 2018.

[2] F. De Angelis, C. D'Arcangelo, R. Angelozzi, and M. Vadini, "Retrospective clinical evaluation of a no-prep porcelain veneer protocol," *The Journal of Prosthetic Dentistry*, 2021, In Press .

[3] A. Johansson, A. K. Johansson, R. Omar, and G. E. Carlsson, "Rehabilitation of the worn dentition," *Journal of Oral Rehabilitation*, vol. 35, no. 7, pp. 548–566, 2008.

[4] A. Johansson and R. Omar, "Identification and management of tooth wear," *The International Journal of Prosthodontics*, vol. 7, no. 6, pp. 506–516, 1994.

[5] B. Keough, "Occlusion-based treatment planning for complex dental restorations: part 1," *The International Journal of Periodontics & Restorative Dentistry*, vol. 23, no. 3, pp. 237–247, 2003.

[6] C. D'Arcangelo, M. Vadini, M. Buonvivere, and F. De Angelis, "Safe clinical technique for increasing the occlusal vertical dimension in case of erosive wear and missing teeth," *Clinical Case Reports*, vol. 9, no. 12, article e04747, 2021.

[7] J. Abduo, "Safety of increasing vertical dimension of occlusion: a systematic review," *Quintessence International*, vol. 43, no. 5, pp. 369–380, 2012.

[8] J. Abduo and K. Lyons, "Clinical considerations for increasing occlusal vertical dimension: a review," *Australian Dental Journal*, vol. 57, no. 1, pp. 2–10, 2012.

[9] R. Ammannato, F. Ferraris, and G. Marchesi, "The "index technique" in worn dentition: a new and conservative approach," *International Journal of Esthetic Dentistry*, vol. 10, no. 1, pp. 68–99, 2015.

[10] I. Moreno-Hay and J. P. Okeson, "Does altering the occlusal vertical dimension produce temporomandibular disorders? A literature review," *Journal of Oral Rehabilitation*, vol. 42, no. 11, pp. 875–882, 2015.

[11] D. Manfredini and C. E. Poggio, "Prosthodontic planning in patients with temporomandibular disorders and/or bruxism: a systematic review," *The Journal of Prosthetic Dentistry*, vol. 117, no. 5, pp. 606–613, 2017.

[12] D. Bartlett and G. Sundaram, "An up to 3-year randomized clinical study comparing indirect and direct resin composites used to restore worn posterior teeth," *The International Journal of Prosthodontics*, vol. 19, no. 6, pp. 613–617, 2006.

[13] J. H. Hastings, "Conservative restoration of function and aesthetics in a bulimic patient: a case report," *Practical Periodontics and Aesthetic Dentistry*, vol. 8, no. 8, pp. 729–736, 1996, quiz 38.

[14] M. Hayashi, K. Shimizu, F. Takeshige, and S. Ebisu, "Restoration of erosion associated with gastroesophageal reflux caused by anorexia nervosa using ceramic laminate veneers: a case report," *Operative Dentistry*, vol. 32, no. 3, pp. 306–310, 2007.

[15] K. W. Hemmings, U. R. Darbar, and S. Vaughan, "Tooth wear treated with direct composite restorations at an increased vertical dimension: results at 30 months," *The Journal of Prosthetic Dentistry*, vol. 83, no. 3, pp. 287–293, 2000.

[16] R. J. Smales and T. L. Berekally, "Long-term survival of direct and indirect restorations placed for the treatment of advanced tooth wear," *The European Journal of Prosthodontics and Restorative Dentistry*, vol. 15, no. 1, pp. 2–6, 2007.

[17] R. C. Spreafico, "Composite resin rehabilitation of eroded dentition in a bulimic patient: a case report," *The European Journal of Esthetic Dentistry*, vol. 5, no. 1, pp. 28–48, 2010.

[18] F. Vailati and U. C. Belser, "Full-mouth adhesive rehabilitation of a severely eroded dentition: the three-step technique. Part 1," *The European Journal of Esthetic Dentistry*, vol. 3, no. 1, pp. 30–44, 2008.

[19] F. Vailati and U. C. Belser, "Full-mouth adhesive rehabilitation of a severely eroded dentition: the three-step technique. Part 2," *The European Journal of Esthetic Dentistry*, vol. 3, no. 2, pp. 128–146, 2008.

[20] F. Vailati and U. C. Belser, "Full-mouth adhesive rehabilitation of a severely eroded dentition: the three-step technique. Part 3," *The European Journal of Esthetic Dentistry*, vol. 3, no. 3, pp. 236–257, 2008.

[21] M. A. Carvalho, P. C. Lazari, M. Gresnigt, A. A. Del Bel Cury, and P. Magne, "Current options concerning the endodontically-treated teeth restoration with the adhesive approach," *Brazilian Oral Research*, vol. 32, article e74, suppl 1, 2018.

[22] T. Weinstein, G. Marano, and R. Aulakh, "Five-to-five clear aligner therapy: predictable orthodontic movement for general

dentist to achieve minimally invasive dentistry," *BMC Oral Health*, vol. 21, no. 1, p. 671, 2021.

[23] J. C. Turp and H. Schindler, "The dental occlusion as a suspected cause for TMDs: epidemiological and etiological considerations," *Journal of Oral Rehabilitation*, vol. 39, no. 7, pp. 502–512, 2012.

[24] Y. Le Bell, T. Jamsa, S. Korri, P. M. Niemi, and P. Alanen, "Effect of artificial occlusal interferences depends on previous experience of temporomandibular disorders," *Acta Odontologica Scandinavica*, vol. 60, no. 4, pp. 219–222, 2002.

[25] P. M. Niemi, Y. Le Bell, M. Kylmala, T. Jamsa, and P. Alanen, "Psychological factors and responses to artificial interferences in subjects with and without a history of temporomandibular disorders," *Acta Odontologica Scandinavica*, vol. 64, no. 5, pp. 300–305, 2006.

[26] B. J. Sessle, "Biological adaptation and normative values," *The International Journal of Prosthodontics*, vol. 16, Suppl, pp. 72–73, 2003, discussion 89–90.

[27] J. Dibbets and C. Tunkel, "Kiefergelenksprobleme und die Stolperstein-Theorie," *Informationen aus Orthodontie und Kieferorthopädie*, vol. 38, no. 3, pp. 185–188, 2006.

[28] C. Caniklioglu and Y. Oztürk, "Patient discomfort: a comparison between lingual and labial fixed appliances," *The Angle Orthodontist*, vol. 75, no. 1, pp. 86–91, 2005.

23

Navigated Recovery of Fractured Dental Injection Needles: Case Report and Suggestions for Management during Pandemic Crises

Lara Schorn, Christoph Sproll, Rita Depprich, Norbert R. Kübler, Majeed Rana, Daman D. Singh, and Julian Lommen

Department of Oral, Maxillofacial and Facial Plastic Surgery, University Hospital Düsseldorf, Düsseldorf, Germany

Correspondence should be addressed to Christoph Sproll; christoph.sproll@med.uni-duesseldorf.de

Academic Editor: Jamil Awad Shibli

Dislocation of a fractured hypodermic needle is a complication requiring immediate and adequate emergency treatment. In this case report, 3D navigation is evaluated for its use to recover a quickly moving fractured needle. The needle was recovered safely, but it could be demonstrated that navigational planning has to be conducted right before surgery and other navigational tools, such as ultrasound, should be considered as well. Furthermore, an approach is suggested for treatment during pandemic crises such as COVID-19.

1. Introduction

In dental surgery, local anesthesia is tremendously important for a painless therapy. It is usually associated with low overall risks and complications [1]. Systemic reactions are for example hypertension, circulatory collapse, and toxic or allergic reactions [2]. Local events like hemorrhage, wound infections, soft tissue damage, nerve irritation, and dislodgement of fractured hypodermic needles can be observed [3]. There are various reasons for needle breakage. Most commonly, fatigue fractures of the needles occur [2]. These incidents, however, have been reduced after the introduction of disposable cannulas in the 1970s. Fractured needles can lead to serious and potentially life-threatening consequences by damaging adjacent vital anatomical structures [4, 5]. Quick extraction of the broken fragment is generally recommended (with very few exceptions). Recovery rates have been reported to be around 95% [2] with little postoperative complications. A recent review of Acham et al. [2] imposed a workflow including 3D navigation as an option for needle removal.

The outbreak of the global pandemic of coronavirus-disease 2019 (COVID-19) is changing medical and surgical procedures. An important task is to reduce the likelihood of infection for patients and medical staff [6]. Dentists, maxillofacial surgeons, and ENT surgeons are particularly exposed due to high viral load in the nasal cavity of infected patients [7]. Since a dislodged dental needle can easily become a life-threatening emergency, an adequate procedure for treatment under pandemic conditions is necessary.

In this case report, 3D navigation is used in a university hospital setting to recover a dislodged fractured needle, and a procedure for pandemic emergencies is suggested.

2. Case Presentation

A 61-year-old, otherwise healthy, male Caucasian patient was referred by his local dentist to our clinic with a 30 G broken needle after anesthesia with inferior alveolar nerve block technique at his local dentist. The patient was stable and did not experience any pain or discomfort. An immediately taken orthopantomogram (OPTG) together with a cephalometric image and cone beam computer tomography (CBCT) showed the needle at the medial side of the ascending ramus close to the mandibular foramen (Figure 1). The patient was planned for removal by an intraoral approach in general anesthesia for the next day. Laboratory testing was done showing no pathological results. No medication was administered. On the morning of the next day, another OPTG was taken to confirm needle position. It showed lateral

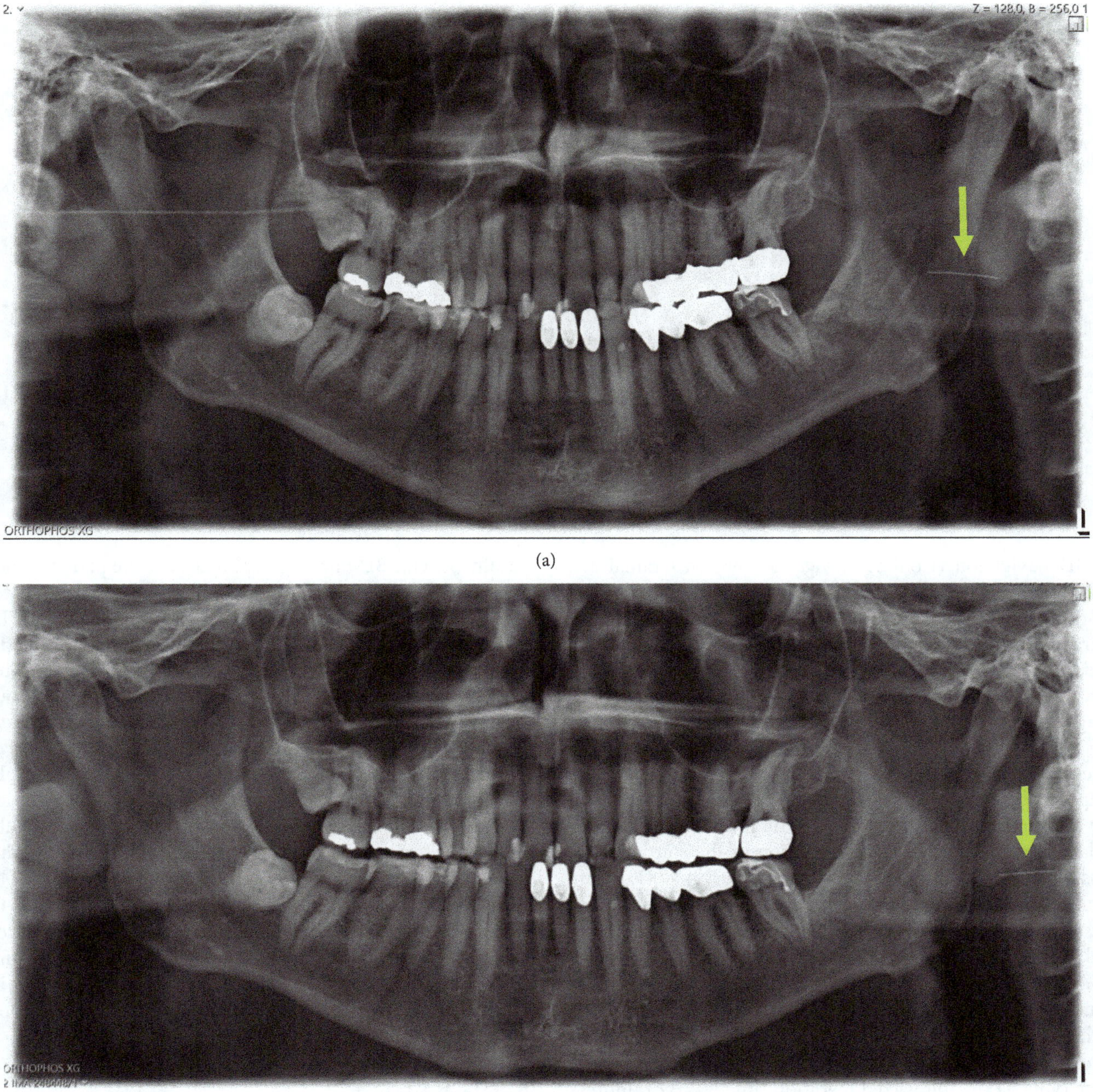

(a)

(b)

FIGURE 1: Orthopantomographic images on the day of initial presentation (a) and one day afterwards (b). The dislodged fractured hypodermic needle is located at the left ascending mandibular ramus and moved by about 1.5 cm after one day.

movement of the needle by around 1.5 cm (Figure 1). Therefore, a CT (SOMATOM Flash CT) with 0.75 mm slice thickness was taken and intraoperative 3D navigation was planned using iPlan 3.0.5 (BrainLab®, Feldkirchen, Germany) (Figure 2). The CT showed needle position to be retroauricular approximately 2 cm dorsal and 1.5 cm below the left ear lobe. Immediately afterwards, the patient was prepped for surgery and told not to move his head. General anesthesia was performed using remifentil (2 mg/Nacl 30 ml/h; Ultiva®, GlaxoSmithKline, Brentford, United Kingdom), propofol 1% 10 mg/ml 160 ml (B. Braun Melsungen AG, Melsungen, Germany), and recuromium bromide 10 mg/ml 30 ml (B. Braun Melsungen AG, Melsungen, Germany). Oral intubation was performed without any complications.

2.1. Surgical Procedure. At first, an incision on the left parietal side of approximately 1.5 cm down to the periosteum was made. Denudation of the calvaria over an area of approximately 1 cm^2 and predrilling with a 5 mm long 1.1 twist drill followed. Then, the scull reference array (tripod) was inserted into the patient's scull and fixed with an 8 mm screw (Medartis AG, Basel, Switzerland). The earlier constructed dental splint with four attached registration screws was inserted. After registration verification, the needle could be located

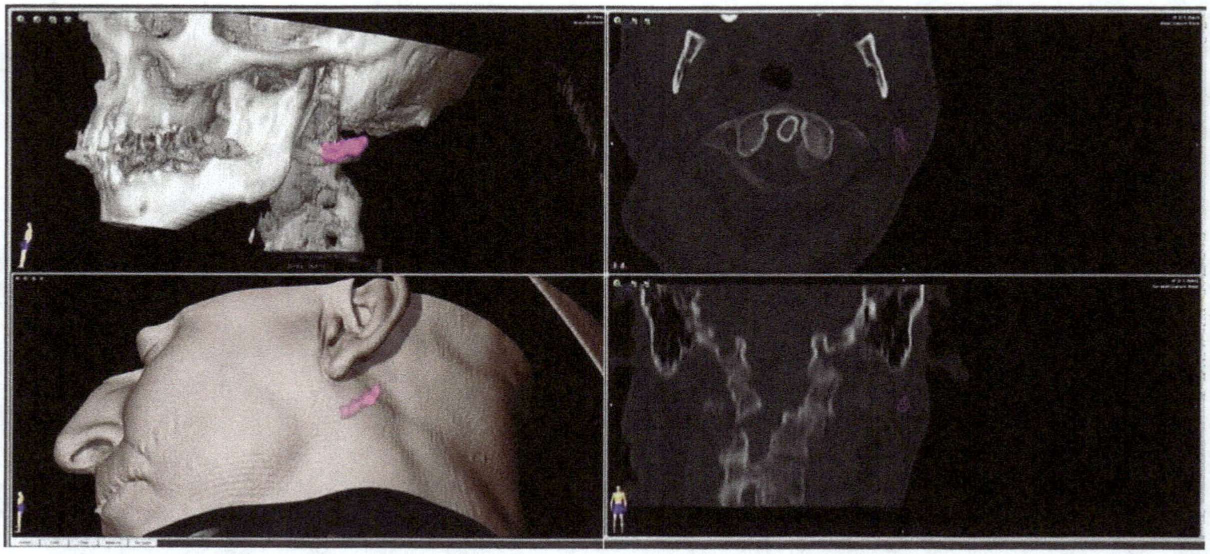

FIGURE 2: 3D-location of the fractured hypodermic needle.

by 3D navigation (Kolibiri Navigation System Cranial 3.0, Brainlab®, Feldkirchen, Germany) with an accuracy of 0.7 mm. The surgical approach was minimally invasive by extraoral incision below the left earlobe. At first, the skin and subcutis, as well as the musculature, were cut using a No. 10-blade scalpel. Hemostasis was performed by electrocoagulation. Then, the parotid capsule was dissected, and the underlying tissue was very carefully dissected layer by layer until the cannula tip could be identified. The 2.1 cm long needle could be fully recovered (Figure 3). Afterwards, the parotid capsule and the musculature injured by the cannula was reconstructed (reconstruction of the sternocleidomastoid muscle and the platysma with Vicryl4 × 0(Ethicon, Johnson & Johnson, Somerville, USA), a multilayer wound closure with Vicryl4 × 0, and finally a simple skin flap plastic with Ethilon5 × 0(Ethicon, Johnson & Johnson, Somerville, USA) were performed). Then, removal of the tripod, reconstruction of the occipitofrontal muscle with Vicryl 3 × 0 (Ethicon, Johnson & Johnson, Somerville, USA), and skin suture with Prolene 3 × 0 (Ethicon, Johnson & Johnson, Somerville, USA) followed. Operation time was 32 minutes.

Postoperatively, the patient showed no signs of complications, in particular no hemorrhage or infection. In a follow-up visit 10 days after the operation, no signs of infection, wound dehiscence, or any other recognizable pathologies could be seen. The sutures were removed, and further follow-up visits were performed by his local dentist. There were no adverse and unanticipated events. Written informed consent was obtained to publish his case.

2.2. Treatment during Pandemics. The case described above happened only one month before the outbreak of COVID-19. During the outbreak, we realized that when fractured needles are recovered as described, the risk of infection for patients and staff is high. We therefore also present a procedure reducing infective transmission to a minimum (Figure 4). The dentist transferring the patient should contact the maxillofacial department before sending the patient and ideally provide 3D imaging. Upon arrival, the patient should be separated, triaged, and tested. Afterwards, needle detection by ultrasound should be tried, using adequate COVID-19 protection gear, such as respirators of a high protection level (FFP3/N99/equivalent), waterproof gowns, eye protection, and gloves [7]. If testing is possible, test results should be awaited. If the needle can be located by ultrasound, sonography-controlled surgical needle recovery should be performed. If the needle cannot be located using sonography, intraoperative 3D visualization such as CT or CBCT should be used in combination with visual exploration, preferably using an extraoral approach. In cases with difficulties finding the needle, 3D navigation by surface scan could follow. If the needle still remains undetectable and/or irremovable, the patient should be closely monitored. Complex highly accurate 3D navigation with dental splints should only be planned if the needle moves towards a potentially life-threatening structure, such as the carotid artery, under strict infection-controlled measures.

3. Discussion

The presented case demonstrates a fractured dental syringe needle advancing from the pterygomandibular space towards the retroauricular region. We applied the treatment algorithm recently suggested by Acham et al. [2] and retrospectively evaluated it for its feasibility during pandemics such as COVID-19. At first, we planned to remove the needle conventionally by intraoral incision, searching for it in its approximate location. After realizing the movement of the needle, we researched the literature for further options. Acham et al. [2] suggest in a recent review an algorithm for needle recovery using 3D navigation. We therefore chose to use computer-assisted surgery to extract the needle. With navigational support, it was very easy to find the needle that had only slightly moved after planning. It could be recovered by a minimally invasive extraoral retromandibular approach. However, the process to enable 3D navigation takes time for

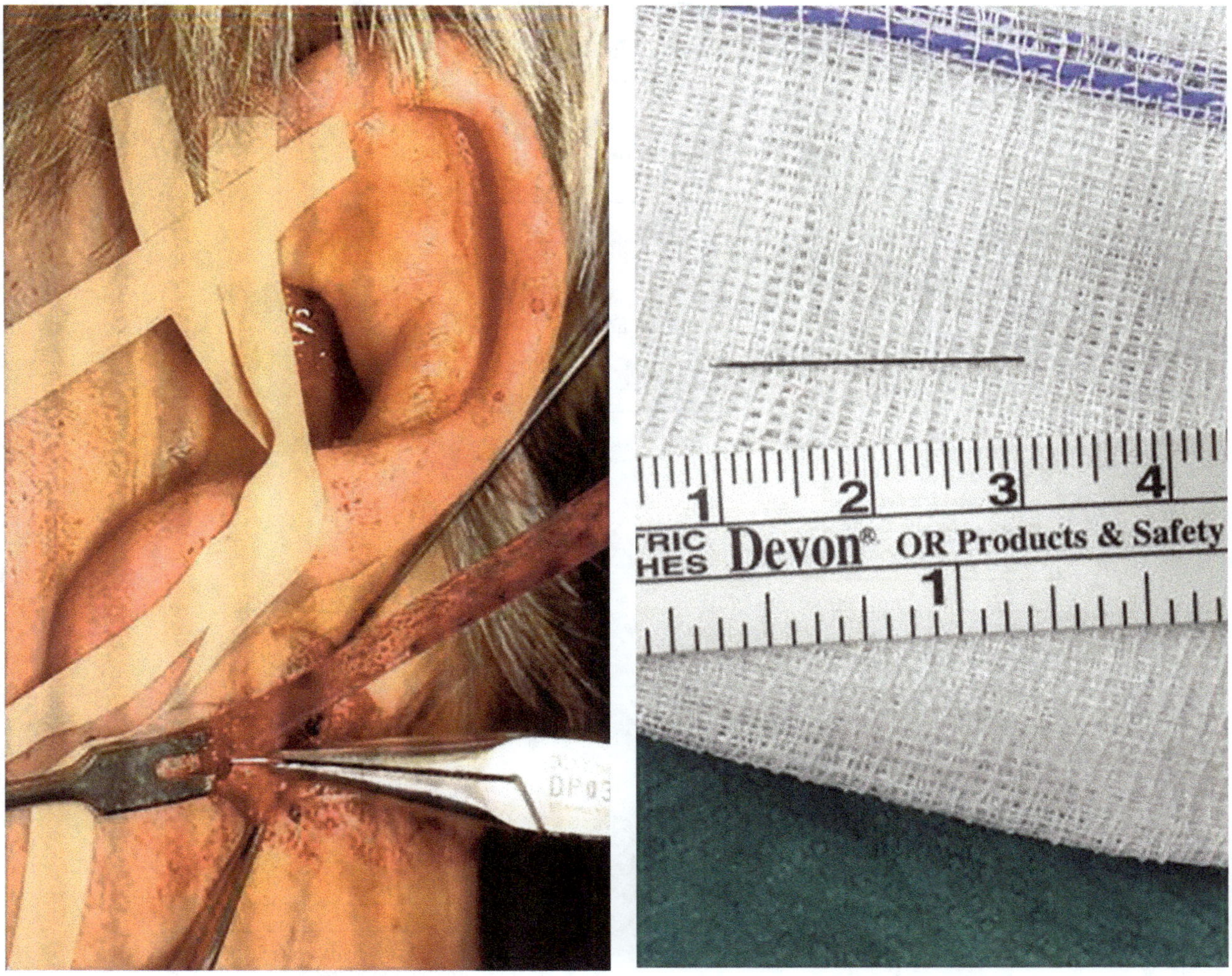

(a) (b)

FIGURE 3: Intraoperative retrieval of the 2.1 cm fractured hypodermic needle (a) and measurement afterwards (b).

the dental splint to be constructed, for additional CT imaging, and for the foreign object to be marked in the software. This takes some time in which the needle can dislocate further. If we had virtually located the needle and planned the navigation after initial imaging, the navigation would have been useless during surgery. It might therefore be helpful to plan navigated extractions only directly before the surgery with the most recent imaging. In only around 50% of reported cases, the needle is removed within one day after the event [2]. In our case, a longer waiting period might have dislocated the needle even further. Brooks and Murphy reported a case in which a dislocated fractured needle had been retrieved from the right internal carotid artery [8]. Luckily, the needle in our case did not damage any vital structures and could be removed with a minimally invasive procedure. In addition, the delay of treatment by one day and preparation for navigation led to hospitalization of the patient in which he had close contact to medical personnel in the emergency unit, the maxillofacial ward, the radiology department, and dental technicians. 3D navigation is not available in every hospital yet, and hardware and software are expensive to obtain. Planning costs and efforts are immense. Additionally, irradiation exposure is high, because when not planned immediately, additional 3D imaging (usually CT) with a dental splint for registration is necessary. Alternatives for 3D navigation suggested in the workflow by Acham et al., when immediate recovery is not possible, are stereotactic localization and visual exploration. Stereotactic options, such as 3D marking by indicator needles, the use of a C-arm, and intraoperative 3D visualization (CT, CBCT) are associated with high irradiation as well. All these expenses may seem like overtreatment in some cases. Visual exploration alone, however, is often confusing and might lead to severe damage. Sonography might be an alternative worth discussing. As it was in our case, the majority of needle fractures occur with inferior alveolar and mandibular nerve block anesthesia, with fragments predominantly situated in the pterygomandibular region [2]. We did not consider using ultrasound for needle location because of sonographic shadowing of the mandibular bone. Besides, applied pressure for sonography might have dislocated the needle further. However, it might be an easy, cheap, and quick intraoperative solution for needle location and should be considered as an additional intraoperative tool especially in cases of fast

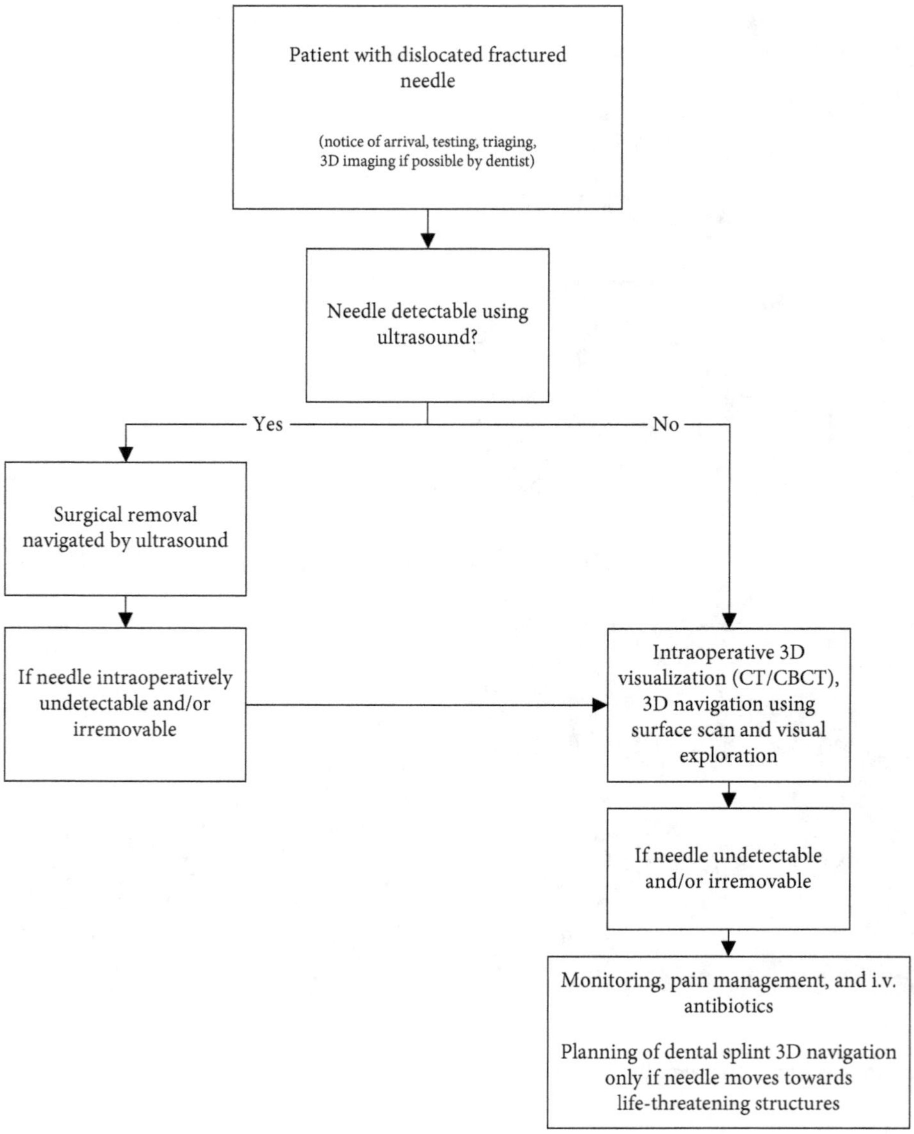

FIGURE 4: Suggestion for treatment during pandemic crises such as COVID-19. Dislocated fractured needle movement usually requires treatment in a department for maxillofacial surgery.

TABLE 1: Eight crucial points for avoiding needle breakage [2].

(1)	Explore the patient-specific anatomy
(2)	Use a sufficiently strong and long canula
(3)	Inspect for damage before use
(4)	Avoid prebending or kinking
(5)	Prepare the patient for puncture and avoid sudden movements
(6)	Do not insert the whole needle
(7)	Puncture only when masticatory musculature is relaxed
(8)	Avoid directional change during needle advancement
(9)	Change the needle for every injection

dislocation. Needles can usually be detected easily within the soft tissue. In difficult cases, intraoperatively navigated 3D-ultrasound, as it is used in neurosurgery, might be advantageous [9]. In times when extra infection precaution procedures have to be applied, procedures should consume as little time and resources as possible and be easy to handle even for less experienced personnel. The suggested treatment plan offers a way around difficult and long planning and can be managed by only one maxillofacial surgeon, limiting the risk of infection. However, it has not yet been tested and requires good sonographic skills. It will be tested as soon as the opportunity presents itself. Other approaches might prove easier and more applicable to daily clinical routines.

The recovery of broken dental needles proves to be very elaborate. Prevention of needle breakage therefore is even more important. Table 1 offers crucial points for avoiding needle breakage. In case a needle breaks and the fragment is still visible, it should immediately be grasped with, e.g., a forceps or a hemostat. The patient should remain as immobile as possible since the visible fragment may disappear with released tissue tension [10].

In conclusion, 3D navigation works well for recovering dislodged fractured hypodermic needles. However, fractured needles can move quickly. Therefore, early recovery is necessary and 3D navigational planning has to be conducted immediately before surgery. Nevertheless, costs, efforts, and risks for infection are high. Other options, such as ultrasound, should be evaluated pre- and intraoperatively, especially during pandemics such as COVID-19.

3.1. Patient's Perspective. The patient denied to offer his full perspective on the case but claims to have felt treated well during the procedure.

References

[1] M. Augello, J. von Jackowski, K. W. Grätz, and C. Jacobsen, "Needle breakage during local anesthesia in the oral cavity—a retrospective of the last 50 years with guidelines for treatment and prevention," *Clinical Oral Investigations*, vol. 15, no. 1, pp. 3–8, 2011.

[2] S. Acham, A. Truschnegg, P. Rugani et al., "Needle fracture as a complication of dental local anesthesia: recommendations for prevention and a comprehensive treatment algorithm based on literature from the past four decades," *Clinical Oral Investigations*, vol. 23, no. 3, pp. 1109–1119, 2019.

[3] M. A. Pogrel, "Broken local anesthetic needles: a case series of 16 patients, with recommendations," *Journal of the American Dental Association (1939)*, vol. 140, no. 12, pp. 1517–1522, 2009.

[4] N. Rahman, M. Clarke, and L. F. Stassen, "Case report: management of broken dental needles in practice," *Journal of the Irish Dental Association*, vol. 59, no. 5, pp. 241–245, 2013.

[5] L. Ribeiro, S. Ramalho, S. Gerós, E. C. Ferreira, A. Faria e Almeida, and A. Condé, "Needle in the external auditory canal: an unusual complication of inferior alveolar nerve block," *Oral Surgery, Oral Medicine, Oral Pathology, Oral Radiology*, vol. 117, no. 6, pp. e436–e437, 2014.

[6] F. Maffia, M. Fontanari, V. Vellone, P. Cascone, and L. G. Mercuri, "Impact of COVID-19 on maxillofacial surgery practice: a worldwide survey," *International Journal of Oral and Maxillofacial Surgery*, vol. 49, no. 6, pp. 827–835, 2020.

[7] M. Zimmermann and E. Nkenke, "Approaches to the management of patients in oral and maxillofacial surgery during COVID-19 pandemic," *Journal of Cranio-Maxillo-Facial Surgery*, vol. 48, no. 5, pp. 521–526, 2020.

[8] J. Brooks and M. T. Murphy, "A novel case of a broken dental anesthetic needle transecting the right internal carotid artery," *Journal of the American Dental Association (1939)*, vol. 147, no. 9, pp. 739–742, 2016.

[9] O. Sergeeva, F. Uhlemann, G. Schackert, C. Hergeth, U. Morgenstern, and R. Steinmeier, "Integration of intraoperative 3D-ultrasound in a commercial navigation system," *Zentralblatt für Neurochirurgie*, vol. 67, no. 4, pp. 197–203, 2006.

[10] N. P. Fuller, R. A. Menke, and W. J. Meyers, "Perception of pain to three different intraoral penetrations of needles," *Journal of the American Dental Association (1939)*, vol. 99, no. 5, pp. 822–824, 1979.

24

Buccal Silicone Granuloma Caused by the Dental Infection

Kazuhiro Murakami, Kazuhiko Yamamoto, Tsutomu Sugiura, and Tadaaki Kirita

Department of Oral and Maxillofacial Surgery, Nara Medical, University, Kashihara City, Nara, Japan

Correspondence should be addressed to Kazuhiro Murakami; murakami@naramed-u.ac.jp

Academic Editor: Andresa Borges Soares

The facial injection of liquid silicone is performed for cosmetic purposes. The use of injectable fillers in facial procedures has become extremely popular over the past decade. Most procedures are performed in the perioral, periocular, and cheek areas of middle-aged women. Even though silicone is biologically inert, its injection can result in the formation of granulomas. Silicone granulomas can result from an inflammatory or autoimmune tissue response. However, the development of silicone granulomas secondary to dental infection has not yet been reported. We report a case of a 73-year-old woman with a right buccal silicone granuloma that developed following a dental infection. Ultimately, this case healed completely after the surgical removal of all lesions. Silicone in the facial region may become infected by a dental infection, and infective silicone develops granulomas and cellulitis. In the context of cosmetic facial silicone injections, it is necessary to improve oral hygiene prior to dental treatment and to maintain a healthy oral environment after surgery. In some cases, surgical treatment using an intraoral approach is effective.

1. Introduction

The use of injectable fillers in facial procedures has become extremely popular over the past decade, with most procedures performed in the perioral, periocular, and cheek areas of middle-aged women [1]. It is aimed at smoothening out wrinkles or creases and at producing an artificial augmentation of lip or cheek volume for cosmetic and rejuvenation purposes [2].

The advantages of liquid silicone implantation include its low cost, stable chemical structure, and low degree of tissue reactivity [3]. However, even though it is biologically inert, silicone injection can result in the formation of granulomas [4]. The severity and frequency of granuloma formation, as well as other immunologic complications, will likely increase if injections are administrated by incautious or unqualified, perhaps unlicensed, practitioners using non-medical-grade silicone [1, 5]. Regardless of the origin and mechanism of silicone dissemination, silicone granulomas can result from an inflammatory or autoimmune tissue response [6]. However, the development of silicone granulomas due to dental infection has not yet been reported.

We report a case of a 73-year-old woman with a right buccal silicone granuloma developed by the dental infection.

2. Case Report

A 73-year-old woman was referred from a private dentist to our department for swelling of the right maxillary premolar buccal gingiva and diffuse swelling of the right cheek. Excision and drainage of the cheek region had been performed with cosmetic surgery a month earlier. Her past medical history was unremarkable except for hypertension. There was a fistula of about 5 mm on the right cheek 10 mm above the oral angle, and pus was discharging from this fistula (Figures 1(a) and 1(b)). Cone beamed computed tomography (CBCT) imaging showed an apical lesion of the second premolar (Figures 1(c) and 1(d)). A bougie was inserted through the fistula and advanced, and it finally reached the apical region of the right upper second premolar. Based on these findings, the lesion was diagnosed as right buccal cellulitis and orofacial external fistula due to apical periodontitis of the right upper second premolar. According to this clinical diagnosis, antibiotics [cefcapene pivoxil (CFPN-PI), 300 mg/day] were administered for three days, and root canal treatment of the right upper first and second premolar was performed. Bacterial examination of pus from the fistula revealed gram-positive *α-streptococcus* (resident bacteria). The administration of antibiotics and root canal treatment

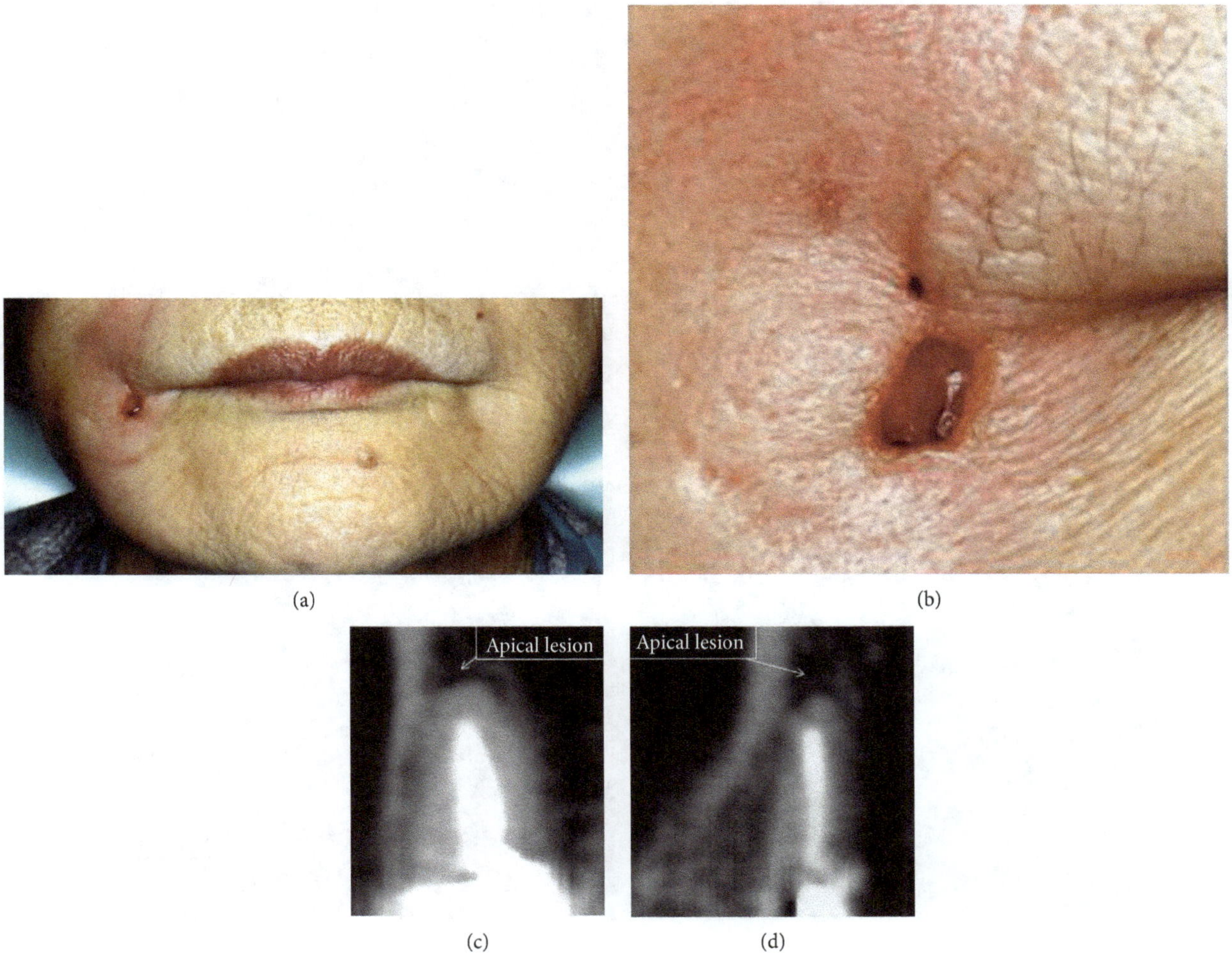

Figure 1: (a) Photograph of the front of the face taken at the first visit. Diffuse swelling of the right cheek was seen. A fistula of about 5 mm was present near the corner of the mouth. (b) Photograph around the fistula. Pus was discharging from the fistula. (c) Cone beamed computed tomography (CBCT) image at the causal tooth in coronal image. (d) CBCT image at the causal tooth in sagittal image. There was an apical lesion of about 3 mm in the root apex of the right maxillary second premolar.

improved the swelling of the right cheek. After the root canal treatment was completed, the external orofacial fistula was removed, and apicoectomy of the right upper first and second premolar was performed. Histological examination of the resected fistula indicated that there were mucus deposition, mucous nodule formation, and foreign body giant cell infiltration in the fat, striated muscle, and fibrous tissue, with mild calcification. AE1/AE3 staining was negative, and no epithelial components were observed. Vimentin staining revealed many positive stromal cells. Histopathological diagnosis suspected a mucin-producing odontogenic tumor or mucinous adenocarcinoma, among other diagnoses (Figures 2(a)–2(c)). Her symptoms had disappeared two months after the surgery. However, swelling of the right cheek and fistula formation developed again at the same site, and bacterial examination and magnetic resonance imaging (MRI) were performed. Bacteriological examination revealed the *Streptococcus anginosus* group. The MRI findings were irregular high signal intensity areas under the subcutaneous tissue on both cheeks on T2-weighted images of fat suppression, and high signal intensity areas were widely distributed on the right side (Figure 3 (a1) and (a2)).

We asked her if she had a past history of injection of any foreign body, but she denied having had liquid silicone injections. Since the *Streptococcus anginosus* group was sensitive for CFPN-PI, it was administered for 28 days. The swelling of the right buccal region disappeared, and there was a reduction of the fistula. However, since a small amount of pus-like effusion was observed from the fistula, minocycline ointment was injected subcutaneously into the fistula. The symptoms disappeared after treatment, but a single subcutaneous nodule, approximately 10×10 mm in size, remained in the cheek, and an extremely small quantity of clear effusion flowed from the fistula. Since the MRI showed a reduction of the nodule six months later, we continued follow-up (Figure 3 (b1) and (b2)). One year later, a swelling with fluctuation developed in the right cheek again, and puncture aspiration of pus was performed. The bacterial examination demonstrated methicillin-sensitive *Staphylococcus aureus* (MSSA), so CFPN-PI was administered. The MRI showed unclear boundary lesions in the high signal area in T2-weighted images and the low signal area in T1-weighted images, and a foreign body-like liquid silicone was suspected again (Figure 3 (c1) and (c2)). When we asked about her past

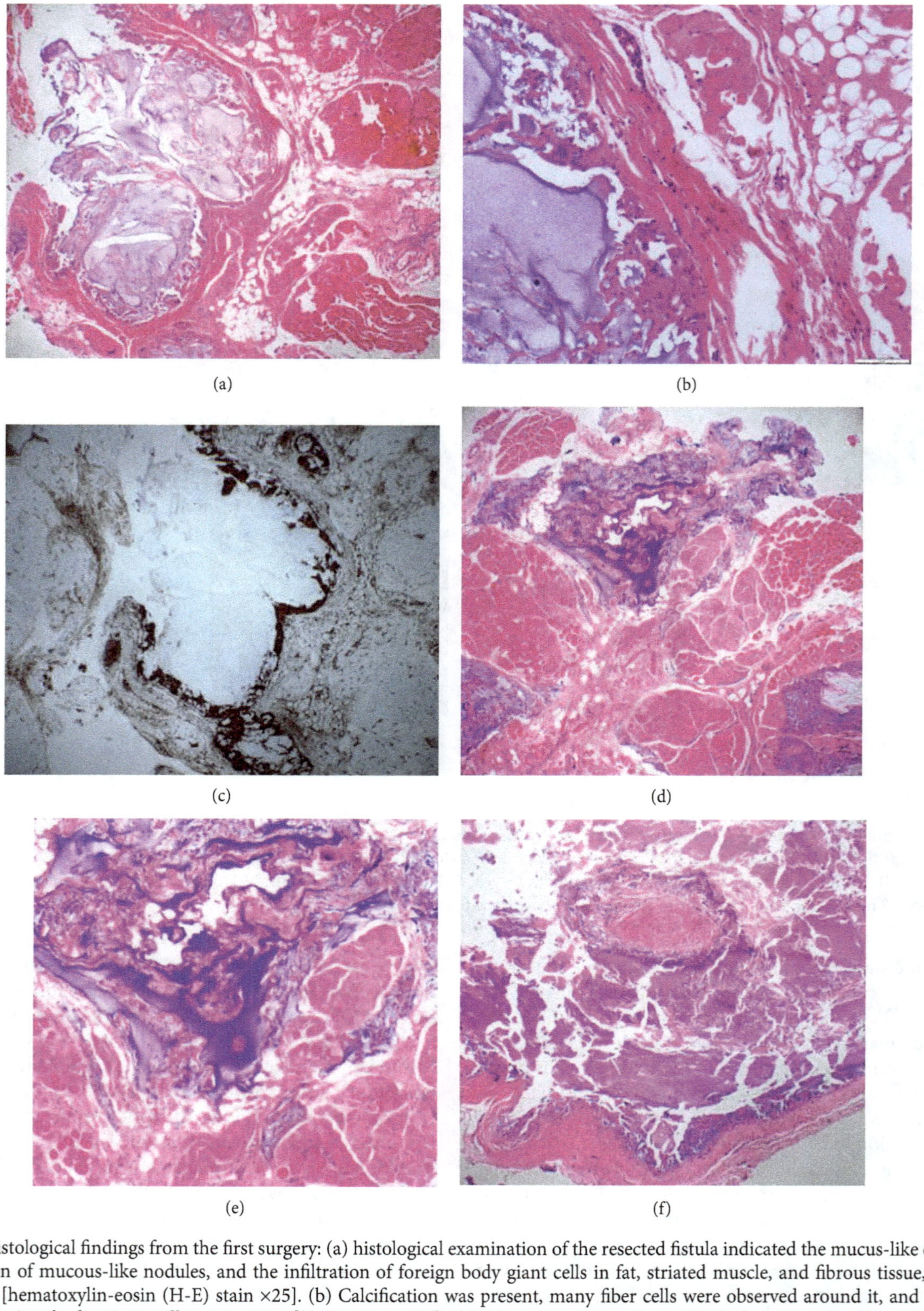

FIGURE 2: Histological findings from the first surgery: (a) histological examination of the resected fistula indicated the mucus-like deposition, the formation of mucous-like nodules, and the infiltration of foreign body giant cells in fat, striated muscle, and fibrous tissue, with mild calcification [hematoxylin-eosin (H-E) stain ×25]. (b) Calcification was present, many fiber cells were observed around it, and vacuolated cells and foreign body giant cells were seen [H-E stain ×100]. (c) Vimentin stain was positive for stromal cells and fibrocytes. Histopathological diagnosis was suspected of mucin-producing odontogenic tumor and mucinous adenocarcinoma, among other diagnoses. Histological findings from the second surgery: (d) histological examination of the removal tumor showed foreign body giant cell, vacuolated cells, fibrous tissue, and striated muscle around calcifications [H-E stain ×25]. (e) H-E stain ×100. (f) Silicone particles, foreign body giant cell, and fibrotic tissue of silicone granuloma [H-E stain ×25].

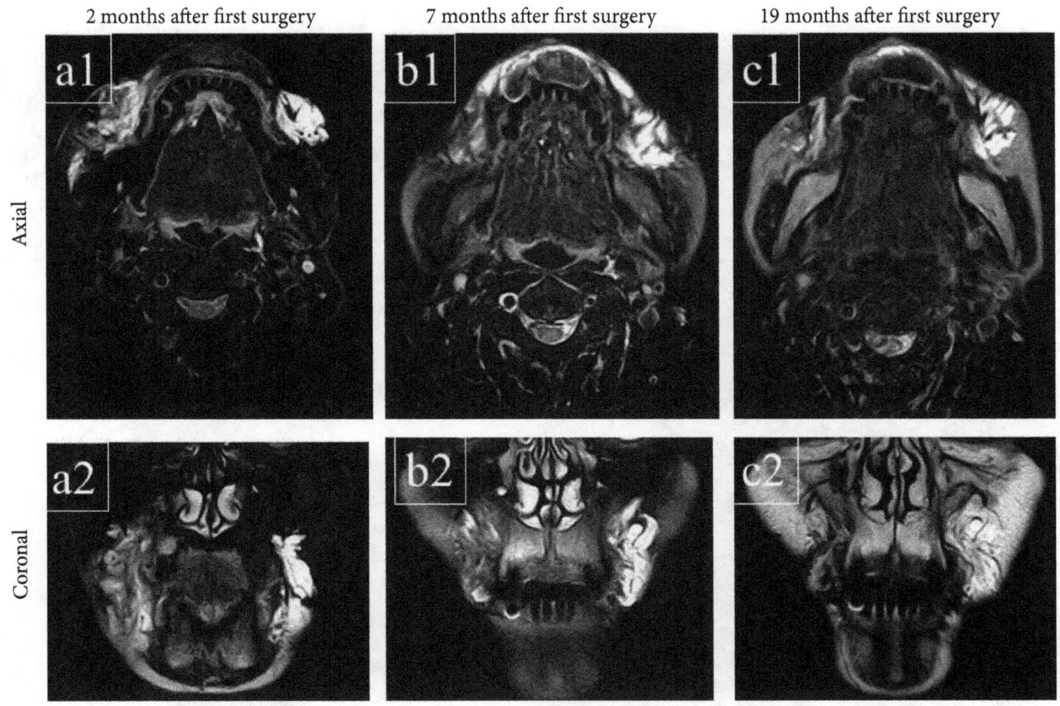

Figure 3: MRI findings. (a1, a2) Axial and coronal images of T2-weighted image of fat suppression two months after the first surgery. Irregular high signal intensity areas under the subcutaneous tissue on both cheeks and high signal intensity areas were widely distributed on the right side. (b1, b2) Axial and coronal images of T2-weighted image of fat suppression seven months after the first surgery. The images showed a reduction of the right nodule compared with those two months after the first surgery. (c1, c2) Axial and coronal images of T2-weighted image 19 months after the first surgery. Unclear boundary lesions showed the high signal area was recognized, and foreign body-like liquid silicone injection was suspected again. The above high signal area on the buccal region was shrinking over time. These findings should develop by loss of silicone from the fistula. The high signal area on the left buccal region had not changed.

medical history again, the patient revealed that liquid silicone had been injected into her cheeks eight years earlier to remove nasolabial folds. Removal of the foreign body was planned for radical treatment. Under local anesthesia, all connective tissue and granuloma, including the silicone from the buccal mucosa, were removed (Figures 4(a) and 4(b)). In the process, bleeding was observed from the upper lip branch of the facial artery, so hemostasis was performed by ablation, and the operation was completed. Histopathologically, the fibrotic hyperplasia was observed in the striated muscles and subcutaneous tissues, and a foreign body granuloma with liquid silicone and foreign body giant cells was identified. Histopathologic diagnoses were the silicone, silicone granuloma, and scar (Figures 2(d) and 2(e)). After the operation, she had no complications, such as facial paralysis or facial deformity (Figures 5(a) and 5(b)). The postoperative course was uneventful, and there were no symptoms for one year after surgery.

3. Discussion

Silicone (polysiloxane) is known widely by general, cosmetic, and surgical dermatologists and is available in gel-filled implants as well as in liquid and solid forms. Liquid and gel implants may be used for tissue augmentation (e.g., breast) and as esthetic fillers [3]. Mostly performed in the perioral, periocular, and cheek areas of middle-aged women, the aim is to smoothen out wrinkles or creases and to produce an artificial augmentation of the lip or cheek volume for cosmetic and rejuvenation purposes [2].

The injection of artificial substances began in the 1950s, and liquid silicone was used up until the early 1960s. However, the U.S. Food and Drug Administration (FDA) banned silicone injections in 1965 due to complications following injection. However, in 1994, purified and sterilized high-viscosity silicone oil made by Adatomed (Munich, Germany) was introduced for ophthalmologic use and was approved by the U.S. FDA for that use. The majority of complications include granulomas, nodularity, migration, and chronic cellulitis [7]. Even though silicone is biologically inert, its injection can result in the formation of granulomas. Silicone granulomas were first described in 1964 as a rare complication that was, and continues to be, a diagnostic challenge. The severity and frequency of granuloma formation, as well as other immunologic complications, will likely increase if injections are administered by incautious or unqualified, perhaps unlicensed, practitioners using non-medical-grade silicone [1]. Although there are several case reports of complications arising from silicone use, the amount of silicone was frequently related in the past with the appearance of granulomas. Impurity from injected liquid silicone can be seen microscopically as translucent, birefringent foreign bodies within the cytoplasm of giant cells [3].

The likelihood of the appearance of silicone granulomas is greater with large volumes of injection. There are reports that pure silicone, administered in small amounts, does not

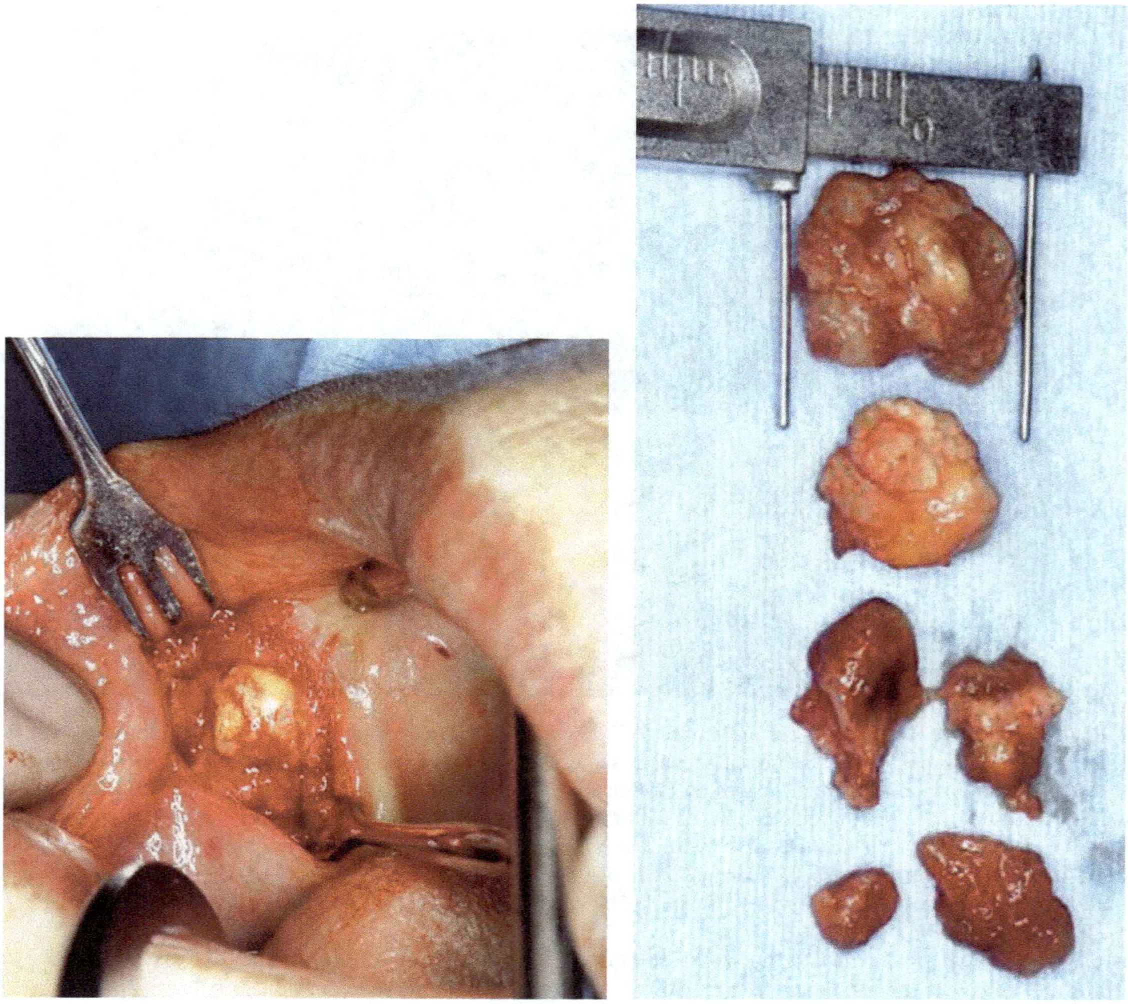

(a) (b)

Figure 4: (a) Intraoperative photograph. (b) Photograph of the removed lesions. Most of the silicone granulomas containing the mass of silicone were removed.

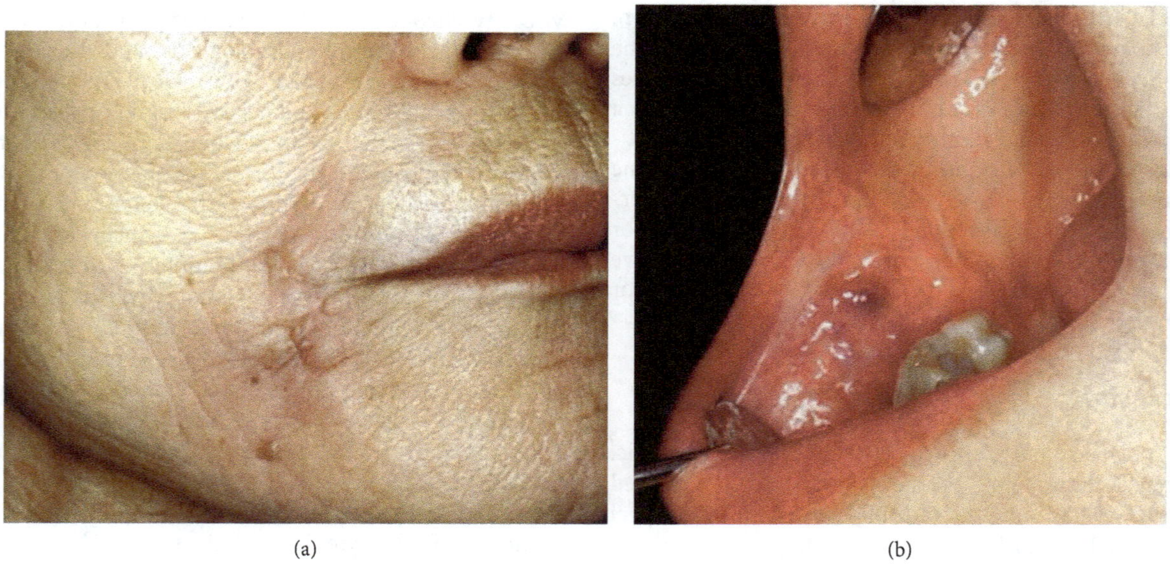

(a) (b)

Figure 5: (a) Extraoral photograph three months after the second surgery. (b) Intraoral photograph three months after the second surgery. Although a slight scar formation was observed around the region where the fistula was present, the healing was completed.

cause granulomas [5]. Liquid silicone is administered with the microdroplet technique, in which very small amounts are injected using a serial puncture technique [1]. Given that there are significant potential benefits to purified, high-viscosity, injectable silicone oil if used correctly, it is important to elucidate the factors that contribute to complications [1]. Although detailed information about the liquid silicone administration method used in this case was not available, it was supposed that the appropriate administration method had probably been performed based on the patient's interview. In this case, it was supposed the silicone granulomas were developed not by immune response reaction of the silicone but by the infection of it. As a cause of that, the cellulitis on the right cheek was initially occurring, a bougie inserted through the fistula reached the apical region of the right upper second premolar, and bacterial examination of pus with silicone particles from the fistula revealed oral resident bacteria. Furthermore, the liquid silicone was injected into the cheeks on both sides; however, cellulitis, fistula, and granuloma formation were observed only on the right side. Therefore, if the silicone injection was done properly, this case was considered to have been caused by a dental infection.

Travis et al. reported the classification into three types: (1) inflow into soft tissues (granulomatous reaction), (2) uptake into lymph nodes, and (3) inflow into blood vessels (human adjuvant disease) [8]. Regardless of the origin and mechanism of silicone dissemination, silicone granulomas can result from an inflammatory or autoimmune tissue response. A systemic manifestation of the inflammatory response to adjuvants, such as silicone, has been termed autoimmune/inflammatory syndrome induced by adjuvants [6]. In this case, no systemic symptoms, such as collagen disease and multiple organ lesions, were observed, and only local inflammation was observed. Silicone granulomas are as prevalent as they have always been, but there is no consensus regarding their treatment. Treatment can be difficult and unsuccessful in many cases. Clinicians should try to individualize treatment for each patient. If surgical excision is deemed necessary, significant scarring can be expected because the silicone itself and the granulomas can migrate throughout multiple layers of soft tissue, often necessitating the removal of thick sections of tissue. In some patients, granulomas will resolve spontaneously without treatment. The more common treatments include systemic and local steroids, minocycline, 5-fluorouracil, isotretinoin, and, for localized granuloma formation, surgical resection. While success has been achieved with steroids, relapse often occurs after a steroid taper. Tetracycline antibiotics, especially minocycline, have been used successfully for their anti-inflammatory and antigranulomatous properties, as well as their mycobacterial coverage. Surgical resection is a good option for localized granulomas, although the resected tissue must be replaced to fill the dead space and minimize postoperative esthetic deformity [1, 9]. The rationale for the administration of minocycline in granulomatous tissue reaction is its anti-inflammatory, immunomodulating, and antigranulomatous effects [9]. After removal of the apical lesion and the external fistula, the facial fistula remained from the infected silicone lesion, so minocycline ointment was administered through the fistula. In this case, the minocycline was locally administered through the fistula and the symptoms improved temporarily, but inflammation occurred again and MSSA was detected in the pus from the fistula. Although it was reported that oral administration of minocycline (100 mg once daily) was effective in a previous report [9], it was unclear whether local administration of minocycline was effective in this case.

The silicone scattered from this region was washed away from the fistula, and the lumped silicone changed the silicone granuloma. It was considered that most of the silicone in the region could be removed, and the healing was actually achieved by removing this granuloma. Facial deformity did not occur in the removal region because it was considered that only a small amount of silicone, which was used for the purpose of smoothing out wrinkles, had been injected. The surgical intervention proved to be effective in this case.

Although artificial materials are injected into many regions of the body in cosmetic surgery, the injection of non-absorbable materials into the facial region has a greater tendency to become infected than other body areas because the facial region is adjacent to the oral tissue. In particular, since the thin facial muscles are present between the subcutaneous tissues of the cheeks and chin and the oral mucosa, an oral infection easily develops into a subcutaneous silicone infection. In esthetic treatments, it is important to have good oral hygiene, and the condition of the oral region, including the teeth and gingiva, needs to be hygienic.

The histologic diagnosis of silicone granuloma is easily interpreted in most cases. However, as in the present case, the patient may fail to report a history of cosmetic surgery. Without a complete clinical history, there is an increased risk of histopathologic misinterpretation [10]. The histology is characterized by multinucleated giant cells as a foreign body reaction. Vacuoles corresponding to the filler material are frequently found, particularly with silicone. With other products, the filler material may not be detected. The differential diagnosis should include erysipelas, allergic contact dermatitis, facial edema with eosinophilia, cheilitis glandularis apostematosa, Ascher's syndrome, orofacial granulomatosis, Crohn's disease, Melkersson-Rosenthal syndrome, and sarcoidosis. Likewise, cutaneous leishmaniasis, leprosy, and tuberculosis can also present as granulomatous inflammations of the skin.[4] Gonçales et al. [10] reported that when the patient denies previous cosmetic procedures, these cases can be misdiagnosed as malignant tumors, such as low-grade liposarcoma. Since the facial silicone granulomas related to esthetics, the patient's pathological history is often concealed. Even in this case, the initial clinical diagnosis, which included mucin-producing odontogenic tumor and mucinous adenocarcinoma, was based on the first histopathologic examination because the patient did not reveal her history. It has been reported that it is necessary to listen closely to the interview [10]. Although the silicone injection was performed properly in this case, it can be considered that the formation of the silicone granuloma was associated with abscess and fistula formation due to an unexpected dental infection. For patients with suspected dental infections, it is desirable for the infection to be resolved and the dental treatment to be completed before silicone injections are performed. Also, it is necessary to maintain good intraoral hygiene after the injections are completed.

4. Conclusion

The facial injection of liquid silicone is performed for cosmetic purposes, but the silicone may become infected by a dental infection, and the infective silicone may develop granulomas and cellulitis. It is necessary to complete preoperative dental treatment to improve oral hygiene and to maintain a clean oral environment after surgery. In some cases, surgical treatment using an intraoral approach is effective.

Authors' Contributions

Kazuhiro Murakami is responsible for the clinical treatment, histological diagnosis, and drafting, critical revision, and approval of the article. Kazuhiko Yamamoto is assigned to the histological diagnosis and also to the drafting, critical revision, and approval of the article. Tsutomu Sugiura and Tadaaki Kirita are also responsible for the critical revision and approval of the article.

Acknowledgments

The authors thank Dr. Akihito Moriyasu, the president of Hattori Memorial Hospital, for the perioperative management of the patient. They also thank Dr. Motokatsu Tsuyuki, the vice president of Hattori Memorial Hospital, and Dr. Junichi Ishida for the histological examination.

References

[1] L. L. Wang, W. W. Thomas, and O. Friedman, "Granuloma formation secondary to silicone injection for soft-tissue augmentation in facial cosmetics: mechanisms and literature review," *Ear, Nose, & Throat Journal*, vol. 97, no. 1-2, pp. E46–E51, 2019.

[2] T. Lombardi, J. Samson, F. Plantier, C. Husson, and R. Küffer, "Orofacial granulomas after injection of cosmetic fillers. Histopathologic and clinical study of 11 cases," *Journal of Oral Pathology & Medicine*, vol. 33, no. 2, pp. 115–120, 2004.

[3] E. Rieder, S. Desai, J. P. Mundi et al., "Granulomatous dermatitis related to silicone implant," *Dermatology Online Journal*, vol. 19, no. 12, p. 20708, 2013.

[4] R. Poveda, J. V. Bagán, J. Murillo, and Y. Jiménez, "Granulomatous facial reaction to injected cosmetic fillers–a presentation of five cases," *Medicina Oral, Patología Oral y Cirugía Bucal*, vol. 11, no. 1, pp. E1–E5, 2006.

[5] R. A. Moscona and L. Fodor, "A retrospective study on liquid injectable silicone for lip augmentation: long-term results and patient satisfaction," *Journal of Plastic, Reconstructive & Aesthetic Surgery*, vol. 63, no. 10, pp. 1694–1698, 2010.

[6] T. A. Chen, C. L. Mercado, K. L. Topping, B. P. Erickson, K. P. Cockerham, and A. L. Kossler, "Disseminated silicone granulomatosis in the face and orbit," *Am J Ophthalmol Case Rep.*, vol. 10, pp. 32–34, 2018.

[7] P. E. Chasan, "The history of injectable silicone fluids for soft-tissue augmentation," *Plastic and Reconstructive Surgery*, vol. 120, no. 7, pp. 2034–2040, 2007.

[8] W. D. Travis, K. Balogh, and J. L. Abraham, "Silicone granulomas: report of three cases and review of the literature," *Human Pathology*, vol. 16, no. 1, pp. 19–27, 1985.

[9] M. J. Arin, J. Bäte, T. Krieg, and N. Hunzelmann, "Silicone granuloma of the face treated with minocycline," *Journal of the American Academy of Dermatology*, vol. 52, 2 Supplement 1, pp. 53–56, 2005.

[10] E. S. Gonçales, A. S. Almeida, S. Soares, and D. T. Oliveira, "Silicone implant for chin augmentation mimicking a low-grade liposarcoma," *Oral Surgery, Oral Medicine, Oral Pathology, Oral Radiology, and Endodontics*, vol. 107, no. 4, pp. e21–e23, 2009.

25

Foreign Body Granuloma in the Tongue by a Pequi Spine

Rafael Martins Afonso Pereira, Patrícia Cristine de Oliveira Afonso Pereira, Vitor Carvalho Rodrigues, Luiz Fernando Braga de Andrade, Elisa Morais de Carvalho, and Helvécio Marangon Júnior

School of Dentistry, University Center of Patos de Minas (UNIPAM), Patos de Minas, Minas Gerais, Brazil

Correspondence should be addressed to Rafael Martins Afonso Pereira; rafaelmap@unipam.edu.br

Academic Editor: Zühre Akarslan

Substances considered foreign to the human organism can penetrate it due to local trauma, initially causing an acute inflammatory response against these substances, involving a neutrophilic infiltrate that, when it fails to deal with these foreign bodies, ends up generating a granulomatous inflammatory response. Granuloma formation has been associated with a variety of conditions. The correct clinical and imaging diagnoses are extremely important for the dentist to choose an appropriate therapeutic approach, aiming at the best possible treatment. This work is aimed at describing a case report of a foreign body granuloma, formed on the tongue, from the penetration of a pequi spine, in a 76-year-old patient, in whom, after an imaging diagnosis with ultrasound, surgical removal of the lesion was performed, and the piece was sent for histopathological examination, which confirmed the initial diagnostic hypothesis of a foreign body granuloma. The initial diagnosis of foreign body granulomas is challenging. For this reason, more sophisticated means of diagnosis such as tomography and magnetic resonance become important in the diagnosis, as they can show with greater clarity and reliability the nature of the lesion and its relationship with adjacent anatomical structures. In the case in question, an ultrasound examination was chosen, which was extremely important as an aid to diagnosis, considerably improving surgical planning. In addition, after surgical removal, the result of the histopathological analysis is essential to determine the definitive diagnosis, as it determines the granulomatous characteristic of the lesion.

1. Introduction

True granulomas are compact microscopic structures, formed by the collection of epithelioid histiocytes, surrounded by inflammatory cells and filled with fibroblasts and collagen fibers, in response to the persistence of some stimulus [1–3]. The presence of multinucleated giant cells, formed by the coalescence of macrophages, can also be observed [2].

A foreign body granuloma can develop from several endogenous or exogenous substances [4]. Endogenous substances, such as cholesterol from cell membranes, keratin, and hair, can originate foreign body granulomas. The introduction of foreign bodies in oral and peribuccal tissues is related to traumatic events, dental procedures, and cosmetic dermatological procedures [5–7]. Amalgam, suture threads, endodontic sealants, and gutta-percha are some examples of dental materials capable of causing a foreign body granulomatous reaction [4].

Granulomatous inflammation in the hard and soft structures of the mouth is an uncommon event [2]. Furthermore, to date, there are no reports in the literature of a case involving the spine of the pequi fruit (*Caryocar brasiliense*) as an etiological factor of the lesion. Thus, the present study is aimed at reporting an unprecedented case of a foreign body granuloma in the tongue caused by pequi spines.

2. Case Report

A 76-year-old male patient sought a maxillofacial surgeon because of difficulty in swallowing and in chewing, pain complaint, and an internal nodule hardened on the tongue. On

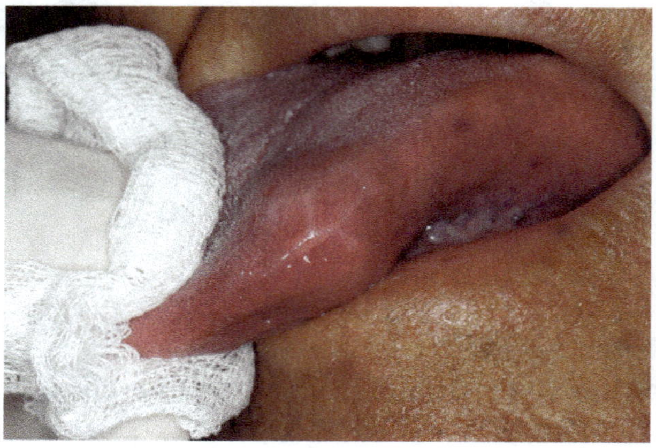

FIGURE 1: Presence of a free, well-defined, rounded nodule, with the tongue showing normal color and an enlarged aspect in the central region on visual clinical examination.

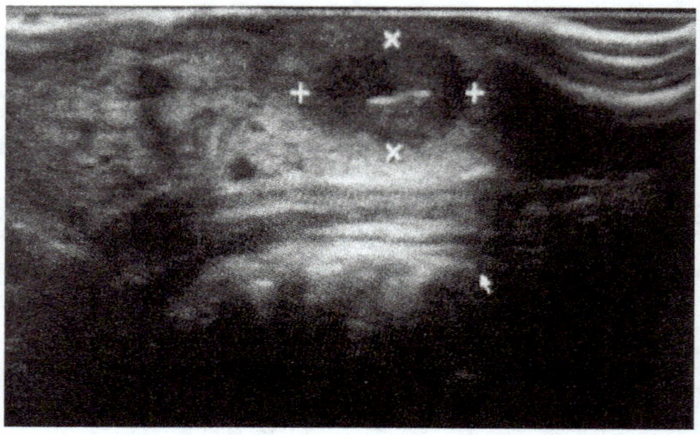

FIGURE 2: Ultrasonography showing a circumscribed nodular lesion. The echographic aspect was suggestive of a foreign body inside, suggesting an image compatible with a thorn, with granuloma formation.

visual and palpatory clinical examination, a free and well-defined rounded nodule was found, with the tongue showing normal color, but with an enlarged aspect in the central region (Figure 1). In the initial clinical interview, the patient did not remember whether he had eaten anything that had hurt his tongue. To assist in the diagnosis and try to elucidate the fact, the patient was asked for a complementary ultrasound examination of the tongue. The ultrasound device was a linear matrix probe, with a frequency of 12 Mhz. In the result, it was possible to observe a 5 mm hyperechoic linear image with a 1.2×0.7 cm granuloma formation. The lesion was located on the left lateral border of the distal third of the patient's tongue, 0.1 cm from the surface.

The echographic aspect suggested a foreign body inside, showing an image compatible with a spine, with granuloma formation (Figure 2). On the patient's return, when asked about the possible spine on the tongue, he recalled that he had eaten pequi a while ago but that he was not sure exactly regarding the time, leading us to a more consistent diagnostic hypothesis of a foreign body granuloma caused by a pequi spine. Complete surgical enucleation of the lesion was then performed, with bilateral anesthetic block of the lingual nerve. Surgical access was performed through a linear incision in the lingual dorsum on the left side, close to the most superficial region of the lesion (Figure 3). The lesion was divulsed, using blunt-tipped instruments, from the adjacent tissue planes, having been cleaved without the rupture of its evident lining capsule (Figure 4). No vascular rupture with subsequent hemorrhagic accident occurred, despite the close proximity of the lesion with lingual arteries and veins. The visualization of these large lingual vessels was perceived by the surgeon during the operation. After total enucleation without compromising the capsule (Figure 5), the synthesis was performed both in deep muscle planes and on the epithelial surface using simple isolated points. The surgical specimen removed by excisional biopsy was sent for anatomopathological examination, which confirmed the initial diagnostic hypothesis of a foreign body granuloma from the penetration of a pequi spine. Histopathological examination revealed a nodule of fibrous tissue well delimited by means of a capsule, with thick collagen fibers richly peripherally vascularized and with sparse chronic inflammatory cells, in addition to numerous macrophages that stand out in the midst of immunoinflammatory cells (Figure 6).

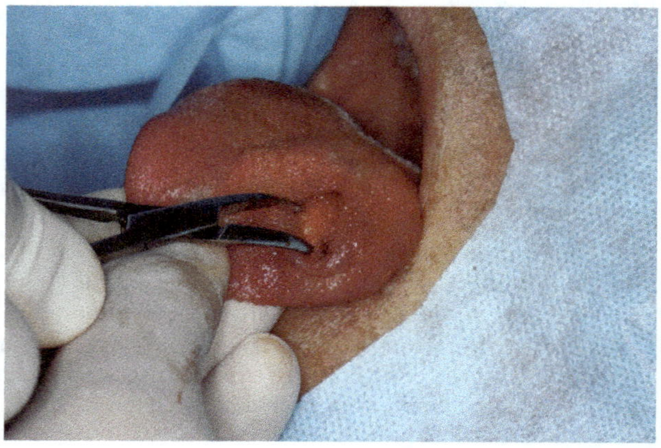

FIGURE 3: Surgical access performed through a linear incision in the lingual dorsum on the left side, close to the most superficial region of the lesion.

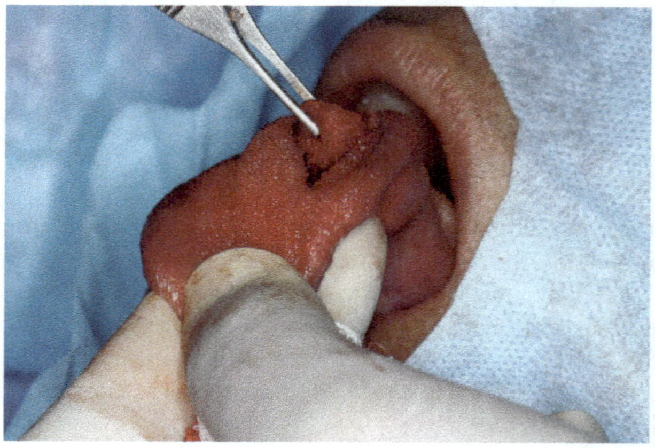

FIGURE 4: Divulsion of the lesion, using blunt-tip instruments, from the adjacent tissue planes, having been cleaved without the rupture of its evident lining capsule.

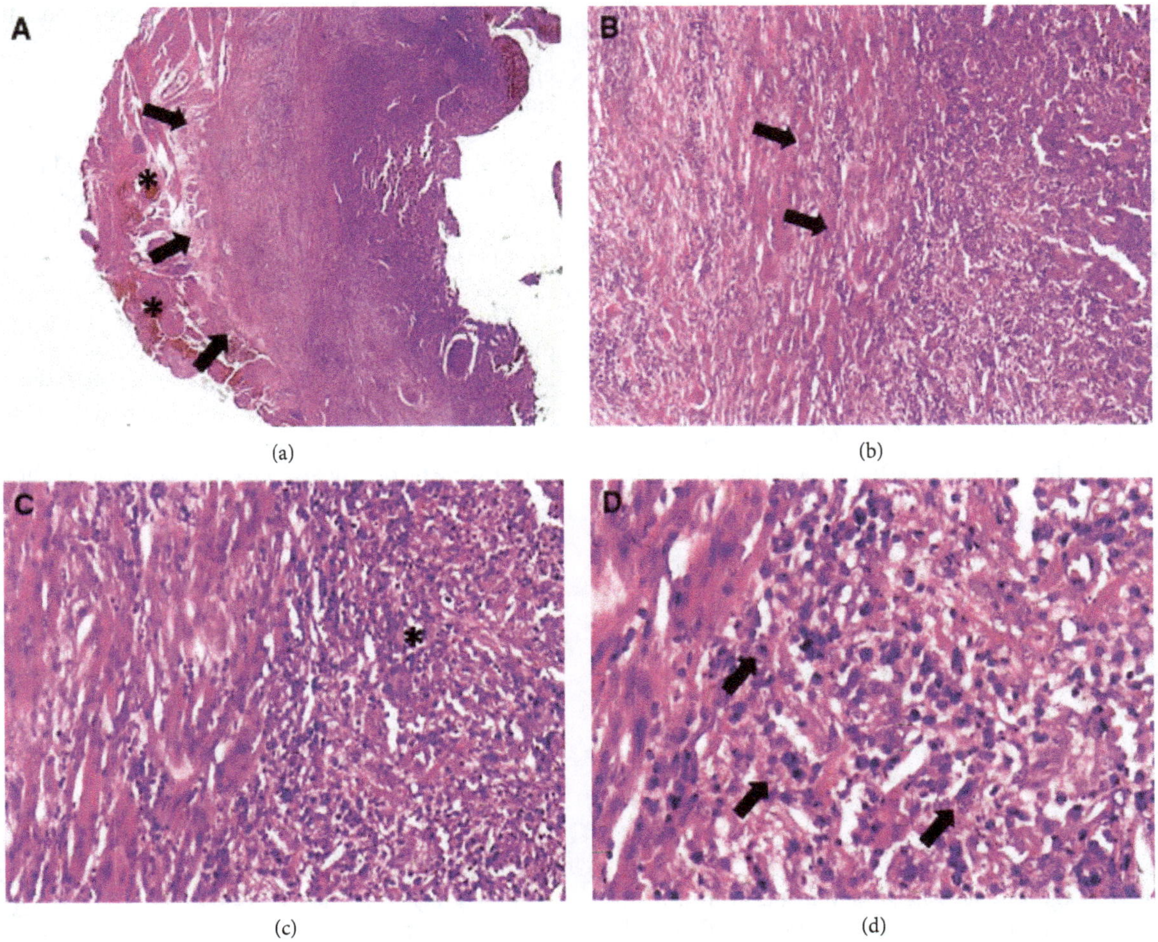

Figure 5: Histopathological examination showing a fragment of a fibrous tissue nodule well delimited by means of a capsule, with thick collagen fibers richly peripherally vascularized and with sparse chronic inflammatory cells, in addition to numerous macrophages that stand out in the midst of immune-inflammatory cells: (a) 50x magnification: the full black arrows represent the outer limit of the fibrous capsule, and the black asterisks represent the peripheral vascular congestion; (b) 100x magnification: the full black arrows represent the bundles of collagen fibers; (c) 200x magnification: the black asterisk represents the chronic inflammatory infiltrate; (d) 400x magnification: the full black arrows represent numerous macrophages in the middle of the chronic inflammatory infiltrate.

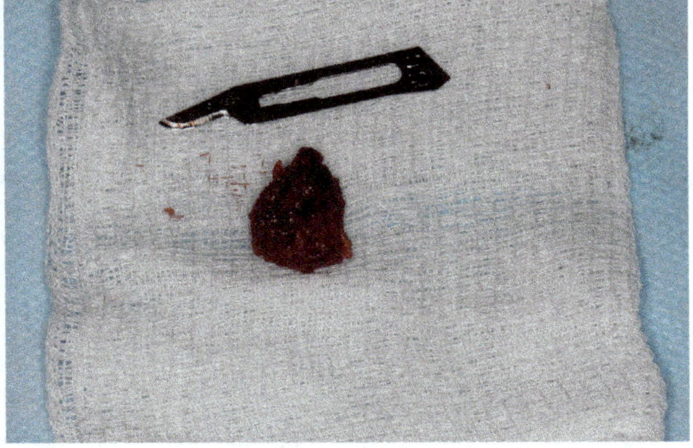

Figure 6: Total enucleation without compromising the capsule.

3. Discussion

There are voluntary and involuntary reasons for foreign substances to penetrate people. Materials for tattoos and aesthetic fillings are included in the first group, while the second is related to substances capable of causing cutaneous trauma and their consequent inclusion in tissues [8], such as glass fragments [9] and bee sting [10]. In the present case, the penetration of the foreign body, pequi spine, happened involuntarily, when the patient was eating. The pequi is a fruit composed of several layers, among them the prickly endocarp, which has the function of protecting the edible seed [11], and, for this reason, it is necessary for people to be cautious during their chewing.

A vegetable foreign body granuloma still has an uncertain etiopathogenesis. However, what is more accepted in the literature is that granulomatous lesions are the result of implantation of foreign bodies of plant origin, which have in their composition an amorphous eosinophilic material surrounded by a hyaline ring [12]. After the foreign body penetrates the tissues, the starch, which constitutes the amorphous material, is rapidly metabolized and eliminated by the human organism, while the hyaline ring, composed of cellulose, remains intact and produces an inflammatory response in the organism [12, 13]. It is common that in these cases, the foreign body of plant origin is associated with other diseases, being of fundamental importance to identify the initial cause of the pathological process [14]. In the present case, as the foreign body granuloma was isolated, that is, being the primary disease, the simple removal of the irritant (pequi spine) was enough for the treatment to be successful.

The time for the appearance of a foreign body granuloma can vary from a few days to years [15], and, clinically, it presents as a local inflammatory reaction, associated or not with purulent secretion, pain [3, 5, 16], material migration [5, 16], slight swelling, ulcerations [4], and color changes, which range from grayish black to bright red [17]. It is rare to find cases in which the foreign body granuloma developed in the oral cavity is asymptomatic [3, 5, 16]. The signs and symptoms found in the case in question confirm what is described in the literature, since the patient had noticeable swelling on the side of the tongue, pain, and difficulty in swallowing.

A foreign body granuloma presents a diagnostic challenge to the dentist [18] and, therefore, requires the association of data collected, during the interview, clinical findings, and complementary imaging tests [16], since these reproduce important characteristics for the diagnosis [19]. The visualization of foreign bodies is related to both the density and the proximity of the tissues, as well as the location in which they are inserted [18]. For the location of foreign bodies in soft tissues, magnetic resonance imaging is a good alternative [18]; however, ultrasonography has proved to be quite effective in identifying foreign body granulomas [20]. To establish the definitive diagnosis, it is necessary to perform a histopathological examination, considered the gold standard technique [16, 21]. In the present case, during the clinical interview, the patient did not present any systemic or local evidence that could explain the genesis of the lingual lesion perceived on physical examination. After the ultrasound result and in view of the ultrasound findings that demonstrated a hyperechoic image at the center of a region compatible with a granulomatous reaction, the hypothesis of a foreign body granuloma was raised, being reinforced, at this moment, by the patient's previous recall that, during his feeding and ingestion of the pequi, an accident had occurred and that inadvertently a spine, contained in the center of the fruit, had pierced his tongue which could have been introduced in a deep tissue plane.

Granulomatous inflammations have different etiopathogenesis; however, they show similar histopathological patterns [17] and great clinical similarities. It is necessary to establish possible differential diagnoses: mucoceles, neoplasms of mesenchymal soft tissues, orofacial granulomatosis, angioedema, and Melkersson-Rosenthal syndrome [5, 22]. In this clinical case, the ultrasound result was very presumptive, demonstrating, therefore, the importance of this complementary imaging exam in helping to clarify the diagnosis in dentistry.

Aesthetic procedures, in an attempt to slow down aging through injectable soft tissue fillers, are increasingly frequent [23]. However, the increasing performance of these procedures, regardless of the type of material used, also causes an increase in the number of side effects [24], the most common being foreign body granulomas [25, 26]. The treatment approach for this type of granulomatous reaction by an exogenous foreign body has good resolvability through intralesional injections of corticosteroids [21, 26]. On the other hand, when foreign body granuloma lesions are caused by other exogenous factors, such as that presented by this clinical case, surgical excision by enucleation of the lesion should be the first option of choice, since this technique can be used both for definitive laboratory diagnosis and for therapy [7, 26, 27].

The surgical treatment adopted, aided by a thorough diagnosis by means of an appropriate complementary imaging exam, selected for the case, allowed for a conservative surgical approach, with a comfortable immediate postoperative period, good recovery, and efficient long-term tissue repair with excellent prognosis, once the cause of the granulomatous inflammatory reaction has been removed.

References

[1] D. O. Adams, "The granulomatous inflammatory response. A review," *The American Journal of Pathology*, vol. 84, no. 1, pp. 164–192, 1976.

[2] F. Alawi, "Granulomatous diseases of the oral tissues: differential diagnosis and update," *Dental Clinics of North America*, vol. 49, no. 1, pp. 203–221, 2005.

[3] T. L. I. Serrano, H. F. Pauna, I. M. Hazboun, A. C. Dal Rio, M. E. P. Correa, and E. M. Nicola, "Foreign body in jugal mucosa," *International Archives of Otorhinolaryngology*, vol. 19, no. 4, pp. 364–366, 2015.

[4] A. A. Alhassani, M. S. Al-Zahrani, and K. H. Zawawi, "Granulomatous diseases: oral manifestations and recommendations," *The Saudi Dental Journal*, vol. 32, no. 5, pp. 219–223, 2020.

[5] B. C. Jham, N. G. Nikitakis, M. A. Scheper, J. C. Papadimitriou, B. A. Levy, and H. Rivera, "Granulomatous foreign-body reaction involving oral and perioral tissues after injection of biomaterials: a series of 7 cases and review of the literature," *Journal of Oral and Maxillofacial Surgery*, vol. 67, no. 2, pp. 280–285, 2009.

[6] H. Rai, M. Shaila, G. Ghosh, and P. D. Suhasini, "Foreign body giant cell granuloma of the mandible subsequent to endodontic surgery," *Journal of Contemporary Dentistry*, vol. 5, no. 3, pp. 178–180, 2015.

[7] J. J. Lee, Y. P. Wang, Y. H. Wu, and J. Y. F. Chang, "Poly-l-lactic acid injection-induced delayed-onset foreign body granuloma," *Journal of the Formosan Medical Association*, vol. 116, no. 5, pp. 402-403, 2017.

[8] L. Requena, L. Cerroni, and H. Kutzner, "Histopathologic patterns associated with external agents," *Dermatologic Clinics*, vol. 30, no. 4, pp. 731–748, 2012.

[9] E. Mazinis, T. Lambrianidis, and J. Margelos, "Detection of a residual foreign body during root canal treatment," *Journal of Endodontia*, vol. 31, no. 9, pp. 691–693, 2005.

[10] K. Yamamoto, Y. Nakayama, Y. Matsusue, M. Kurihara, T. Yagyuu, and T. Kirita, "A foreign body granuloma of the buccal mucosa induced by honeybee sting," *Case Reports in Dentistry*, vol. 2017, Article ID 7902978, 4 pages, 2017.

[11] F. D. Araujo, "A review of Caryocar brasiliense (Caryocaraceae)—an economically valuable species of the central Brazilian cerrados," *Economic Botany*, vol. 49, no. 1, pp. 40–48, 1995.

[12] A. A. Talacko and B. G. Radden, "The pathogenesis of oral pulse granuloma: an animal model," *Journal of Oral Pathology & Medicine*, vol. 17, no. 3, pp. 99–105, 1988.

[13] H. P. Philipsen and P. A. Reichart, "Pulse or hyaline ring granuloma. Review of the literature on etiopathogenesis of oral and extraoral lesions," *Clinical Oral Investigations*, vol. 14, no. 2, pp. 121–128, 2010.

[14] S. Patil, R. S. Rao, A. T. Raj et al., "Insights into the pathogenesis and clinicopathological spectrum of oral vegetable granuloma. Case series with literature review," *Clinics and Practice*, vol. 7, no. 4, 2017.

[15] V. A. Silveira, E. D. De Carmo, C. E. Colombo, A. S. Cavalcante, and Y. R. Carvalho, "Intraosseous foreign-body granuloma in the mandible subsequent to a 20-year-old work-related accident," *Medicina Oral, Patología Oral y Cirugía Bucal*, vol. 13, p. e657, 2008.

[16] D. Puliyel, A. Balouch, S. Ram, and P. P. Sedghizadeh, "Foreign body in the oral cavity mimicking a benign connective tissue tumor," *Case Reports in Dentistry*, vol. 2013, 3 pages, 2013.

[17] L. Tettamanti, L. Azzi, A. Grimaldi et al., "An unusual green macular lesion of the gingiva: a foreign-body granulomatous reaction," *Oral Surgery, Oral Medicine, Oral Pathology, Oral Radiology*, vol. 117, no. 1, pp. e65–e69, 2014.

[18] S. Joyce, B. R. Sripathi, M. O. Mampilly, and C. F. Nyer, "Foreign body granuloma," *Journal of Oral and Maxillofacial Surgery*, vol. 13, no. 3, pp. 351–354, 2014.

[19] G. C. Felin, J. P. De Carli, M. E. Flores, J. L. B. Pretto, L. C. Dogenski, and F. de Conto, "Foreign body reaction simulating mandibular osteosarcoma — case report," *International Journal of Surgery Case Reports*, vol. 60, pp. 58–62, 2019.

[20] F. R. Grippaudo, M. Di Girolamo, M. Mattei, E. Pucci, and C. Grippaudo, "Diagnosis and management of dermal filler complications in the perioral region," *Journal of Cosmetic and Laser Therapy*, vol. 16, no. 5, pp. 246–252, 2014.

[21] C. E. P. Alcântara, M. S. Noronha, J. F. Cunha, I. L. Flores, and R. A. Mesquita, "Granulomatous reaction to hyaluronic acid filler material in oral and perioral region: a case report and review of literature," *Journal of Cosmetic Dermatology*, vol. 17, no. 4, pp. 578–583, 2018.

[22] M. R. de Souza Quirino, A. C. C. Neves, M. S. Campos, A. A. H. Brandão, and A. L. Anbinder, "Oral granuloma formation after injection of cosmetic filler," *Journal of Cranio-Maxillo-Facial Surgery*, vol. 40, no. 7, pp. e194–e197, 2012.

[23] T. Daley, D. D. Damm, J. A. Haden, and M. T. Kolodychak, "Oral lesions associated with injected hydroxyapatite cosmetic filler," *Oral Surgery, Oral Medicine, Oral Pathology, Oral Radiology*, vol. 114, no. 1, pp. 107–111, 2012.

[24] J. Kunjur and H. Witherow, "Long-term complications associated with permanent dermal fillers," *The British Journal of Oral & Maxillofacial Surgery*, vol. 51, no. 8, pp. 858–862, 2013.

[25] M. El-Khalawany, S. Fawzy, A. Saied, M. Al Said, A. Amer, and B. Eassa, "Dermal filler complications: a clinicopathologic study with a spectrum of histologic reaction patterns," *Annals of Diagnostic Pathology*, vol. 19, no. 1, pp. 10–15, 2015.

[26] P. Tamiolakis, E. Piperi, P. Christopoulos, and A. Sklavounou-Andrikopoulou, "Oral foreign body granuloma to soft tissue fillers. Report of two cases and review of the literature," *Journal of Clinical and Experimental Dentistry*, vol. 10, article e177, 2018.

[27] S. B. Aregbesola and V. I. Ugboko, "Unusual foreign bodies in the orofacial soft tissue spaces: a report of three cases," *Nigerian Journal of Clinical Practice*, vol. 16, no. 3, pp. 381–385, 2013.

26

A Case of Cytomegalovirus-Induced Oral Ulcer in an Older Adult Patient with Nephrotic Syndrome due to Membranous Nephropathy

Shinichi Sato,[1,2] Masato Takahashi,[1] and Tetsu Takahashi[2]

[1]*Oral and Maxillofacial Surgery, Japan Community Health Care Organization Sendai Hospital, 3-16-1 Tsutsumimachi, Aoba-ku, Sendai 981-8501, Japan*
[2]*Division of Oral and Maxillofacial Surgery, Tohoku University Graduate School of Dentistry, 4-1, Seiryo-machi, Aoba-Ku, Sendai 980-8575, Japan*

Correspondence should be addressed to Shinichi Sato; sato-shinichi@sendai.jcho.go.jp

Academic Editor: Junichi Asaumi

We report a case of cytomegalovirus- (CMV-) induced buccal ulcer in a patient with nephrotic syndrome. An 82-year-old man with membranous nephropathy was on immunosuppressive therapy presented with an ulcer in the oral cavity and was hospitalized. Intraoral examination revealed an inflamed and painful ulcer on the left buccal mucosa. Blood test results showed CMV positivity, and histopathological examination confirmed the diagnosis. Anti-CMV therapy (ganciclovir) was initiated from the third day of hospitalization. However, he developed dyspnea on the 14th day. Computed tomography images of the chest revealed the presence of ground-glass opacities, and noninvasive positive pressure ventilation was initiated under the provisional diagnosis of pneumocystis pneumonia caused by ganciclovir-associated myelosuppression and/or steroid-induced immunocompromised state. The patient died of pneumocystis pneumonia on the 21st day. The patient had received immunosuppressive therapy for renal dysfunction. Immunocompromised patients with CMV infection should be treated with caution, as drugs for CMV may themselves cause myelosuppression, deteriorating the prognosis of the patient.

1. Introduction

Cytomegalovirus (CMV) is a genus of viruses of the order Herpesvirales, which is estimated to infect approximately 90% of adults at some point in their lives. CMV infection is usually subclinical and can persist in this manner for the entire life span of an infected individual [1–3]. It is also an opportunistic pathogen [2] and can affect multiple organs, leading to pneumonia, peptic ulcers, retinitis, and/or encephalitis in immunocompromised hosts, including patients who have undergone allogeneic hematopoietic stem cell transplantation [4, 5], allogeneic bone marrow transplantation [6, 7], and/or organ transplantation [8] and patients infected with the human immunodeficiency virus (HIV) [9].

To date, however, few reports have documented the manifestations of CMV infection in the oral cavity [10–12]. Here, we report a case of CMV infection of the buccal mucosa in an immunocompromised patient.

2. Case Presentation

An 82-year-old man was referred to our hospital from another clinic on June 11, 2019; at that time, he had low total protein (4.8 g/dL)/albumin levels (1.6 g/dL) and high protein-creatinine ratio (7.3) and was thus admitted to our department of nephrology. His medical history revealed frequent tonsillitis in childhood and two episodes of hemorrhagic gastric ulcers at the age of 76 years. He was not positive for HIV, and no family history of renal failure or history of consanguineous marriage was reported.

He was diagnosed with membranous nephropathy based on the findings of a renal biopsy and was treated according to the standard treatment protocol [13], which included

Table 1: The extent of kidney damage in terms of creatinine level of blood, estimated glomerular filtration rate (eGFR), protein-creatinine ratio, uric acid (UA), blood urea nitrogen (BUN), blood sodium, potassium, and chloride levels and serum phosphorus level at the start of treatment, midtreatment (8 days), and posttreatment (18 days).

	8/5/19 Start of treatment	8/13/19 Midtreatment (8 days)	8/23/19 Posttreatment (18 days)
Creatinine level of blood (mg/dL)	2.0	1.5	3.7
eGFR	25.9	34.6	13.2
Protein-creatinine ratio	3.0	4.4	1.5
UA (mg/dL)	6.3	4.6	13.0
BUN (mg/dL)	54.0	39.0	134.0
Blood sodium level (mEq/L)	125.0	130.0	144.0
Blood potassium level (mEq/L)	4.8	4.6	4.4
Blood chloride level (mEq/L)	96.0	99.0	109.0
Serum phosphorus level (mg/dL)	3.9	2.4	7.9
Urinary creatinine (mg/dL)	105.9	77.6	74.0

prednisolone (30 mg) and cyclosporine A (100 mg). Steroid pulse therapy was not initiated, and he was discharged from the hospital on July 9 (Table 1).

On July 26, he started experiencing pain and difficulty in chewing due to pain in the entire oral cavity, and on August 5, he was admitted to our hospital on an emergency basis due to the presence of a severely painful lesion in the mouth.

At the time of admission on August 5, 2019, his height and weight were 160 cm and 62.9 kg, respectively. Results of blood tests revealed the following: albumin concentration, 1.3 g/dL; C-reactive protein concentration, 1.39 mg/dL; total protein concentration, 4.1 g/dL; platelet count, $14.7 \times 10^4/\mu$ L; and leukocyte count, $35.9 \times 10^2/mm^3$. The results of further antibody tests revealed that he was positive for CMVpp65 antigens (C10, C11) 546/434. His β-D glucan concentration was 40.2 pg/mL, suggesting a strong possibility of CMV infection.

On August 6, 2019, the patient presented with a painful intraoral ulcer; intraoral examination revealed ulcers on the left buccal mucosa and generalized inflammation of the gingiva. Moreover, erosion was observed on the left side of the tongue (Figure 1). No ulceration or erosion was observed on the right buccal mucosa or the right side of the tongue.

A clinical diagnosis of ulcer on the left buccal mucosa was made, and the attending physician requested a biopsy of the ulcer for a definitive diagnosis. An incisional biopsy was performed, and the specimen was sent for a pathological examination.

Histopathological findings revealed a prominent ulcerative lesion containing numerous CMV-positive vascular endothelial cells scattered at the fundus of the ulcer (Figures 2 and 3). Based on these findings, the diagnosis of CMV infection was confirmed.

The pain persisted even after admission, and the patient was prescribed an azulene sodium sulfonate gargle containing 4% xylocaine. A 10-day course of anti-CMV medication (ganciclovir) was initiated on August 7, 2019.

The C-reactive protein concentration on August 5 was 1.39 mg/dL, and ganciclovir was administered from August 7; however, on August 9, the C-reactive protein concentration had increased to 1.78 mg/dL. Nonetheless, his condition gradually improved to a status of 3/3 CMV antigenemia. Oral findings on August 16, after the start of ganciclovir therapy on August 7, are shown in Figure 4. A persistent ulcer on the left buccal mucosa was noted, and the inflammation was less severe. However, he developed dyspnea on August 18, and blood test results revealed increases in his C-reactive protein concentration and leukocyte count to 24.78 mg/dL and $89.4 \times 10^2/mm^3$, respectively (Figure 5). Computed tomography images of the chest revealed the presence of ground-glass opacities, and noninvasive positive pressure ventilation was initiated under the provisional diagnosis of pneumocystis pneumonia caused by ganciclovir-associated myelosuppression and/or steroid-induced immunocompromised state.

On August 18, his estimated glomerular filtration rate (eGFR) was 25.80 mL/min and blood urea nitrogen (BUN) was 60 mg/dL, while on August 19, eGFR decreased to 19.42 mL/min and BUN increased to 73 mg/dL. A rapid decline in his renal function was evident. Sulfamethoxazole-trimethoprim (10 mL/day) was initiated from August 20. However, the patient died due to respiratory failure on August 25, 2019.

Before his death, the patient provided written informed consent for the publication of his images and case details. The requirement for ethical approval was waived by the appropriate institutional review board.

3. Discussion

The potential routes of CMV infection include vertical transmission via the placenta, birth canal, and/or breast milk; horizontal transmission via the saliva, urine, semen, blood, and/or cervical and vaginal discharge; or organ transplantation. In many cases, CMV infection occurs during the perinatal period or infancy, and many infected individuals are asymptomatic [1]. However, the adrenal glands, lungs, gastrointestinal tract, and/or retinas of immunocompromised

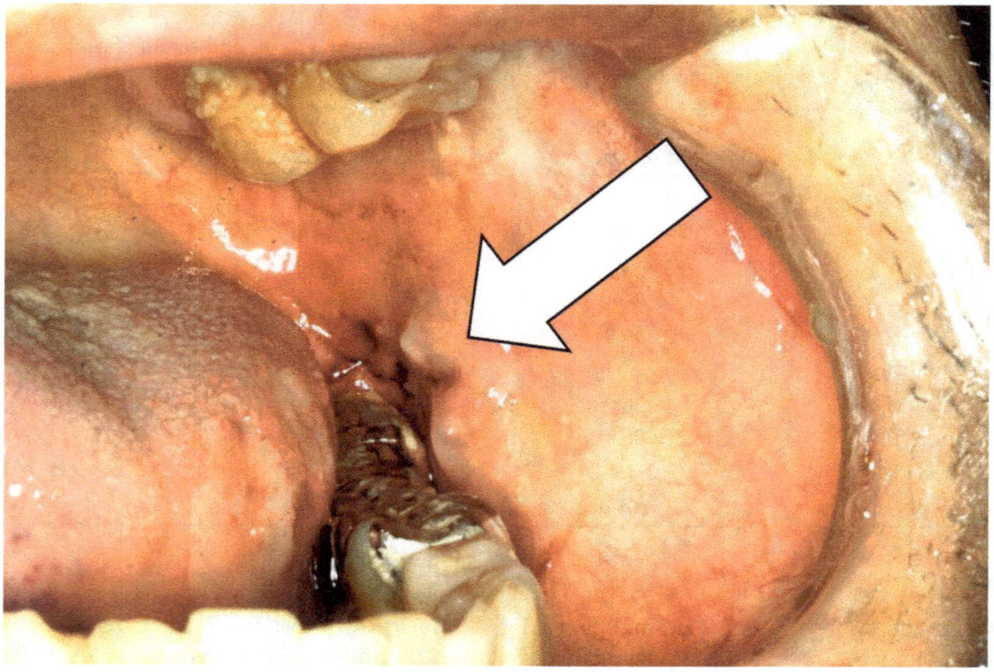

FIGURE 1: Oral findings in the patient at the initial visit. Ulcers are visible on the left buccal mucosa. Moreover, an erosion is seen on the tongue. Open arrow: cytomegalovirus-associated ulcer.

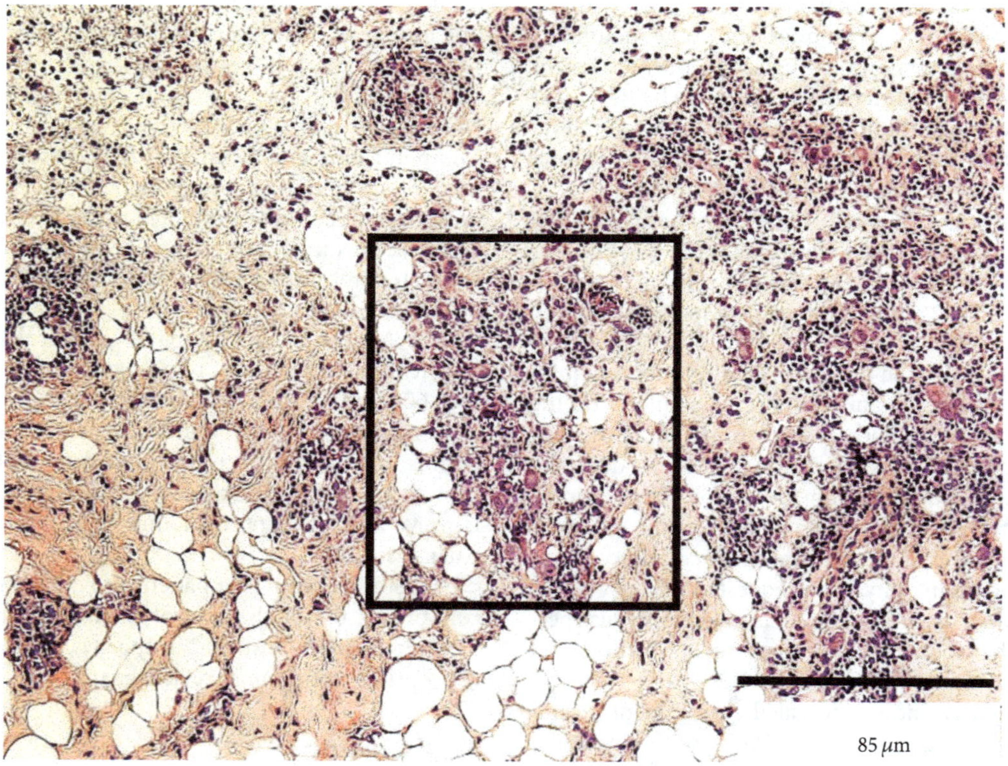

FIGURE 2: Histopathological findings of the specimen obtained from the biopsy of the ulcer. The black box shows vascular endothelial cells containing enlarged nuclei with intranuclear inclusions (hematoxylin-eosin staining). Bar: 85 μm.

hosts could be infected. Occasionally, CMV infection may be associated with serious and potentially fatal CMV-related manifestations, such as pneumonia, peptic ulcer, retinitis, and/or encephalitis.

A few reports of intraoral CMV infection [4, 14] in the form of nonspecific ulcers on the lips, palate, tongue, and gingiva [14] have been documented. Moreover, several cases of CMV infection associated with HIV infection, malignant

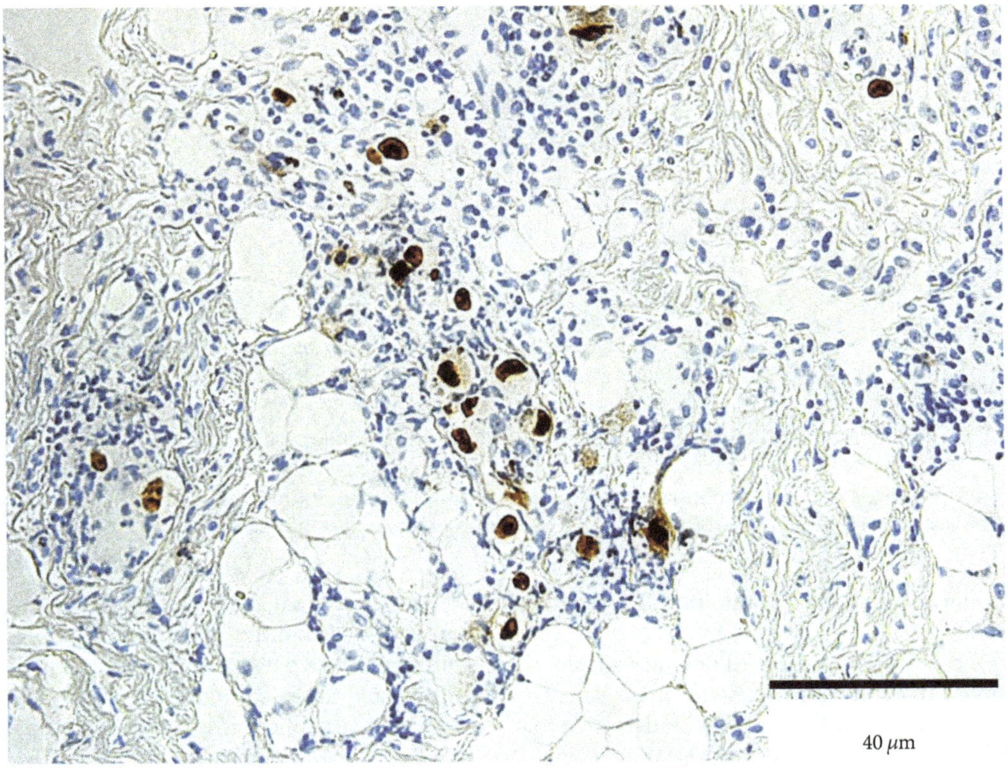

FIGURE 3: Findings from immunohistochemical staining of the specimen obtained from ulcer biopsy. Anticytomegalovirus antibodies are detected in the nuclei of infected cells. Bar: 40 μm.

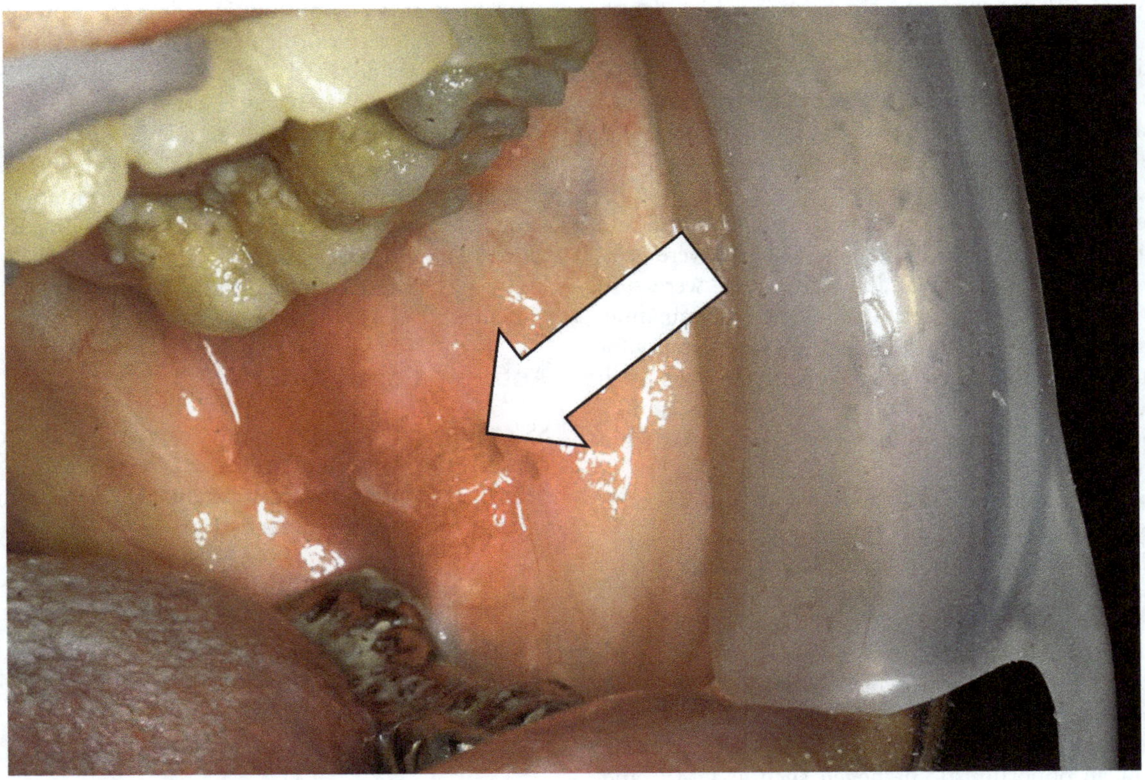

FIGURE 4: Oral findings on day 9 after initiation of ganciclovir therapy. A persistent ulcer on the left buccal mucosa is visible, with reduced signs of inflammation. Open arrow: cytomegalovirus-associated ulcer.

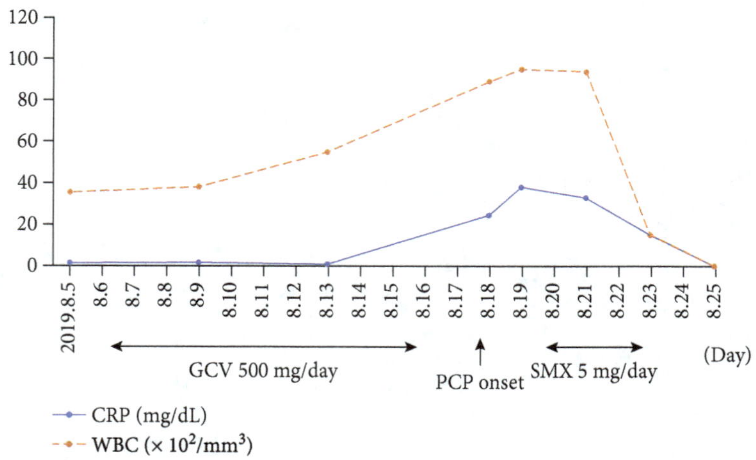

FIGURE 5: CRP and WBC levels and the administered medications during hospitalization are shown. CRP: C-reactive protein; WBC: leukocytes; GCV: ganciclovir; PCP: pneumocystis pneumonia; SMX: sulfamethoxazole-trimethoprim.

lymphoma, organ transplantation, and autoimmune diseases have been reported.

In contrast, few reports have described oral ulcers caused by CMV in patients with adult nephrotic syndrome, presenting with fatigue, edema, and proteinuria [15], rather than in patients with graft-versus-host disease [16], HIV, or malignant lymphoma. The oral findings in this case included generalized inflamed gingiva and an ulcer on the left buccal mucosa.

A diagnosis of CMV infection can be confirmed by virus isolation; the presence of antigenemia, which detects polymorphonuclear leukocytes that are positive for the viral antigen pp65 [17, 18]; polymerase chain reaction, which detects viral DNA; nucleic acid sequence-based amplification, which detects viral mRNA; and CMV-specific immunoglobulin M antibody analysis. However, in the present case, a histopathological assessment was performed, because infected endothelial cells and fibroblasts could be observed easily in the samples obtained from the ulcer.

In the specimen obtained from our patient, the nuclei and cytoplasm of hematoxylin and eosin-stained cells were positive for the viral antigens, and positive cells were also observed during the immunohistopathological examination. Particularly, vascular endothelial cells show high affinity for CMV and harbor the virus [19]. The infected cells swell and rupture, impeding blood flow and leading to ulceration. Our patient was immunocompromised owing to steroid treatment for membranous nephropathy, and the swelling of the vascular endothelial cells caused by intranuclear inclusions may have led to the circulatory disturbance.

In principle, antiviral medications such as ganciclovir are indicated for CMV infections (e.g., interstitial pneumonia, retinitis, and/or enteritis) [9, 19, 20]. As a result, CMV antigenemia improved from 546/434 to 3/3.

The patient presented with renal dysfunction and developed pneumocystis pneumonia after the onset of the clinical CMV infection. Pneumocystis pneumonia is a serious manifestation of an opportunistic pathogen such as CMV, and previous reports have documented concurrent CMV infection and pneumocystis pneumonia in patients with HIV [21].

The dose and duration of ganciclovir therapy with respect to immune dysfunction were appropriate. The susceptibility of the patient to pneumocystis pneumonia could be attributed to the steroid therapy initiated for the original membranous nephropathy and the myelosuppression as a side effect of ganciclovir therapy.

Our findings also show the relationship between CMV infection and pneumocystis pneumonia. Potentially, the pneumocystis pneumonia in our patient may have been related to the immunocompromised state induced by the steroid use and/or myelosuppression, which is an adverse reaction associated with ganciclovir therapy. Myelosuppression can be prevented by preemptive administration of ganciclovir, which can result in significant dose reduction compared to the normal dose [21].

In conclusion, we report a case of oral ulcer caused by CMV infection in a patient with membranous nephropathy, which was severe and showed atypical manifestations. CMV infections in the oral cavity are not common. However, close collaboration with medical departments is essential when an immunocompromised patient with oral CMV infection is encountered, considering the possibility of a negative outcome.

Authors' Contributions

SS conceived this report, drafted the article, and revised it critically for important intellectual content. TM and TT helped in drafting the manuscript. All authors have read and approved the final manuscript.

Acknowledgments

We would like to express our sincere thanks for Dr. Daiki Ito of JCHO Sendai Hospital Renal Center for his advice on the patient's general condition.

References

[1] A. C. Jones, P. D. Freedman, J. A. Phelan, R. A. Baughman, and S. M. Kerpel, "Cytomegalovirus infections of the oral cavity,"

Oral Surgery Oral Medicine Oral Pathology, vol. 75, no. 1, pp. 76–85, 1993.

[2] A. D. Friedman, W. G. Maurer, M. C. Byrd, J. R. Cook, and R. R. Lorenz, "A cytomegalovirus-associated mass presenting with laryngeal obstruction," *Archives of Otolaryngology-Head & Neck Surgery*, vol. 132, no. 12, pp. 1375–1378, 2006.

[3] J. E. Grundy, "Virologic and pathogenetic aspects of cytomegalovirus infection," *Review of Infectious Diseases*, vol. 12, Supplement_7, pp. S711–S719, 1990.

[4] S. Palmason, "How do we manage oral infections in allogeneic stem cell transplantation and other severely immunocompromised patients?," *Oral & Maxillofacial Surgery Clinics of North America*, vol. 23, no. 4, pp. 579–599, 2011.

[5] T. Mori, S. Mori, Y. Kanda et al., "Clinical significance of cytomegalovirus (CMV) antigenemia in the prediction and diagnosis of CMV gastrointestinal disease after allogeneic hematopoietic stem cell transplantation," *Bone Marrow Transplantation*, vol. 33, no. 4, pp. 431–434, 2004.

[6] M. Boeckh, R. A. Bowden, J. M. Goodrich, M. Pettinger, and J. D. Meyers, "Cytomegalovirus antigen detection in peripheral blood leukocytes after allogeneic marrow transplantation," *Blood*, vol. 80, no. 5, pp. 1358–1364, 1992.

[7] J. F. Apperley and J. M. Goldman, "Cytomegalovirus: biology, clinical features and methods for diagnosis," *Bone Marrow Transplantation*, vol. 3, no. 4, pp. 253–264, 1988.

[8] P. Ljungman, P. Griffiths, and C. Paya, "Definitions of cytomegalovirus infection and disease in transplant recipients," *Clinical Infectious Diseases*, vol. 34, no. 8, pp. 1094–1097, 2002.

[9] F. Brown, L. Banken, K. Saywell, and I. Arum, "Pharmacokinetics of valganciclovir and ganciclovir following multiple oral dosages of valganciclovir in HIV- and CMV-seropositive volunteers," *Clinical Pharmacokinetics*, vol. 37, no. 2, pp. 167–176, 1999.

[10] N. Besbas, U. S. Bayrakci, G. Kale et al., "Cytomegalovirus-related congenital nephrotic syndrome with diffuse mesangial sclerosis," *Pediatric Nephrology*, vol. 21, no. 5, pp. 740–742, 2006.

[11] J. E. Vidal, R. F. Dauar, A. C. Penalva de Oliveira, J. F. G. S. Coelho, and D. L. M. Lins, "Cerebral mass lesion due to cytomegalovirus in a patient with AIDS: case report and literature review," *Revista do Instituto de Medicina Tropical de São Paulo*, vol. 45, no. 6, pp. 333–337, 2003.

[12] F. G. LeVeque, V. Ratanatharathorn, M. E. Dan, B. Orville, D. N. Coleman, and S. Turner, "Oral cytomegalovirus infection in an unrelated bone marrow transplantation with possible mediation by graft-versus-host disease and the use of cyclosporin-A," *Oral Surgery Oral Medicine Oral Pathology*, vol. 77, no. 3, pp. 248–253, 1994.

[13] M. Yamaguchi, M. Ando, R. Yamamoto et al., "Patient age and the prognosis of idiopathic membranous nephropathy," *PLoS One*, vol. 9, no. 10, article e110376, 2014.

[14] M. Boeckh, T. A. Gooley, D. Myerson, T. Cunningham, G. Schoch, and R. A. Bowden, "Cytomegalovirus pp65 antigenemia-guided early treatment with ganciclovir versus ganciclovir at engraftment after allogeneic marrow transplantation: a randomized double-blind study," *Blood*, vol. 88, no. 10, pp. 4063–4071, 1996.

[15] J. B. Epstein, C. H. Sherlock, and R. A. Wolber, "Oral manifestations of cytomegalovirus infection," *Oral Surgery, Oral Medicine, Oral Pathology*, vol. 75, no. 4, pp. 443–451, 1993.

[16] M. Boeckh, W. Leisenring, S. R. Riddell et al., "Late cytomegalovirus disease and mortality in recipients of allogeneic hematopoietic stem cell transplants: importance of viral load and T-cell immunity," *Blood*, vol. 101, no. 2, pp. 407–414, 2003.

[17] for Fukuoka Blood and Marrow Transplant Group (FBMTG), K. Takenaka, T. Eto et al., "Oral valganciclovir as preemptive therapy is effective for cytomegalovirus infection in allogeneic hematopoietic stem cell transplant recipients," *International Journal of Hematology*, vol. 89, no. 2, pp. 231–237, 2009.

[18] J. Alcami, T. Barzu, and S. Michelson, "Induction of an endothelial cell growth factor by human cytomegalovirus infection of fibroblasts," *Journal of General Virology*, vol. 72, no. 11, pp. 2765–2770, 1991.

[19] D. J. Winston, L. R. Baden, D. A. Gabriel et al., "Pharmacokinetics of ganciclovir after oral valganciclovir versus intravenous ganciclovir in allogeneic stem cell transplant patients with graft-versus-host disease of the gastrointestinal tract," *Biology of Blood and Marrow Transplantation*, vol. 12, no. 6, pp. 635–640, 2006.

[20] M. M. Polaczek, J. Zych, K. Oniszh, J. Szopiński, J. Grudny, and K. Roszkowski-Śliż, "Pneumocystis pneumonia in HIV-infected patients with cytomegalovirus co-infection. Two case reports and a literature review," *Pneumonologia i Aalergologia Polska*, vol. 82, no. 5, pp. 458–466, 2014.

[21] T. Mori, S. Okamoto, R. Watanabe et al., "Dose-adjusted preemptive therapy for cytomegalovirus disease based on real-time polymerase chain reaction after allogeneic hematopoietic stem cell transplantation," *Bone Marrow Transplantation*, vol. 29, no. 9, pp. 777–782, 2002.

27

Trefoil System for the Treatment of Mandibular Edentulism: A Case Report with 30 Months Follow-Up

Andrea E. Borgonovo, Simone L. M. Galbiati, and Dino Re

Department of Aesthetic Dentistry, University of Milan, Istituto Stomatologico Italiano, Milan, Italy

Correspondence should be addressed to Simone L. M. Galbiati; simone.galbiati92@gmail.com

Academic Editor: Jamil Awad Shibli

The purpose of this work is to describe a clinical case of full-arch mandible rehabilitation with a fixed prosthesis on three implants. The chosen protocol is the Trefoil system by Nobel (Nobel Biocare, Zurich, Switzerland) that allows to realize a mandibular fixed rehabilitation on three particularly designed fixtures through the use of prefabricated surgical guides and a preassembled bar on which the prosthesis is built. Both surgical and prosthetic procedures were completed without complications, and after 30 months, the rehabilitations are in good health conditions. The patient is able to maintain a good level of hygiene and is satisfied with the work from an aesthetic and functional point of view.

1. Introduction

After tooth loss, which occurs more often in senior people, when the rehabilitation involves a fixed prosthesis on implants, the ideal solution would be alveolar ridge regeneration [1–4]. This kind of surgery is aimed at restoring the correct bone anatomy and allows the insertion of more implants, particularly in the molar region, thus creating a prosthesis without distal cantilever and orthopedic resin gingiva. The survival rate of dental implants is high, regardless of the bone augmentation technique chosen, but such procedures require great operator skills and a long healing period [5, 6]. Moreover, they imply high morbidity and treatment costs, and they need strong patient compliance to achieve clinical success.

The economic aspect of the rehabilitation often guides patients in their choice and, when it is possible, they prefer fixed rehabilitations instead of removable. The aim of modern dentistry is, therefore, to develop minimally invasive rehabilitations that ensure function, aesthetics, comfort, and cost containment.

In the case of edentulous mandible, the Branemark protocol with five axial fixtures between the two mandibular foramina has undergone several changes over the years. Immediate loading has almost routinely replaced conventional loading protocols with long-term predictability and success rate [7, 8]. Malò and Rangert introduced the greatest innovation regarding the number of implants thanks to his all-on-four concept. This technique consists of the insertion of two axial implants in the lateral incisor/canine area and two fixtures just anterior to the foramina intentionally tilted distally about 30° relative to the occlusal plane which thus merging at the second premolar position. This arrangement allows for good implant anchorage, short cantilever length, and large interimplant distance [9]; moreover, it can also be used with six implants.

The implants number is further decreased in the Branemark Novum Concept with only three fixtures. This protocol involves prefabricated components, elimination of the impression procedure, and attachment of the permanent fixed bridge on the day of implant placement [10–12].

The Trefoil system by Nobel Biocare (Nobel Biocare, Zurich, Switzerland) is an evolution of the Branemark Novum Concept. Three particularly designed fixtures are placed in the anterior part of the mandible using drilling templates and then immediately splinted with a prefabricated titanium bar. This bar simplifies the creation of the final acrylic prosthesis and saves time for both the clinician and the laboratory. It is anatomically designed for the natural curvature of the mandible, it features adaptable joints that adjust to compensate for horizontal, and vertical and angular deviations from the ideal implant position and allow passive fit of the final prosthesis. The aim of this work is to show a clinical case realized with this technique.

2. Case Presentation

A male patient aged 65 and in good health conditions required a complete rehabilitation of the jaw. As it can be observed in the orthopantomography (Figure 1), he was completely edentulous and used two conventional removable prosthesis. It was decided to rehabilitate his lower jaw with Nobel Trefoil system surgical protocol.

After locoregional anesthesia into the vestibular and lingual mucosa of the mandible, a crestal incision connecting the two first molar regions was performed, and the alveolar ridge was exposed. The lingual flap was then sutured with a 2/0 silk suture in order to facilitate surgical proceedings and improve visibility.

Once the vestibular and the lingual mucosa had been protected with retractors, the surgeon regularized the alveolar ridge with an osteotomy drill. The aim of this step is to obtain a flat surface and an adequate thickness on the ridge for the application of the surgical guides and the following implant insertion (Figure 2).

With a pilot drill, the surgeon performed a guide bore in the center of the mandible and verified the correct orientation in occlusion with a parallelism pin. After that, the first surgical guide was positioned and fixed with a pin in the cavity previously drilled. The same guide has two other bores where the two distal implants will be placed. In these positions with the pilot drill, two new guide perforations were performed and used to fix the surgical guide. The first pin was thence removed and with the help of metal bushings of increasing diameter (from 3.00 mm to 5.00) mounted in the center bore on the guide the operator prepared the first implant site and inserted the fixture (Nobel Trefoil Implant 5.00 × 13 mm, Nobel Biocare, Zurich, Switzerland) (Figure 3).

The surgical guide was removed and a new one was initially fixed on the implant. This second guide differs from the first because of the presence of two further bores next to the central one which is used to lock the guide and prevent it from rotating. Once this guide was completely locked even with appropriate pins in the cavities described, the bores in correspondence of the distal implants were, therefore, free and ready for the site preparation. A surgical template with metal bushings on its ends, different from that used for the first implant, was applied on the surgical guide and used to prepare the distal implants sites (Figure 4).

When the insertion of the distal fixtures (Nobel Trefoil Implant 5.00 × 13 mm, Nobel Biocare, Zurich, Switzerland) was completed even, the second guide was removed, and the prefabricated titanium bar was screwed onto the implants to check its fitting (Figure 5).

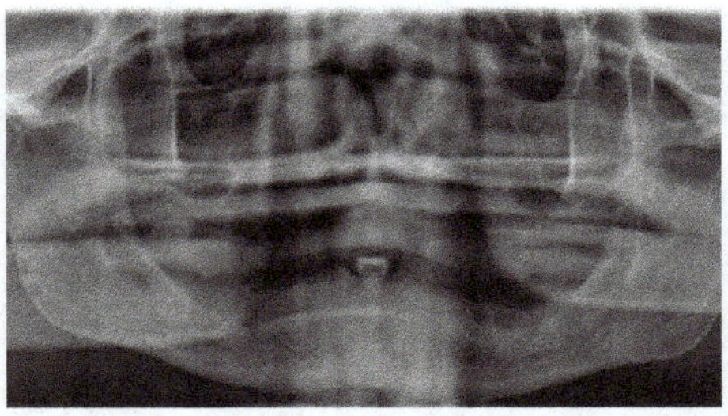

Figure 1: Preoperatory panoramic radiograph.

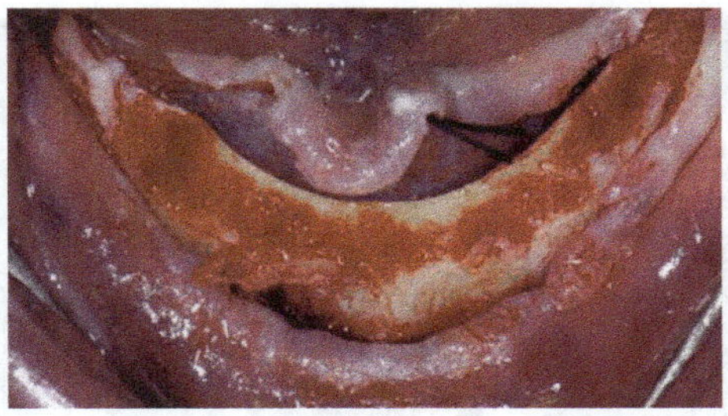

Figure 2: The alveolar ridge after the osteotomy: the flat surface is necessary for the application of the surgical templates.

Next, the bar was substituted with the healing caps so that the surgeon could suture the flap around them with 4/0 resorbable thread (Figure 6).

As a last step, the transfers were placed on the implants and splinted together with composite in order to give the technician the right position of the fixture to build the prosthesis on the titanium bar (Figure 7).

About four hours after the surgery, the prosthesis was screwed on the implants and functionalized in occlusion (Figure 8).

The patient underwent a follow-up program and orthopantomographies were taken at six, eighteen, and thirty months after the surgery (Figure 9). The fixtures and the prosthesis appeared in good health both clinically and radiographically during the last control visit.

3. Discussion

The aim of reducing the number of implants in full arch fixed rehabilitations is to avoid complex and invasive surgeries such as bone augmentation and/or gingival grafts, improve hygiene maintenance, and reduce costs [13].

According to some reviews, full-arch fixed dental prosthesis in mandible supported by 2 to 4 implants exhibit a low rate of failures for implants and prostheses, a low rate of MBL, and a low rate of biomechanical and biological complications. One of these works, particularly, states that fixed prosthesis on three implants, when analyzed separately, has the lowest cumulative survival rates compared to the other group even if it is anyway high (95.5%). No statistically significant difference has been found in outcomes (implant and prosthesis survival) for full-arch FDPs in the mandible supported by less than five implants when compared to five or more implants. However, using 4–6 implants is a well-

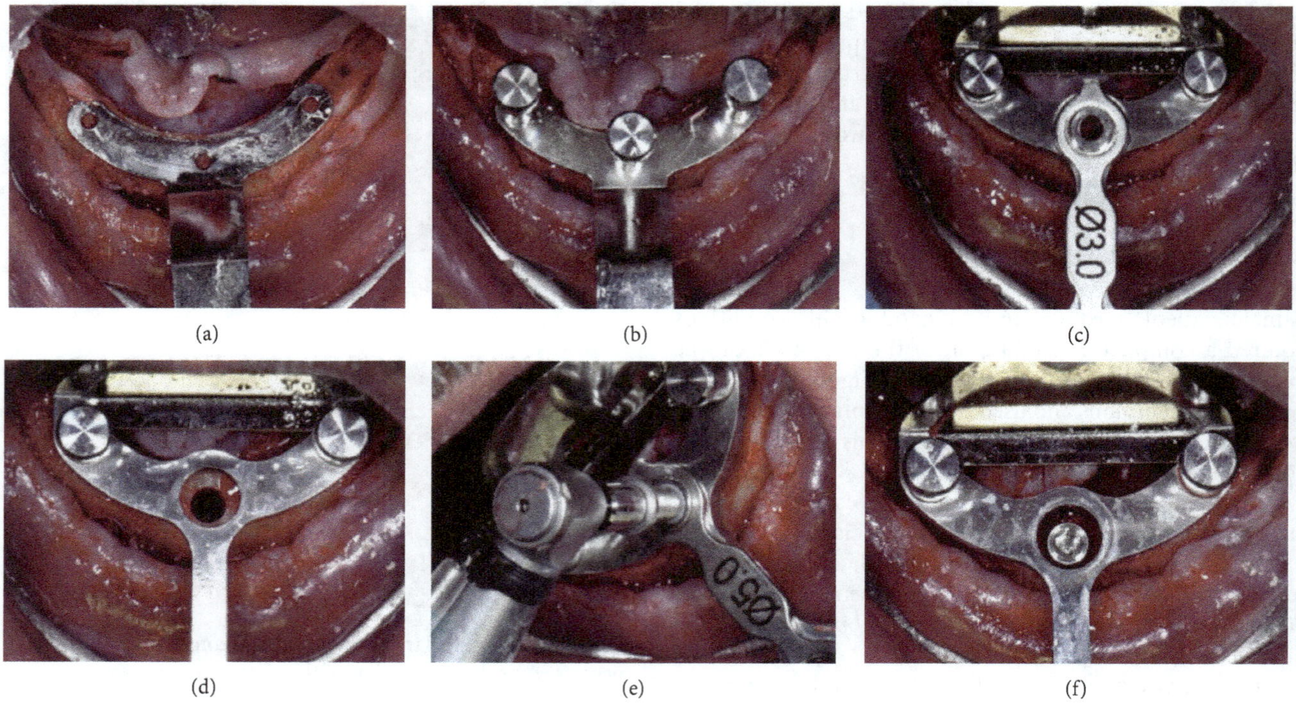

FIGURE 3: Intraoral view of the surgical steps (1): the first surgical guide is placed (a) and fixed (b), the central implant site is prepared thanks to metal bushings of increasing diameter (c, d), and the fixture is inserted (e, f).

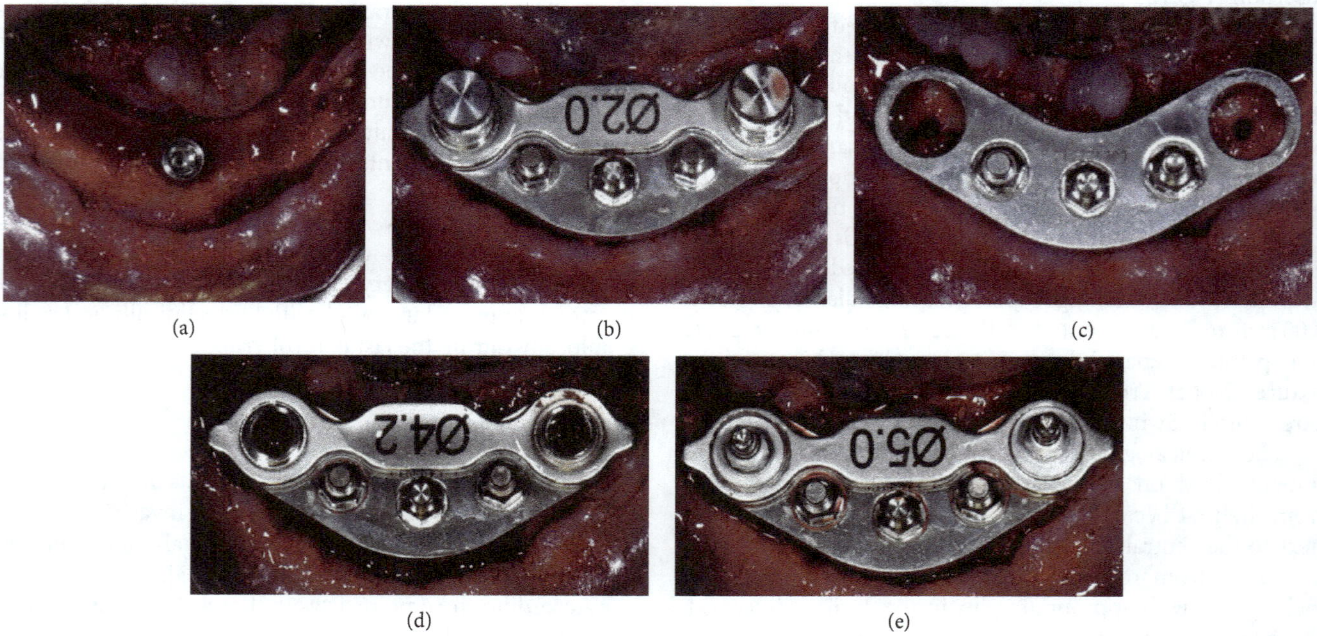

FIGURE 4: Intraoral view of the surgical steps (2): the first surgical guide is removed (a) and the second is placed and fixed (b, c), the distal implants sites are prepared thanks to metal bushings of increasing diameter (d), and the fixtures are inserted (e).

documented treatment option with high estimated 5-year survival of the construction, whereas it is unclear whether three implants for supporting a FAFDP will achieve similar survival rates [4, 13, 14].

The use of only three fixtures to support a full arch rehabilitation is not yet, therefore, confirmed in literature with specific systematic reviews or meta-analysis. Preliminary results of a recent study suggest that immediately loaded cross-arch prostheses can be supported by only three dental implants at least up to 1-year postloading but the Authors stated that longer follow-ups are needed to properly evaluate this therapeutic option [15].

Other works about all-on-three implants rehabilitation, like Branemark Novum Concept protocol, of which Trefoil

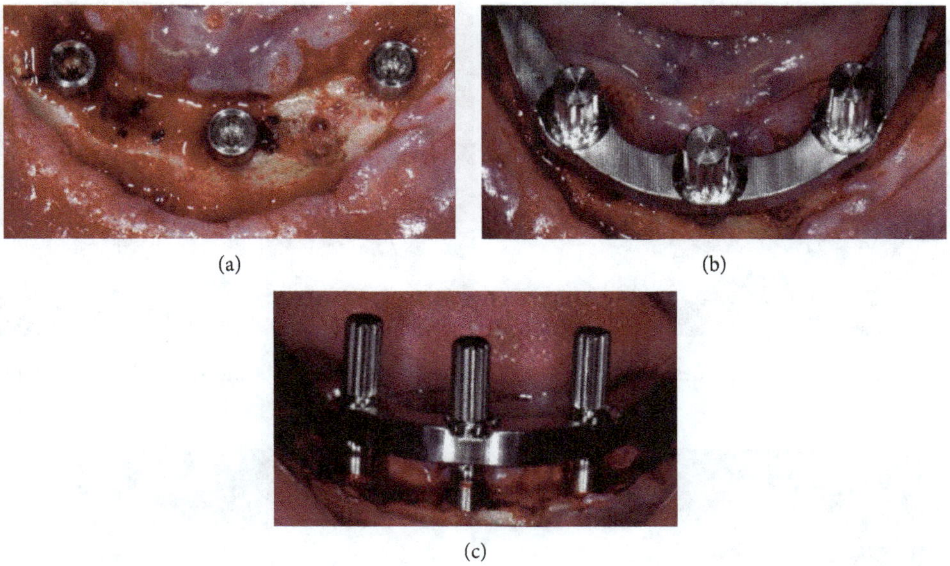

Figure 5: All the implants are placed (a), and the prefabricated titanium bar is screwed on the fixtures (b, c).

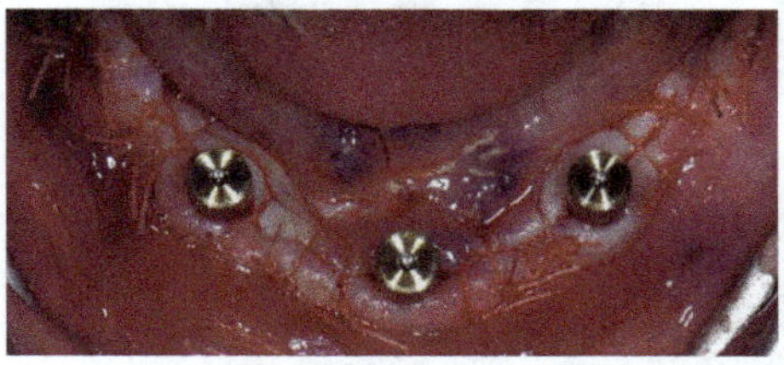

Figure 6: The surgical flap is sutured around the healing caps.

represents the evolution, reported promising and encouraging outcomes with high survival rates both for implants and prosthesis but immediate loading seemed to be associated with lower survival of individual fixtures [10, 11]. A retrospective study with a 5-year follow-up about three implants (all-on-three) supporting a delayed loaded fixed prosthesis, indeed, showed that no implants were lost, giving a 100% success rate. The Authors stated that within the limits of the small group clinical study (24 patients and 72 implants), the high survival rate of the all-on-three protocol with delayed loading may be a viable concept [16].

A recent study with a long follow-up period (16 years) demonstrated very good long-term outcomes for the Branemark Novum protocol. No implant failed (CSR 100%) and no prosthesis needed to be substituted (CSR 100%). Only one biologic complication was detected on a central implant (crater-form bone destruction), and several prosthodontic complications occurred during the 16 years (fractures of resin or teeth), the majority of which were registered on the same parafunctional patient [12].

In the Authors' opinion, the Trefoil system is a valid therapeutic solution for the treatment of mandibular edentulism not only from the economic point of view. Fewer implants together with prefabricated components help to reduce cost and also to save time. The estimate of the active working time is in fact about six hours from the beginning of the surgery to the screwing of the prosthesis on the same day. It should be emphasized that the protocol suggested by Nobel provides for the immediate realization of the final prosthesis while usually in full arch rehabilitation cases a provisional one is needed. This leads to time-saving in the treatment plan of about 3-6 months.

On the other hand, the surgical protocol is not as simple as it may appear and the clinician must be well trained in order to manage any complication during the surgery such as proximity to the mental foramen which can lead to an intraoperative change of strategy. Moreover, it seems to be indicated for specific cases with a particular mandibular shape not very widespread in Italy and Europe but, particularly, in South America. At last, similar rehabilitations can be realized nowadays thanks to different technologies at our disposal. Digital, for example, allows us to plan the intervention and realize the prosthesis even before implant insertion with good reliability and similar savings in costs and time but with less complexity in the surgical phase.

4. Conclusion

In the realization of this particular clinical case, the Trefoil system proved to be a good surgical protocol and, after 30 months follow-up, the rehabilitation appeared in good health both for fixtures and the prosthesis. Moreover, the patient was satisfied with the work from an aesthetic, functional, and hygienic maintenance point of view.

In our opinion, this protocol can be useful in edentulous patients who present not only economic needs in the treatment plan but also short realization times. Both requests are achieved thanks to the use of prefabricated components.

Nevertheless, a wider number of cases with a long follow-up period are needed to provide a more correct assessment of the protocol.

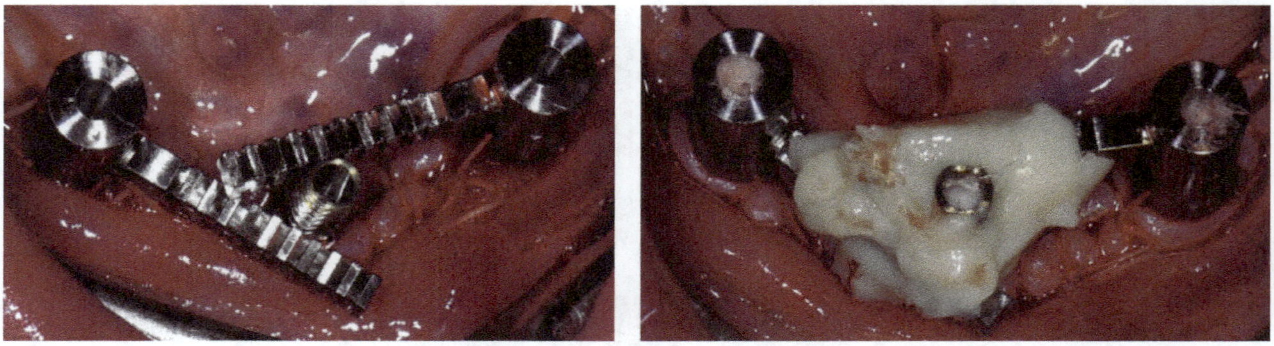

Figure 7: Three particularly designed transfers are screwed on the implants and splinted with composite.

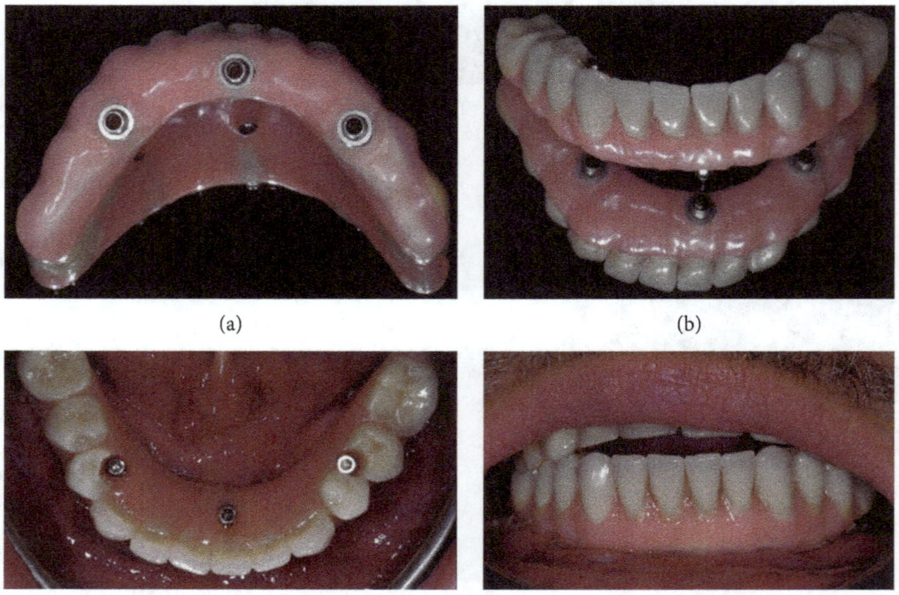

(a) (b) (c) (d)

Figure 8: Extraoral view of the prosthesis before its insertion (a, b) and intraoral occlusal (c) and buccal (d) view once it has been screwed.

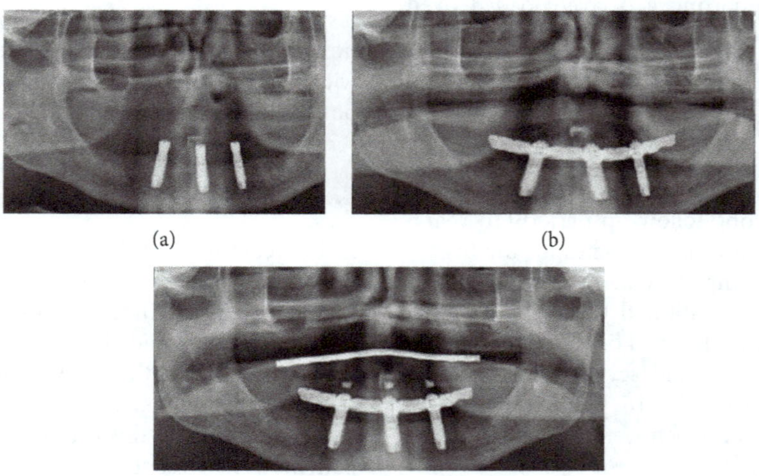

(a) (b) (c)

Figure 9: The OPT was taken immediately after the surgery (a), at six months (b), and during the last control visit (30 months).

References

[1] N. U. Zitzmann, E. Hagmann, and R. Weiger, "What is the prevalence of various types of prosthetic dental restorations in Europe?," *Clinical Oral Implants Research*, vol. 18, Supplement 3, pp. 20–33, 2007.

[2] N. U. Zitzmann, C. P. Marinello, E. Zemp, P. Kessler, and U. Ackermann-Liebrich, "Tooth loss, dental restorations and dental attendance in Switzerland," *Schweizer Monatsschrift fur Zahnmedizin= Revue mensuelle suisse d'odonto-stomatologie= Rivista mensile svizzera di odontologia e stomatologia*, vol. 111, pp. 1288–1294, 2001.

[3] N. U. Zitzmann, K. Staehelin, A. W. G. Walls, G. Menghini, R. Weiger, and E. Zemp Stutz, "Changes in oral health over a 10-yr period in Switzerland," *European Journal of Oral Sciences*, vol. 116, no. 1, pp. 52–59, 2008.

[4] G. Heydecke, M. Zwahlen, A. Nicol et al., "What is the optimal number of implants for fixed reconstructions: a systematic review," *Clinical Oral Implants Research*, vol. 23, Supplement 6, pp. 217–228, 2012.

[5] B. Elnayef, A. Monje, G. Albiol, P. Galindo-Moreno, H. L. Wang, and F. Hernández-Alfaro, "Vertical ridge augmentation in the atrophic mandible: a systematic review and meta-analysis," *The International Journal of Oral & Maxillofacial Implants*, vol. 32, no. 2, pp. 291–312, 2017.

[6] R. J. de Groot, M. A. E. M. Oomens, T. Forouzanfar, and E. A. J. M. Schulten, "Bone augmentation followed by implant surgery in the edentulous mandible: a systematic review," *Journal of Oral Rehabilitation*, vol. 45, no. 4, pp. 334–343, 2018.

[7] P. Papaspyridakos, C. J. Chen, S. K. Chuang, and H. P. Weber, "Implant loading protocols for edentulous patients with fixed prostheses: a systematic review and meta-analysis," *The International Journal of Oral & Maxillofacial Implants*, vol. 29, Supplement, pp. 256–270, 2014.

[8] M. Del Fabbro, T. Testori, V. Kekovic, F. Goker, M. Tumedei, and H. L. Wang, "A systematic review of survival rates of osseointegrated implants in fully and partially edentulous patients following immediate loading," *Journal of Clinical Medicine*, vol. 8, no. 12, p. 2142, 2019.

[9] P. Maló, B. Rangert, and M. Nobre, ""All-on-Four" immediate-function concept with Brånemark System® implants for completely edentulous mandibles: a retrospective clinical study," *Clinical Implant Dentistry and Related Research*, vol. 5, Supplement 1, pp. 2–9, 2003.

[10] P. I. Brånemark, P. Engstrand, L. O. Ohrnell et al., "Brånemark Novum: a new treatment concept for rehabilitation of the edentulous mandible. Preliminary results from a prospective clinical follow-up study," *Clinical Implant Dentistry and Related Research*, vol. 1, no. 1, pp. 2–16, 1999.

[11] P. Engstrand, K. Grondahl, L. O. Öhrnell, P. Nilsson, U. Nannmark, and P. I. Branemark, "Prospective follow-up study of 95 patients with edentulous mandibles treated according to the Branemark Novum concept," *Clinical Implant Dentistry and Related Research*, vol. 5, no. 1, pp. 3–10, 2003.

[12] M. Menini, F. Bagnasco, P. Pera, T. Tealdo, and P. Pesce, "Brånemark Novum immediate loading rehabilitation of edentulous mandibles: case series with a 16-year follow-up," *The International Journal of Periodontics & Restorative Dentistry*, vol. 39, no. 5, pp. 729–735, 2019.

[13] V. Moraschini, G. Velloso, D. Luz, D. M. Cavalcante, and E. . S. P. Barboza, "Fixed rehabilitation of edentulous mandibles using 2 to 4 implants," *Implant Dentistry*, vol. 25, no. 3, pp. 435–444, 2016.

[14] D. Morton, G. Gallucci, W. S. Lin et al., "Group 2 ITI consensus report: prosthodontics and implant dentistry," *Clinical Oral Implants Research*, vol. 29, Supplement 16, pp. 215–223, 2018.

[15] G. Cannizzaro, I. Loi, P. Viola et al., "Immediate loading of two (fixed-on-2) versus three (fixed-on-3) implants placed flapless supporting cross-arch fixed prostheses: one-year results from a randomised controlled trial," *European Journal of Oral Implantology*, vol. 9, pp. 143–153, 2016.

[16] J. Oliva, X. Oliva, and J. D. Oliva, "All-on-three delayed implant loading concept for the completely edentulous maxilla and mandible: a retrospective 5-year follow-up study," *The International Journal of Oral & Maxillofacial Implants*, vol. 27, no. 6, pp. 1584–1592, 2012.

28

A Case of a Stafne Bone Defect Associated with Sublingual Glands in the Lingual Side of the Mandible

Kamichika Hayashi,[1] **Takeshi Onda**,[1] **Takahiro Iwasaki**,[1] **Mitsuru Takata**,[2] **Kiyotaka Mori**,[2] **Hiroyuki Matsuda**,[2] **Shinya Watanabe**,[2] **Hidetoshi Tamura**,[2] **Takahiko Shibahara**,[1] **and Masayuki Takano**[1]

[1]*Department of Oral and Maxillofacial Surgery, Tokyo Dental College, Tokyo, Japan*
[2]*Oral and Maxillofacial Surgery, Kameda General Hospital, Chiba, Japan*

Correspondence should be addressed to Kamichika Hayashi; hayashikamichika@tdc.ac.jp

Academic Editor: Pia L. Jornet

A Stafne bone defect from the mandibular anterior to the premolar region is an extremely rare case. A case of a Stafne bone defect extending from the mandibular anterior to the premolar region was presented. Computed tomography (CT) and magnetic resonance imaging (MRI) suggested that salivary gland tissue connected to the sublingual glands was involved in the formation of the cavity. The patient was a 68-year-old man who was examined at our hospital's emergency outpatient department after a traffic accident. He was referred to our department for the treatment of contusions of the lips and oral cavity. A bone defect in the lingual side of the mandible from the right anterior to the right premolar region was incidentally detected on CT. CT showed a rounded cavity in the lingual side of the mandible that had a lingual opening, was monocystic, and had a cortical margin. The margin of the cavity was relatively dull and regular. MRI showed that the tissue filling the cavity in the lingual side of the mandible had similar signal intensity as the sublingual glands and was contiguous with the normal sublingual glands. Based on these findings, the bone defect was diagnosed as a Stafne bone defect filled with salivary gland tissue connected to the sublingual gland tissue.

1. Introduction

The first case of a Stafne bone defect was reported by Stafne in 1942 [1]. Stafne bone defect are also known as the so-called Stafne bone cavity or static bone defect [2, 3]. A Stafne bone defect is a cavity in the lingual side of the mandible in the vicinity of the mandibular angle that is filled with salivary gland tissue, adipose tissue, lymphatic tissue, or other tissues. It is generally asymptomatic and is usually incidentally detected by oral-maxillofacial radiography [2]. Radiography depicts this condition as a unilocular radiolucent area with a clear boundary and a smooth margin. It is sometimes suspected to be a cyst or tumor in the jawbone [4]. Usually, a Stafne bone defect is found inferior to the mandibular canal from the mandibular molars to the mandibular angle [5]. A case with a Stafne bone defect from the mandibular anterior to the premolar region that appeared to be filled with salivary gland tissue connected to the sublingual glands is reported, along with a short discussion of the literature.

2. Case Presentation

Fully informed consent for publication of clinical information relating to this case was obtained from the patient.

The patient was a 68-year-old man who was examined at our hospital's emergency outpatient department after his face was struck by the steering wheel during a traffic accident. The emergency room doctor performed computed tomography (CT), which showed no abnormalities of the internal organs or brain. That same day, he was referred to our department for the treatment of contusions of the lips and oral cavity. No abnormal findings in his medical history or family history were noted. When he arrived at the hospital, he was in pain and bleeding from the contusions, but there were no signs of nerve paralysis or infection. The contusions of the lips and oral mucosa were debrided and sutured.

The CT performed in the emergency department showed no fractures anywhere. However, it showed a cavity in the lingual side of the mandible from the right anterior to the premolar region. CT in hard tissue mode showed a high-density line, suggesting cortical bone on the margin of the cavity in the lingual side of the mandible (Figure 1). The lingual cortical bone was recessed from the lingual side to the buccal side and, at the most recessed point, was contiguous with the buccal cortical bone (Figure 2). There was no continuity between the apex of the adjacent #27 and the cavity in the lingual side of the mandible, and a high-density line suggested the presence of bony tissue between the apex of #27 and the cavity in the lingual side of the mandible. There was no continuity between the cavity in the lingual side of the mandible and the mandibular canal. CT in soft tissue mode showed that the inside of the cavity in the lingual side of the mandible had similar soft tissue density (CT number, 40–70 Hounsfield units (HU)) to the sublingual glands (CT number, 40–60 HU) and was contiguous with the sublingual glands (Figure 3). Based on these CT findings, our presumed diagnosis was a Stafne bone defect.

In 3 months after the first examination, magnetic resonance imaging (MRI) was performed to examine the tissue inside the cavity in the lingual side of the mandible. The area exhibited greater hyperintensity than the muscle and similar signal intensity to the sublingual gland tissue on T1-weighted and T2-weighted images and was filled with soft tissue contiguous with the sublingual glands. Short T1 inversion recovery images showed no signs of tumors or inflammation in the surrounding area. A final diagnosis of a Stafne bone defect was established based on the presence of a cavity in the lingual side of the mandible from the right anterior to the premolar region that was filled with salivary gland tissue connected to the sublingual gland tissue (Figures 4 and 5). Subsequently, regular imaging was performed, and the patient was followed up.

Abnormal findings had not been observed 12 months after the first examination.

3. Discussion

In general, static bone cavities are often observed near the mandibular angle starting posterior to the mandibular molars. In panoramic radiographs, the cavity usually appears as a single cystic bone defect with a distinct round boundary surrounded by radiolucent tissue. Cavities are often detected incidentally [5]. The probability rate of incidentally discovering a Stafne bone defect in panoramic radiography is 0.08%–0.7%, which is predominantly observed in men in their 40s or 50s [4]. In addition, static bone cavities are less common in the front teeth and premolar areas. The probability rate of discovering a monocystic radiolucent area with a distinct boundary around the front teeth or premolars in panoramic radiography is 0.009% [5]. Schneider proposed a diagnostic algorithm for static bone cavities in panoramic radiographs, but this is not considered suitable for static bone cavities around the anterior region because of the narrow tomographic area in panoramic radiographs in this area, the overlapping shadows of the cervical spine, and other factors [6].

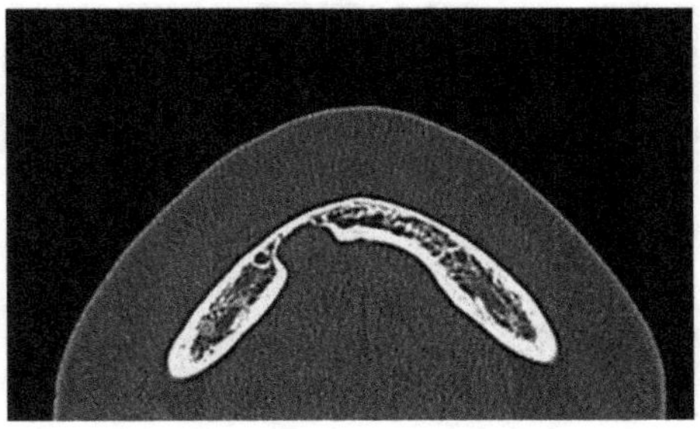

FIGURE 1: Computed tomography image, horizontal cross section, hard tissue mode. A rounded cavity is observed in the lingual side of the mandible from the right anterior to the premolar region. The margin of the cavity in the lingual side of the mandible is a high-density line, suggesting cortical bone, and is smooth. The mandibular canal is not connected with the cavity.

CT and MRI are useful for diagnosing static bone cavities[2]. CT is particularly effective for morphological evaluations of the mandible. Some studies have considered CT to be the most effective tool for diagnosing static bone cavities [7], whereas others have found that CT is insufficient and MRI is the most effective tool [8]. CT is generally the first choice if abnormal findings are observed in radiographs [9]. CT findings of a Stafne bone defect include a rounded cavity in the lingual side of the mandible that has a lingual opening, is monocystic, and has a cortical margin. The margin of the cavity is relatively dull and regular. A Stafne bone defect can be diagnosed when these findings are observed, and no additional tests are considered necessary [5, 10]. CT-sialography is more useful than plain CT when investigating connections with the major salivary glands [11]. However, because it is difficult to selectively contrast the sublingual glands to examine associated lesions, CT-sialography is considered inappropriate.

Compared to CT, MRI involves no radiation exposure and has higher histological resolution and is thus suitable for depicting the properties of tissue filling the cavity in the lingual side of the mandible [12, 13]. MRI is particularly useful for examining tissue filling the cavity in the lingual side of the mandible. If MRI suggests that the tissue is normal, additional tests that are surgically invasive can be avoided [12]. Furthermore, MRI can visualize the cortical bone and marrow of the mandible. In the present case, it was confirmed that the cavity in the lingual side of the mandible had a cortical margin, and because the signal intensity of the tissue in the cavity in the lingual side of the mandible was similar to that of the sublingual gland tissue, the presence of a tumorous lesion was unlikely, and it was considered normal salivary gland tissue. Combining CT and MRI improves the reliability in diagnosing a Stafne bone defect [2].

The exact pathogenesis has not been clarified yet. Previous theories of the origins of static bone cavities include those

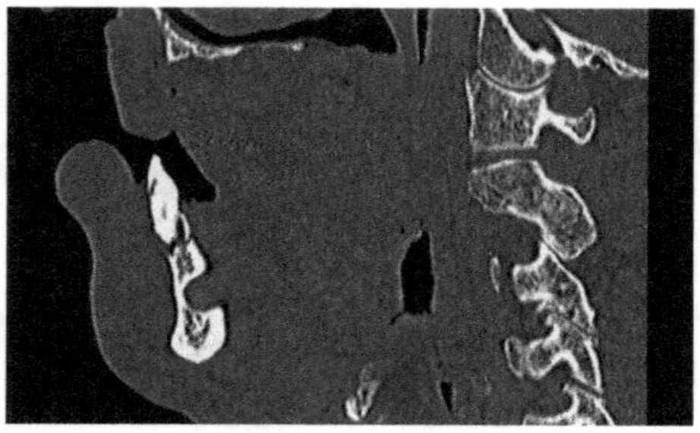

FIGURE 2: Computed tomography image, sagittal cross section, hard tissue mode. The lingual cortical bone recessed from the lingual to the buccal side is contiguous with the buccal cortical bone at the deepest point of the cavity. There is no connection of the apex of the adjacent #27 with the cavity in the lingual side of the mandible, and a high-density line suggests the presence of bony tissue between the apex of #27 and the cavity in the lingual side of the mandible.

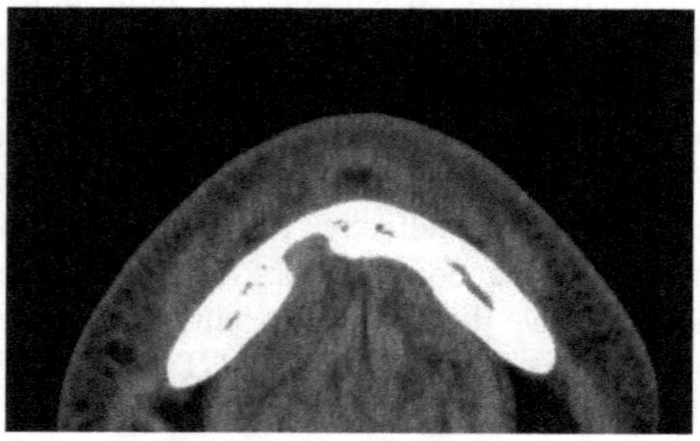

FIGURE 3: Computed tomography (CT) image, horizontal cross section, soft tissue mode. The inside of the cavity in the lingual side of the mandible has similar soft tissue density (CT number, 40–70 Hounsfield units (HU)) to the sublingual glands (CT number, 40–70 HU), with findings that suggest continuity with the sublingual glands.

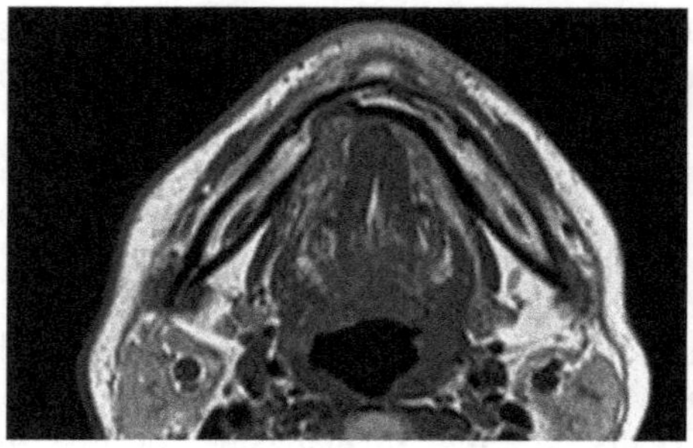

FIGURE 4: Magnetic resonance imaging, horizontal cross section, T1-weighted imaging. A rounded cavity is observed in the lingual side of the mandible from the right anterior to the premolar region. The margin of the cavity in the lingual side of the mandible exhibits a cortical bone structure, and the cavity's margin is smooth. A layer of myeloid tissue is observed in the cavity between the lingual cortical bone and the buccal cortical bone. The tissue in the cavity in the lingual side of the mandible has similar signal intensity to the sublingual glands and is contiguous with the sublingual gland tissue.

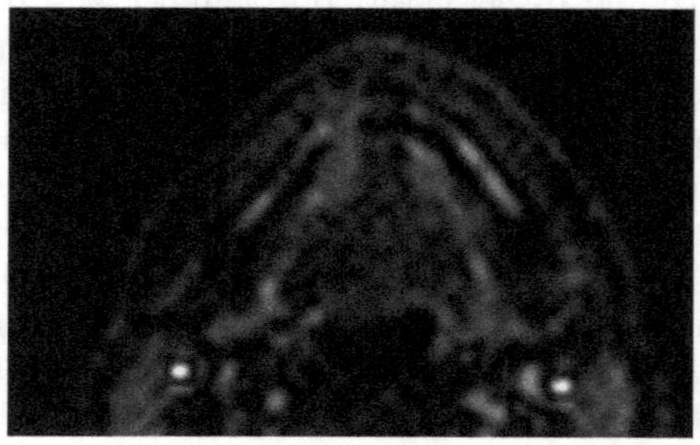

FIGURE 5: Magnetic resonance imaging, horizontal cross section, short T1 inversion recovery. There are no signs of tumors or inflammation.

of Fordyce [14], Rushton and Cantab [15], Thoma [16], Choukas and Toto [3], and Harvey and Noble [17]. A Stafne bone defect is currently considered to occur when postnatal mandibular bone absorption creates a cavity due to pressure from salivary gland tissue and the surrounding soft tissue [5, 8, 12, 18]. That is, the most widely accepted view is that the cavities develop as a result of a localized pressure atrophy of the lingual surface of the mandible from the adjacent salivary gland [19]. In the present case, both CT and MRI showed recessed sublingual gland tissue contiguous with the salivary gland tissue from the mandibular anterior to the premolar region, indicating that the Stafne bone defect formed postnatally due to pressure from the sublingual gland tissue in the lingual side of the mandible.

The differential diagnostic of Stafne bone defect includes odontogenic cystic, salivary gland tumors, fibro-osseous lesions, central giant cell lesions, hyperparathyroidism, ameloblastoma, eosinophilic granuloma, hemangioma of the bone, myxoma, aneurismal bone cyst, multiple myeloma, and benign neurogenic tumors [4, 19, 20].

In the present case, CT showed a rounded cavity in the lingual side of the mandible that had a lingual opening, was monocystic, and had a cortical margin. The margin of the cavity was relatively dull and regular, and the CT number of the tissue filling the cavity in the lingual side was similar to that of the sublingual glands. As was observed on CT, MRI also showed a rounded cavity in the lingual side of the mandible that had a lingual opening, was monocystic, and had a cortical margin, with a relatively dull and regular margin. MRI also confirmed that the signal intensity of the tissue inside the cavity in the lingual side of the mandible was similar to that of the sublingual glands, that the cavity was filled with tissue contiguous with the normal sublingual glands, and that tumors or inflammatory findings were not observed in the surrounding area. Based on these CT and MRI findings, a final diagnosis of a Stafne bone defect with a cavity in the lingual side of the mandible from the right anterior to the premolar region that was filled with salivary gland tissue connected to the sublingual gland tissue was established.

Static bone cavities do not require aggressive treatment in the absence of functional disorders or subjective symptoms. Clinicians rarely perform additional imaging or surgical procedures on cases that are diagnosed by CT or MRI and usually opt for follow-up. Although biopsies and other surgically invasive tests are important for establishing a definitive diagnosis, considering the pathology of static bone cavities, performing thorough imaging examinations and establishing a diagnosis noninvasively should be prioritized. Whereas static bone cavities are rare, there have been reports of an increasing trend [21] and of detecting pleomorphic adenoma in the cavity area [22]. Therefore, the determination of stasis in a case diagnosed as Stafne bone defect should not be made based on a single time point, but through follow-up observations. In either case, surgical treatments can be selected if follow-up shows that the shape of the Stafne bone defect is increasing in size or that the properties of the tissue filling the cavity in the lingual side of the mandible are changing. Data on more cases need to be accumulated to determine the proper intervals and durations for follow-up.

4. Conclusion

A case of a Stafne bone defect extending from the mandibular anterior to the premolar region was presented. CT and MRI suggested that salivary gland tissue connected to the sublingual glands was involved in the formation of the cavity.

Consent

Fully informed consent was obtained from the patient for the use of clinical information relating to this case.

Acknowledgments

The authors would like to thank the staff of Kameda General Hospital Dental Center for editing this manuscript.

References

[1] E. C. Stafne, "Bone cavities situated near the angle of the mandible," *The Journal of the American Dental Association*, vol. 29, no. 17, pp. 1969–1972, 1990.

[2] T. Schneider, K. Filo, M. Locher et al., "Stafne bone cavities: systematic algorithm for diagnosis derived from retrospective data over a 5-year period," *British Journal of Oral and Maxillofacial Surgery*, vol. 52, no. 4, pp. 369–374, 2014.

[3] N. C. Choukas and P. D. Toto, "Etiology of static bone defects of the mandible," *Journal of Oral Surgery, Anesthesia, and Hospital Dental Service*, vol. 18, no. 1, pp. 16–20, 1960.

[4] A. T. Assaf, M. Solaty, T. A. Zrnc et al., "Prevalence of Stafne's bone cavity–retrospective analysis of 14,005 panoramic views," *In Vivo*, vol. 28, no. 6, pp. 1159–1164, 2014.

[5] H. P. Philipsen, T. Takata, P. A. Reichart, S. Sato, and Y. Suei, "Lingual and buccal mandibular bone depressions: a review based on 583 cases from a world-wide literature survey, including 69 new cases from Japan," *Dentomaxillofacial Radiology*, vol. 31, no. 5, pp. 281–290, 2002.

[6] S. Venkatraman, J. S. Gowda, and N. Kamarthi, "Unusual ghost image in a panoramic radiograph," *Dentomaxillofacial Radiology*, vol. 40, no. 6, pp. 397–399, 2011.

[7] C. Quesada-Gómez, E. Valmaseda-Castellón, L. Berini-Aytés, and C. Gay-Escoda, "Stafne bone cavity: a retrospective study of 11 cases," *Medicina Oral Patologia Oral Y Cirugia Bucal*, vol. 11, no. 3, pp. E277–E280, 2006.

[8] J. He, J. Wang, Y. Hu, and W. Liu, "Diagnosis and management of Stafne bone cavity with emphasis on unusual contents and location," *Journal of Dental Sciences*, vol. 14, no. 4, pp. 435–439, 2019.

[9] M. Kuroda, K. Ohmori, and M. Yamasaki, "A case of static bone cavity," *Oral Radiology*, vol. 9, no. 2, pp. 25–29, 1993.

[10] E. Ariji, N. Fujiwara, O. Tabata et al., "Stafne's bone cavity: classification based on outline and content determined by computed tomography," *Oral Surgery, Oral Medicine and Oral Pathology*, vol. 76, no. 3, pp. 375–380, 1993.

[11] G. Baker, "A radiolucency of the ascending ramus of the mandible associated with invested parotid salivary gland material and analogous with a Stafne bone cavity," *British Journal of Oral and Maxillofacial Surgery*, vol. 26, no. 1, pp. 81–84, 1988.

[12] B. F. Branstetter, J. L. Weissman, and S. B. Kaplan, "Imaging of a Stafne bone cavity: what MR adds and why a new name is needed," *American Journal of Neuroradiology*, vol. 20, no. 4, pp. 587–589, 1999.

[13] K. Minowa, N. Inoue, T. Sawamura, A. Matsuda, Y. Totsuka, and M. Nakamura, "Evaluation of static bone cavities with CT and MRI," *Dentomaxillofacial Radiology*, vol. 32, no. 1, pp. 2–7, 2003.

[14] G. L. Fordyce, "The probable nature of so-called latent haemorrhagic cysts of the mandible," *British Dental*, vol. 101, pp. 40–42, 1956.

[15] M. H. Rushton and B. C. Cantab, "Solitary bone cysts in the mandible," *British Dental Journal*, vol. 81, no. 2, pp. 37–49, 1946.

[16] K. H. Thoma, "Case report of a so-called latent bone cyst," *Oral Surgery, Oral Medicine and Oral Pathology*, vol. 8, no. 9, pp. 963–966, 1955.

[17] W. Harvey and N. W. Noble, "Defects on the lingual surface of the mandible near the angle," *British Journal of Oral Surgery*, vol. 6, no. 2, pp. 75–83, 1968.

[18] Y. Sisman, O. Miloglu, A. E. Sekerci, A. B. Yilmaz, O. Demirtas, and T. T. Tokmak, "Radiographic evaluation on prevalence of Stafne bone defect: a study from two centres in Turkey," *Dentomaxillofacial Radiology*, vol. 41, no. 2, pp. 152–158, 2012.

[19] A. P. Münevveroğlu and K. C. Aydın, "Stafne bone defect: report of two cases," *Case Reports in Dentistry*, vol. 2012, 5 pages, 2012.

[20] K. Turkoglu and K. Orhan, "Stafne bone cavity in the anterior mandible," *Journal of Craniofacial Surgery*, vol. 21, no. 6, pp. 1769–1775, 2010.

[21] H. Shibata, N. Yoshizawa, and T. Shibata, "Developmental lingual bone defect of the mandible. Report of a case," *Journal of Oral and Maxillofacial Surgery*, vol. 20, no. 6, pp. 328-329, 1991.

[22] W. Simpson, "A Stafne's mandibular defect containing a pleomorphic adenoma: report of case," *Journal of Oral Surgery*, vol. 23, pp. 553–556, 1965.

29

Cardiopulmonary Arrest with Airway Obstruction due to Postoperative Bleeding

Kenichi Sato, Mami Chikuda, Yoshihisa Miyamae, and Miwako Kan

Division of Dental Anesthesiology, Department of Reconstructive Oral and Maxillofacial Surgery, School of Dentistry, Iwate Medical University, 19-1 Uchimaru, Morioka, Iwate 020-8505, Japan

Correspondence should be addressed to Kenichi Sato; satoken@iwate-med.ac.jp

Academic Editor: Michael J. Wahl

An 84-year-old woman underwent soft palate resection and skin grafting with tie-over under general anesthesia. Fourteen years previously, she had undergone aortic valve replacement and coronary artery bypass grafting followed by lifelong warfarin and aspirin anticoagulation. We terminated the two drugs 8 and 6 days, respectively, before the present surgery and substituted intravenous heparin (10,000 units/day), which was terminated 6 h preoperatively. The surgery was uneventful. Heparin was restarted 2 days postoperatively but without warfarin potassium or aspirin because of postoperative soft palate bleeding, which continued for 10 days despite compression hemostasis. On day 10, she exhibited a suffocating large hemorrhagic mass, leading to cardiopulmonary arrest. Emergency consultation with medical doctors and dental anesthetists resulted in pulmonary resuscitation and tracheal intubation. After confirming spontaneous circulation/respiration, she was transferred to the intensive care unit. We now consider it essential that all medical/surgical/anesthesia specialists managing patients under anticoagulant therapy collaborate perioperatively.

1. Introduction

Today's aging society has produced a growing population of patients on antithrombotic drugs for cerebrovascular and/or cardiovascular disease who are undergoing dental procedures. Guidelines [1] for anticoagulant and antiplatelet therapy for cardiovascular diseases recommend that antithrombotic drugs be changed to heparin sodium for perioperative management. We have often had difficulty, however, with perioperative hemostasis when administering treatments that themselves cause bleeding in patients taking antithrombotic drugs [2, 3]. Discontinuing or reducing anticoagulants (e.g., warfarin potassium) to avoid bleeding complications increases coagulation ability, thereby increasing the risk of developing thrombosis and/or embolism [4].

Because reducing the dosage of antithrombotic drugs or discontinuing them entirely, even for a short time, increases the risk of thrombogenesis, we must shorten the interruption period as much as possible or maintain anticoagulant conditions by other means [5]. The Iwate Medical University guidelines [6] recommend that the antithrombotic drugs in use be changed to heparin sodium to allow perioperative management for patients in whom postoperative bleeding would normally be expected. Some patients in whom the antithrombotic drug was changed to heparin sodium during the perioperative period, however, had to continue on heparin because of unremitting postoperative bleeding, precluding the switch back to their usual antithrombotic drug. We report such a patient in whom the situation led to airway obstruction and cardiopulmonary arrest because of hemorrhaging from the surgical wound 10 days after the surgery.

2. Case Presentation

The patient was an 84-year-old woman (height 148 cm, weight 39 kg). Left-palate tumor resection was scheduled under general anesthesia. Her history included the following events.

(i) At age 60: percutaneous transluminal coronary angiography for angina

(ii) At age 65: plastic surgery for internal carotid artery stenosis; resection of a tongue tumor

(iii) At age 70: coronary artery bypass and aortic valve replacement for aortic valve stenosis; surgery for varicose veins in the lower limbs; cataract surgery

(iv) At age 84 (currently): under surveillance for a thoracic aortic aneurysm and a goiter mass

She was currently taking the following oral medications: aspirin, warfarin potassium, spironolactone, isosorbide nitrate, nitroglycerin, etizolam, and eszopiclone.

Electrocardiography showed complete right bundle branch block and left atrial enlargement. Echocardiography revealed mitral valve reflux disease and tricuspid valve dysplasia. The ejection fraction was 71%. Other hematologic tests, respiratory function tests, and chest radiography showed no abnormalities. She exhibited no chest pain or symptoms of heart failure, and her heart function was judged to be good.

The oral surgeon consulted her primary doctor and received instructions to discontinue the aspirin 8 days and the warfarin 6 days before the planned surgery. Thus, at the time of discontinuing the warfarin, we initiated heparin sodium (10,000 units/day) using a 24 h continuous drip, which was discontinued 6 h before commencing the operation [6]. On the day of surgery, the prothrombin time-international normalized ratio (PT-INR) was 1.02, and the activated partial thromboplastin time (APTT) was 36.0 s.

Rapid induction of anesthesia was undertaken with fentanyl citrate, midazolam, and rocuronium, followed by oral intubation. The anesthesia was maintained with air, oxygen, and sevoflurane. The surgical procedure involved the left side of the hard palate, soft palate, and cheek mucosa. The front and rear portions were sewn down, the central portion was implanted with Terdermis® (Terumo, Tokyo, Japan), and terramycin ointment gauze was placed on the Terdermis and the distal end of the soft palate. The tie-over was then completed. The operation time was 115 min, anesthesia time was 245 min, and the bleeding volume was 26 g.

During the operation, the patient's blood pressure occasionally dropped, and we took measures to increase it, as appropriate. After the patient awakened and wound hemostasis was confirmed, the tracheal tube was removed, and she was returned to the ward. On the day after the operation, however, continuous bleeding was apparent, and she was treated with compression hemostasis because her blood pressure and hematologic tests were normal. On postoperative day (POD) 2, after confirming wound hemostasis, heparin sodium (10,000 units/day) administration was resumed. Although bleeding from the wound again became evident, warfarin potassium (1.75 mg) was resumed on POD 3 and aspirin (100 mg) on POD 4. Because the bleeding had not stopped by POD 5, however, the warfarin and aspirin were discontinued. Heparin sodium (10,000 units/day in a sustained drip) was resumed, but continuous bleeding was seen through PODs 6–10, even though the patient was still being treated with compression hemostasis. Her APTT and PT-INR had been assessed both preoperatively and perioperatively (Table 1).

On POD 10, the oral surgeon, who routinely performed disinfection procedures on the dental unit of the ward, found a large amount of clotted blood in our patient that was obstructing her airways and making it difficult to breathe. There was an immediate emergency call, and experts from the medical emergency and dental anesthesia departments responded. Respiratory arrest occurred 7 min after discovering the clotted blood, and cardiopulmonary arrest was confirmed 10 min afterward. Cardiopulmonary resuscitation was started. A large amount of clotted material was found in the oral cavity, making tracheal intubation difficult. It was finally performed using the McGrath® apparatus, and 3 ampoules of adrenaline were administered intravenously.

The first rhythm check after tracheal intubation confirmed self-initiated resumption of the heartbeats and 100% SpO_2 with auxiliary breathing using an ambu bag. Her blood pressure was 181/99 mmHg. Electrocardiography showed sinus rhythm, complete right bundle branch block, and obvious ST changes. The right pupil was 2.5 mm and the left was 3.0 mm. Light reflection was left and right quickly. Consciousness, according to the Glasgow Coma Scale, was 3 (eye opening 1, verbal response 1, and motor response 1), and she was transferred to the intensive care unit. At this point, heparin sodium administration was discontinued. Communication became possible on POD 14.

Because bleeding from the wound continued, tracheotomy was performed, and hemostatic sutures were placed under general anesthesia on POD 15. She was discharged from the hospital in good condition 5 months after the original surgery.

3. Discussion and Conclusion

Dental surgeons treating patients who are on antithrombotic medications should ensure that the patient undergoes preoperative coagulation function tests under the direction of the primary physician. Informed decisions can then be made on the basis of the laboratory results, the dental treatment proposed, and a thorough evaluation of the methods available for hemostasis.

One study reported that about 1% of cases of severe cerebral infarction occurred due to only a 1 h interruption of warfarin potassium administration [7]. The incidence of cerebral infarction was 3.4 times higher than usual if an aspirin regimen to prevent recurrence was interrupted [8]. In general, it is necessary to switch to heparin sodium therapy when the risk of thrombosis is high in a patient for whom the operation is predicted to cause a large amount of hemorrhaging and warfarin potassium administration cannot be interrupted.

The Iwate Medical University guidelines [6] for anticoagulant and antiplatelet therapy in patients with a cardiovascular disease who are undergoing major surgery are as follows. Warfarin potassium should be discontinued 3–5 days prior to surgery and changed to heparin sodium, which has a short half-life. The dosage should be adjusted, so the partial thromboplastin time extends to 1.5–2.5 times the normal control value. The heparin sodium is stopped 4–6 h before surgery

Table 1: APTT and PT-INR values the day before, the day of, and several days after the operation.

	Day before operation 1	Day of operation Before op.	Days after operation 2	3	5	8	10
APTT	100.9	36.0	85.6	68.0	72.3	53.0	57.1
PT-INR	1.05	1.02	0.98	0.93	0.97	0.91	0.98

The results for APTT measurements are expressed in seconds. APTT: activated partial thromboplastin time; PT-INR: prothrombin time-international normalized ratio.

or heparin sodium with protamine sulfate just before surgery. After the operation, warfarin potassium is resumed whenever possible, and heparin sodium administration continues until the PT-INR value is restored to within the proper range. Oral maxillofacial surgeons and other medical doctors refer to this Iwate Medical University guideline [6], which was designed with reference to the guidelines [1] established for anticoagulant and antiplatelet therapy for cardiovascular diseases.

Recent publications have indicated that perioperative heparin bridging anticoagulation increased the bleeding risk without decreasing the thromboembolic risk in patients. It has been reported that low-dose heparin bridging anticoagulation is unlikely to affect either bleeding or thromboembolic risks in patients undergoing major abdominal surgery for a malignancy [9]. It has also been reported that bridging with heparin in patients with atrial fibrillation is associated with a significant bleeding risk compared with not bridging [10]. Thus, bridging therapy seems controversial as it may not lower the risk of bleeding or thromboembolism.

Table 1 shows the APTT and PT-INR values on POD 1, the day of the operation, and PODs 2, 3, 5, 8, and 10. Thus, although our patient's APTT and PT-INR were measured every morning from the time of her hospitalization 7 days prior to the incident until POD 10, we failed to assess and cope with adequately what the results had suggested. Proper monitoring and assessment might have improved the outcome.

In the present case, when the warfarin potassium was switched to heparin sodium during the perioperative period, blood clotting occurred due to airway obstruction, leading to cardiopulmonary arrest due to postoperative hemorrhage. It was thought that aggressive hemostatic treatment was necessary at an early stage when continuous bleeding was confirmed from the start of heparin sodium administration. The cause of the postoperative bleeding was eliminated from the soft palate to the cheek mucosa by implementing a tie-over technique, while maintaining the range of motion. Although the soft palate and part of the cheek mucosa had not completely healed, there was sufficient hemostasis. Despite continuous bleeding, however, it was treated only with compression hemostasis, so blood clots were more likely to flow into the pharynx, blocking the airway and causing breathing difficulty. Fortunately, routine morning disinfection treatment by an oral surgeon identified a blood clot causing airway obstruction and difficult breathing. An emergency call from the oral surgeon gathered emergency doctors and dental anesthesiologists for a rapid response.

Oral surgeons must always keep in mind that a postoperative bleeding surgical site in the upper respiratory tract can lead to serious airway obstruction or breathing difficulty [2, 11], which requires appropriate management. To prevent such complications as postoperative bleeding, it is important for all those involved with a patient undergoing upper respiratory tract surgery to work together to plan careful perioperative management. As oral surgery for patients undergoing antithrombotic therapy continues to increase, oral surgeons must work closely with their patients' primary physicians and dental anesthesiologists to perform appropriate perioperative management, thereby preventing complications associated with postoperative bleeding.

We experienced a case of airway obstruction and cardiopulmonary arrest due to continuous postoperative bleeding after resecting a soft palate tumor. During the perioperative period, the patient's antithrombotic drugs had been replaced by sodium heparin. For patients at risk of bleeding complications, oral surgeons, physicians, and dental anesthesiologists should work together to ensure adequate perioperative management.

Additional Points

Summary. (i) An 84-year-old woman with a history of cardiac problems—and thus on a lifelong warfarin and aspirin regimen—required dental surgery that entailed palatal resection and skin grafting. (ii) Soft palate bleeding continued up to 10 days postoperatively because her anticoagulant regimen was problematic. (iii) On POD 10, an oral surgeon—routinely performing disinfection procedures on the dental unit of the ward—found that the patient had accumulated blood clots that were suffocating her, which led to cardiopulmonary arrest.

Consent

Written consent for publication was obtained from the patient.

Acknowledgments

We thank Nancy Schatken, BS, MT (ASCP), from Edanz Group (https://en-author-services.edanzgroup.com/), for editing a draft of this manuscript.

References

[1] Japanese Circulation Society, Japanese Coronary Association, Japanese Association for Thoracic Surgery et al., "Guidelines for anticoagulant and antiplatelet therapy for cardiovascular disease," 2009, http://www.j-circ.or.jp/guideline/pdf/JCS2009_hori_h.pdf.

[2] K. Oga, S. Satsuka, H. Nishizawa, R. Serita, and T. Kitabashi, "A case of obstruction from airway swelling due to abnormal bleeding after partial lysis of the tongue," *Journal of Japanese Dental Society of Anesthesiology*, vol. 42, no. 2, pp. 216-217, 2013.

[3] T. Matsuoka, K. Inoue, M. Katsura et al., "Examination of surgical cases of antithrombotic therapy during the perioperative period replaced with heparin," *Acta urolgica Japonica*, vol. 58, no. 5, pp. 223–226, 2012.

[4] T. Kataoka, S. Kumasaka, S. Morita et al., "A study of 12 cases of general anesthesia oral surgery in patients under anticoagulant therapy," *Journal of Japanese Society of Dentistry for Medically Compromised Patient*, vol. 17, no. 3, pp. 173–179, 2008.

[5] Japanese Society of Dentistry for Medical Compromised Patient, Japanese Society of Oral and Maxillofacial Surgeons, and Japanese Society of Gerodontology, *Guidelines for tooth loss in patients with antithrombotic therapy based on scientific evidence*, Gakujutsusha, Tokyo, 1st edition, 2015.

[6] Iwate Medical University, *Guide to discontinuing oral anticoagulants and antiplatelet drugs Medical Safety Manual*, Iwate Medical University, 13th edition, 2014.

[7] M. J. Wahl, "Dental surgery in anticoagulated patients," *Archives of Internal Medicine*, vol. 158, no. 15, pp. 1610–1616, 1998.

[8] B. M. Alexadre, C. B. Daniel, M. Patrik, and B. Julien, "Effects of discontinuing aspirin therapy on the risk of brain ischemic stroke," *Archives of Internal Medicine*, vol. 62, no. 8, pp. 1217–1220, 2005.

[9] K. Ono, H. Hidaka, Y. Koyama et al., "Effects of heparin bridging anticoagulation on perioperative bleeding and thromboembolic risks in patients undergoing abdominal malignancy surgery," *Journal of Anesthesia*, vol. 30, no. 4, pp. 723–726, 2016.

[10] C. L. Garwood, B. Korkis, D. Grande, C. Hanni, A. Morin, and L. R. Moser, "Anticoagulation bridge therapy in patients with atrial fibrillation: recent updates providing a rebalance of risk and benefit," *Pharmacotherapy*, vol. 37, no. 6, pp. 712–724, 2017.

[11] H. Kobe, M. Sasahara, K. Koga et al., "A case of emergency tracheotomy after jawbone reconstruction by free fibula transplantation with vascular pattern," *Journal of Japanese Dental Society of Anesthesiology*, vol. 39, no. 2, pp. 210-211, 2011.

30

A Rare Case of Plasma Cell Granuloma

Archana P. Kanteti[1] **W. Patrick Kelsey**[2] **and Ernesto Martinez Duarte**[1]

[1]*Department of Pathology and Microbiology, University of Nebraska Medical Center, USA*
[2]*Creighton University School of Dentistry, USA*

Correspondence should be addressed to Ernesto Martinez Duarte; e.martinezduarte@unmc.edu

Academic Editor: Sukumaran Anil

Plasma cell granulomas (PCGs) or inflammatory pseudotumors are nonneoplastic lesions that consist of predominantly antibody-secreting plasma cells and innate immune cells such as neutrophils, macrophages, and eosinophils. Unlike in multiple myeloma, the plasma cells are polyclonal and present in a spindly fibroblast-rich stromal background. These lesions mainly occur in the lungs; however, they can arise in other organs. PCGs from the gingiva are extremely rare, and a proper diagnosis is crucial to treat these patients further. These tumors have an increased number of plasma cells that are immunoreactive with CD138 and are polyclonal for kappa and lambda light chains, confirming these proliferations' nonneoplastic nature. Surgical resection with clear margins, when possible, is the primary choice of treatment. Radiation and anti-inflammatory steroid therapy are other therapeutic approaches. Critical and careful examination by a pathologist is necessary to rule out plasma cell neoplasms. Here, we report a rare occurrence of gingival PCG in an elderly male.

1. Introduction

Plasma cell granulomas (PCGs) are benign inflammatory growths that commonly occur in the lungs and are rarely found in the oral cavity [1, 2]. They typically consist of a mass collection of polyclonal plasma cells [2]. In the oral cavity, plasma cell granuloma occurring in the gingiva is rare [2]. Mass-forming gross disease can mimic a malignant process. Accurate diagnosis is based on gross, radiographic, morphologic, and immunophenotypic characteristics [3]. We present and discuss the underlying pathology in the general context of PCGs.

2. Case History

The patient is a 71-year-old male with a past medical history significant for prediabetes, hyperlipidemia, and gastroesophageal reflux disease. He presented for a periodontal consultation due to an inflamed gingival swelling in the #8-9 interproximal space. The patient reported minimal to no discomfort but was aware that the site bled profusely when he flossed. He believed he was able to remove a fragment of debris from the area, which temporarily improved the swelling, but over time, the swelling and bleeding did not completely resolve. The patient does brush and floss regularly and did not note any recent trauma. Upon physical examination, the soft tissues between teeth #8-9 were erythematous. The lesional tissue had a sessile base and was soft but not fluctuant to pressure (Figure 1). The lesion was 5 mm wide and 6 mm tall and extended through the interdental papilla space. There was an open contact between the gold onlay restoration at #9 and the tooth at #8. The lesion appeared to be a reactive process due to irritation, possibly from the open contact, such as a pyogenic granuloma. Periapical radiographs showed 1-2 mm of horizontal bone loss between teeth #8-9 (Figure 2). The patient was advised to use 0.12% chlorhexidine gluconate rinse three times per day for thirty-second intervals, focus on interproximal plaque removal for three weeks, and then return for follow-up. After three weeks of home treatment, minimal improvement of the gingival lesion was noted. The patient underwent an excisional biopsy with complete removal and degranulation of the papillary tissues.

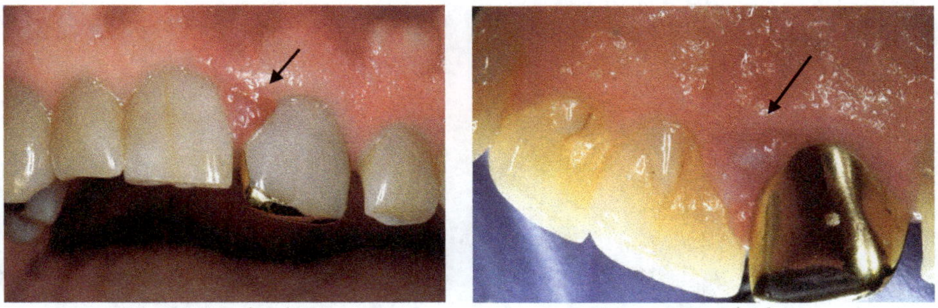

Pre-operative facial view

(a)

Pre-operative palatal view

(b)

FIGURE 1

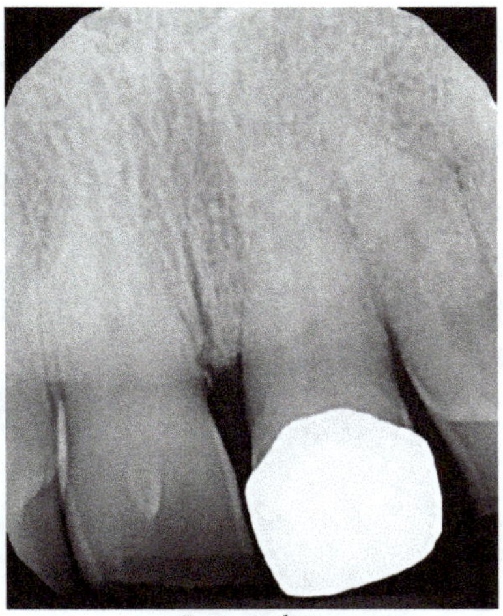

Periapical x-ray

FIGURE 2

The dentist recommended using salt water rinses, to reduce plaque formation in the interproximal space.

Microscopic examination by H&E showed benign squamous epithelium with underlying submucosa filled with sheets of numerous bland-appearing plasma cells (Figure 3). The plasma cells have a characteristic eccentrically placed nucleus with a nuclear Hoff (Figure 3(b)). Lymphocytes and histiocytes are also present infiltrating the stroma. Characteristic Russel bodies are present in the cytoplasm of the plasma cells (Figure 3(c)).

Immunohistochemical staining for CD138, a plasma cell marker, was diffusely positive in the lesional tissue highlighting the abundance of plasma cells (Figure 4(a)). Kappa and lambda light chain expression by in situ hybridization showed polytypic plasma cells (Figures 4(b) and 4(c)). The following findings were all consistent with a diagnosis of plasma cell granuloma.

The patient returned for postoperative follow-up at two weeks and eight weeks (Figure 5). Over two weeks (Figure 5(a)), the soft tissues between teeth #8 and #9 began to granulate via secondary intention. By eight weeks (Figure 5(b)), a more normal-appearing, much thinner, interdental papilla was visible with some residual inflammation. Probing with a UNC 15 mm probe revealed resistance at 4 mm deep with minimal bleeding. The patient was instructed to return to his general dentist for regular recall prophylaxis and exam appointments and referral request if the lesion recurred.

3. Discussion

Plasma cell granuloma (PCG) is also known as "inflammatory pseudotumor" [4]. It is an infrequent nonneoplastic lesion of uncertain etiology [5]. Zoon first recognized it in 1952 as balanitis plasmacellularis, or plasma cell balanitis [6]. The first use of the term PCG occurred in 1950 and 1960. It was first reported as an entity in the gingiva in 1968 [7, 8] and described as an inflammatory pseudotumor in 1973 by Bahadori and Liebow [7]. It is also known as inflammatory myofibrohistiocytic proliferation, inflammatory myofibroblastic tumor, and xanthomatous pseudotumor [8, 9].

The pathogenesis of PCG is still unclear. It is thought to be reactive and associated with periodontitis, periradicular inflammation due to a foreign body's presence, or the presence of a foreign antigen such as EBV and HHV8 [10–12]. Amlodipine and cyclosporines are known causative agents for plasma cell granulomas [10, 13, 14].

PCG most commonly arises from the lungs, although it can present in various other organs in the body [8, 15]. In the head and neck regions, it accounts for fewer than 5% of all extrapulmonary cases [10, 16]. The orbit is the most common location, followed by the meninges, paranasal sinuses, infratemporal fossa, and soft tissues [16, 17]. The temporal bone, skull base, and facial nerve are rarely involved [10].

It also involves the oral cavity, with the gingiva being the most commonly affected area with an equal rate of involvement of the maxillary and mandibular gingiva [18, 19]. Early lesions of nonneoplastic plasma cell infiltrate of the oral cavity were called atypical gingivostomatitis, idiopathic gingivostomatitis, and allergic gingivostomatitis [19]. They were considered secondary to chewing gum, dentifrices, or foreign oral substances [19].

While relatively benign, these tumors may simulate malignancy, become symptomatic secondary to size or location, and present a diagnostic challenge to clinicians, pathologists, and radiologists [5]. Reports of recurrences are few, hence the importance of thinking about the diagnosis and treating it properly [20, 21].

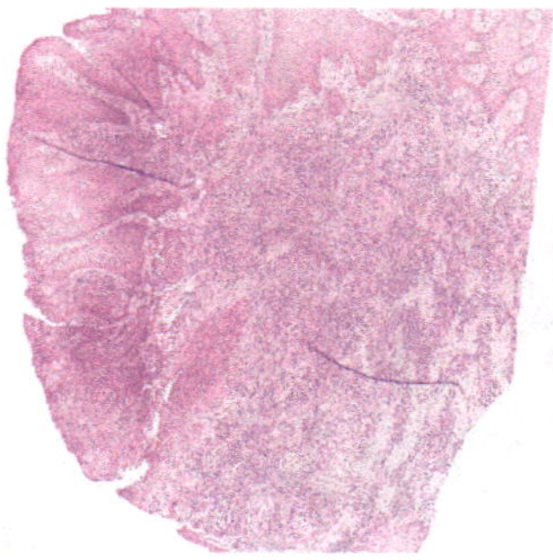
H&E (4×)
(a)

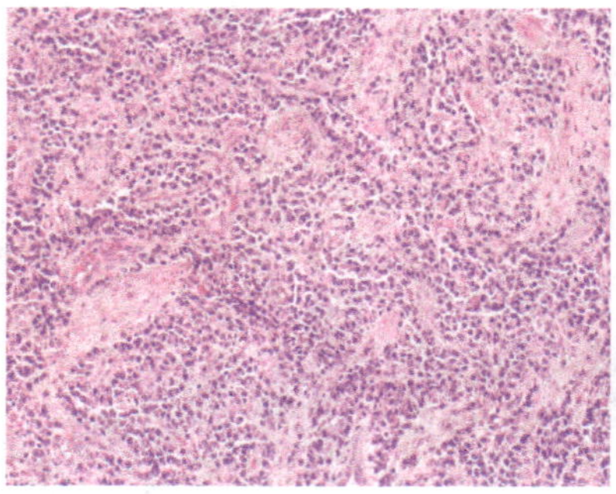
H&E (20×)
(b)

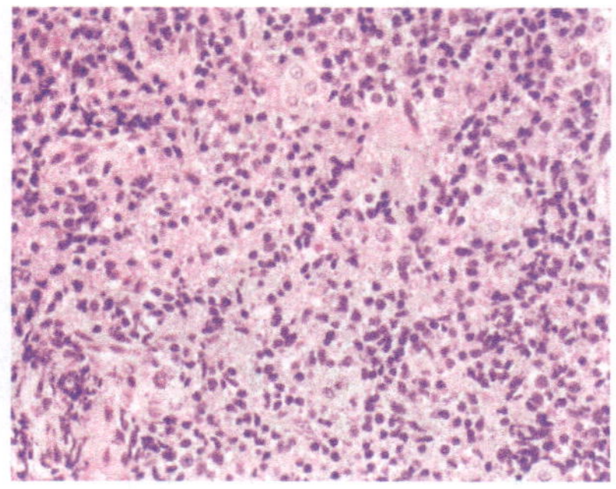
H&E (40×)
(c)

FIGURE 3

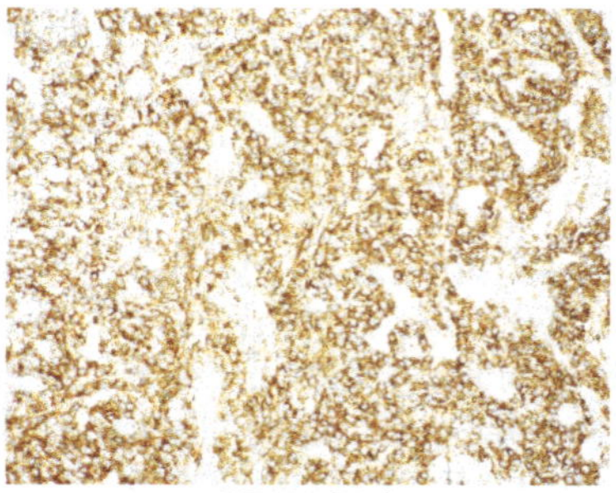
CD138 (20×)
(a)

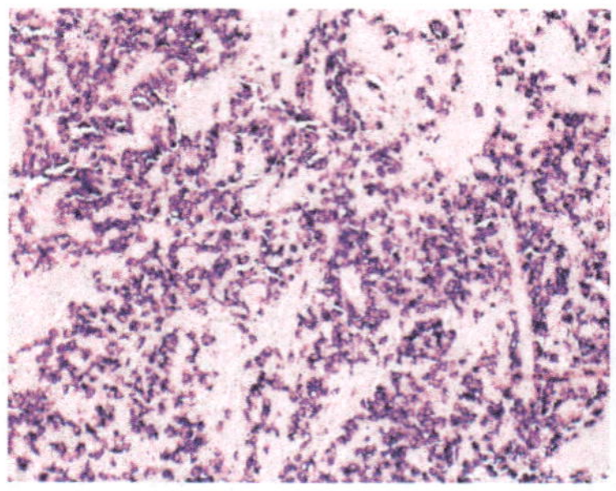
ISH kappa (20×)
(b)

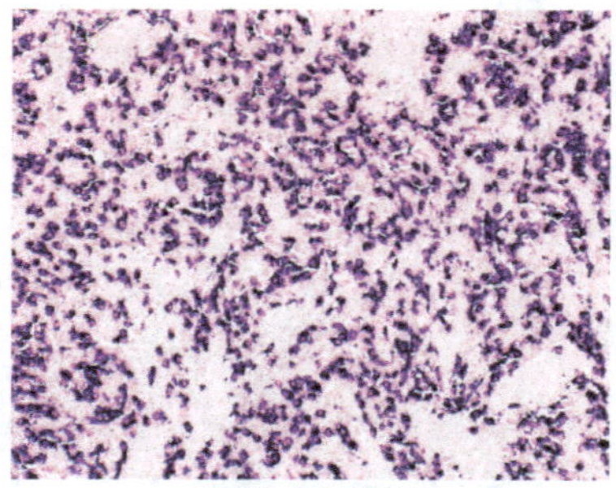
ISH lamda (20×)
(c)

FIGURE 4

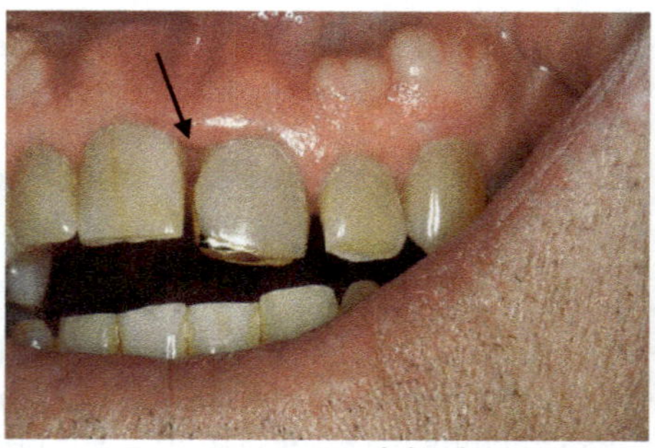
Post-operative 2 week facial view
(a)

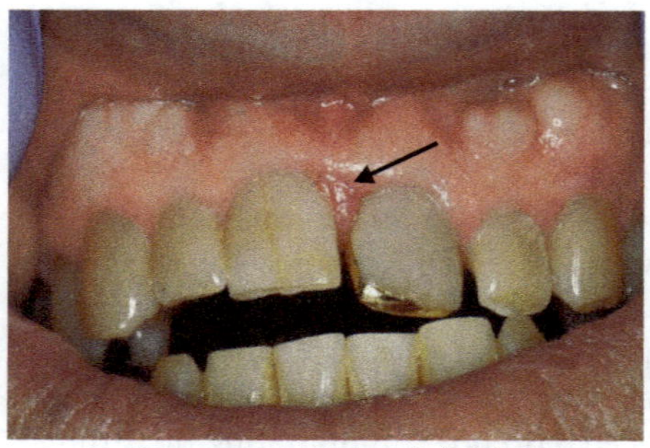
Post-operative 1-month facial view
(b)

FIGURE 5

PCG does not have an age preference [22]. Even though they can present as multiple simultaneous lesions, they are most commonly solitary [22]. More often than not, these lesions are asymptomatic and detected incidentally during routine dental evaluations [10, 15]. The alveolar mucosa is not usually involved, and subsequent bone loss depends on the lesion's etiology and chronicity. The patient can complain of bleeding and an inability to maintain oral hygiene [15, 23].

Microscopically, they are composed of a mixture of inflammatory cells, predominantly a polyclonal population of plasma cells, admixed with neutrophils and lymphocytes [18, 23]. The plasma cells show the classic eccentric nuclei, with clear, perinuclear Hoffs and numerous cytoplasmic Russell-Fuchs bodies [19]. The stroma tends to be fibrotic with areas of spindled, reactive fibroblastic proliferation [2, 5]. Russell bodies are large, eosinophilic, homogeneous immunoglobulin-containing inclusions in the plasma cell [8]. The presence of these bodies further supports the reactive nature of the plasma cell infiltrates [15].

Immunohistochemistry studies show that the plasma cells are positive for CD138 [24, 25]. The plasma cells are polyclonal illustrated by positive reactivity for both kappa and lambda light chains by immunohistochemistry or in situ hybridization [24, 25].

Treatment of the lesion depends on the size and associated symptomatology. It includes scaling, excisional biopsy, or possible extraction of the adjacent tooth if involved [26]. A few cases have reported the use of steroid therapy and spontaneous regression [27–29]. Due to these tumors' unencapsulated nature, surgical excision with wide margins is necessary to prevent recurrence [10, 26, 30].

The differential diagnosis of plasma cell infiltrates in the oral cavity includes plasma cell mucositis, plasma cell gingivitis, multiple myeloma, solitary myeloma, and plasmacytomas [2, 31]. Multiple myeloma and solitary myeloma are frequently solitary bone tumors, whereas plasmacytoma and plasma cell granulomas primarily affect the soft tissues [18, 32]. Differentiating the type of soft tissue tumor is crucial, as plasma cell granuloma is a benign growth, whereas plasmacytoma can represent the early stages of multiple myeloma [32].

Morphology and basic immunostains are enough to differentiate plasma cell mucositis, gingivitis, and plasmacytomas. Plasma cell granuloma will show a plasma cell-rich inflammatory infiltrate composed of polyclonal plasma cells [33].

Other rare entities that can affect the oral cavity are oral fibroma, peripheral giant cell reparative granulomas, and pyogenic granulomas. All these lesions show a fibrous or vascular rich stroma instead of a plasma cell predominant infiltrate [3].

References

[1] G. A. Agrons, M. L. Rosado-de-Christenson, W. M. Kirejczyk, R. M. Conran, and J. T. Stocker, "Pulmonary inflammatory pseudotumor: radiologic features," *Radiology*, vol. 206, no. 2, pp. 511–518, 1998.

[2] A. Acevedo and J. E. Buhler, "Plasma-cell granuloma of the gingiva," *Oral Surgery, Oral Medicine, and Oral Pathology*, vol. 43, no. 2, pp. 196–200, 1977.

[3] D. M. S. Andrade, S. J. Martins, O. Paz, J. B. Cardozo, A. E. Novaes, and M. B. Santiago, "Inflammatory pseudotumor: a diagnostic dilemma," *European Journal of Internal Medicine*, vol. 17, no. 7, pp. 514–516, 2006.

[4] K. A. Batich, E. William St Clair, R. E. McLendon, and J. H. Sampson, "Complete response to steroids in dural inflammatory pseudotumor associated with Still's disease," *Journal of Clinical Neuroscience*, vol. 20, no. 10, pp. 1445–1448, 2013.

[5] J. Forcucci, S. Butler-Williams, N. Miller, and J. Lazarchick, "Plasma cell granuloma: an entity within the spectrum of IgG4-related disease," *Annals of Clinical and Laboratory Science*, vol. 45, no. 3, pp. 340–343, 2015.

[6] J. J. Zoon, "Balanoposthite chronique circonscrite bénigne à plasmocytes," *Dermatologica*, vol. 105, no. 1, pp. 1–7, 1952.

[7] M. Bahadori and A. A. Liebow, "Plasma cell granulomas of the lung," *Cancer*, vol. 31, no. 1, pp. 191–208, 1973.

[8] F. Ide, T. Shimoyama, and N. Horie, "Plasma cell granuloma of the oral mucosa with angiokeratomatous features: a possible analogue of cutaneous angioplasmocellular hyperplasia," *Oral Surgery, Oral Medicine, Oral Pathology, Oral Radiology, and Endodontics*, vol. 89, no. 2, pp. 204–207, 2000.

[9] A. Vahedi, A. Moya-Plana, S. Guyot, and G. Touré, "Plasma cell granuloma of the jaw and the infratemporal fossa: a clinical case," *Journal of Oral and Maxillofacial Surgery*, vol. 76, no. 2, pp. 363–367, 2018.

[10] D. V. Ajibade, I. K. Tanaka, K. V. Paghda, N. Mirani, H. J. Lee, and R. W. Jyung, "Inflammatory pseudotumor (plasma cell granuloma) of the temporal bone," *Ear, Nose, & Throat Journal*, vol. 89, no. 7, pp. E1–13, 2010.

[11] A. Fukunaga, K. YOSHIDA, M. OTANI et al., "Plasma cell granuloma extending from the extracranial to the intracranial space associated with Epstein-Barr virus infection," *Neurologia Medico-Chirurgica (Tokyo)*, vol. 38, no. 5, pp. 292–296, 1998.

[12] D. A. Arber, O. W. Kamel, M. van de Rijn et al., "Frequent presence of the Epstein-Barr virus in inflammatory pseudotumor," *Human Pathology*, vol. 26, no. 10, pp. 1093–1098, 1995.

[13] B. Vishnudas, Z. Sameer, B. Shriram, and K. Rekha, "Amlodipine induced plasma cell granuloma of the gingiva: a novel case report," *Journal of Natural Science, Biology and Medicine*, vol. 5, no. 2, pp. 472–476, 2014.

[14] S. S. Kim, D. W. Eom, J. R. Huh et al., "Plasma cell granuloma in cyclosporine-induced gingival overgrowth: a report of two cases with immunohistochemical positivity of interleukin-6 and phospholipase C-gamma1," *Journal of Korean Medical Science*, vol. 17, no. 5, pp. 704–707, 2002.

[15] N. Akdogan, B. Yalçın, G. G. Aksoy, E. E. Tuna, and D. T. Ünal, "A case of plasma cell granuloma located on the gingiva," *The American Journal of Dermatopathology*, vol. 39, no. 5, pp. 393–396, 2017.

[16] E. Ballesteros, B. M. Osborne, and A. Y. Matsushima, "Plasma cell granuloma of the oral cavity: a report of two cases and review of the literature," *Modern Pathology*, vol. 11, no. 1, pp. 60–64, 1998.

[17] M. Kilinc, İ. Ö. Ertürk, H. Uysal, K. Birler, T. Evrenkaya, and B. B. Akkalyoncu, "Multiple plasma cell granuloma of the central nervous system: a unique case with brain and spinal cord involvement. Case report and review of literature," *Spinal Cord*, vol. 40, no. 4, pp. 203–206, 2002.

[18] J. Laco, K. Kamarádová, R. Mottl et al., "Plasma cell granuloma of the oral cavity: a mucosal manifestation of immunoglobulin G4-related disease or a mimic?," *Virchows Archiv*, vol. 466, no. 3, pp. 255–263, 2015.

[19] B. Manohar and S. Bhuvaneshwari, "Plasma cell granuloma of gingiva," *Journal of Indian Society of Periodontology*, vol. 15, no. 1, pp. 64–66, 2011.

[20] D. J. Balsarkar, N. U. Ranadive, M. A. Gore, and M. A. Joshi, "Recurrent inflammatory pseudotumor of small bowel mesentery presenting as perforative peritonitis," *Indian Journal of Gastroenterology*, vol. 21, no. 2, pp. 79-80, 2002.

[21] B. A. Garcia, S. Tinsley, T. Schellenberger, and G. C. Bobustuc, "Recurrent inflammatory pseudotumor of the jaw with perineural intracranial invasion demonstrating sustained response to rituximab," *Medical Oncology*, vol. 29, no. 4, pp. 2452–2455, 2012.

[22] A. Brage-Varela, P. E. Boullosa, J. P. Otero, M. B. Rodríguez, M. L. Novoa, and F. A. Monreal, "Multifocal hepatic inflammatory pseudotumor: spontaneous regression in a diabetic patient," *Revista Española de Enfermedades Digestivas*, vol. 102, no. 8, pp. 507–509, 2010.

[23] P. Jeyaraj, T. K. Bandyopadhyay, N. Naresh, and N. K. Sahoo, "Value of immunohistochemistry in diagnosing a rare case of maxillofacial plasma cell granuloma masquerading as a gingival epulis," *Journal of Maxillofacial and Oral Surgery*, vol. 14, no. 1, pp. 40–45, 2015.

[24] A. M. Buccoliero, A. Caldarella, M. Santucci et al., "Plasma cell granuloma–an enigmatic lesion: description of an extensive

intracranial case and review of the literature," *Archives of Pathology & Laboratory Medicine*, vol. 127, no. 4, pp. e220–e223, 2003.

[25] J. Deb, A. D. Chaudhuri, R. Saha, and S. Chakraborty, "Plasma cell granuloma of lung," *Journal of the Indian Medical Association*, vol. 105, no. 2, pp. 92–3, 98, 2007, 98.

[26] L. Piroth, P. Menecier, L. Charvillat, A. Naouri, and J. P. Kisterman, "Diagnosis and treatment of pulmonary plasma cell granuloma. A propos of a case successfully treated by antibiotics," *La Revue de Médecine Interne*, vol. 17, no. 8, pp. 670–674, 1996.

[27] E. Biecker, A. Zimmermann, and J. F. Dufour, "Spontaneous regression of an inflammatory pseudotumor of the liver," *Zeitschrift für Gastroenterologie*, vol. 41, no. 10, pp. 991–994, 2003.

[28] K. C. Brown, V. P. McCarthy, and T. Gaines, "Spontaneous resolution of a plasma cell granuloma in a 9-year-old," *Journal of the Association for Academic Minority Physicians*, vol. 9, no. 2, pp. 31–34, 1998.

[29] A. Bush, M. N. Sheppard, U. Wahn, and J. O. Warner, "Spontaneous arrest of growth of a plasma cell granuloma," *Respiratory Medicine*, vol. 86, no. 2, pp. 161–164, 1992.

[30] C. H. Chen, W. C. Huang, H. C. Liu, C. H. Chen, and T. Y. Chen, "Surgical outcome of inflammatory pseudotumor in the lung," *The Thoracic and Cardiovascular Surgeon*, vol. 56, no. 4, pp. 214–216, 2008.

[31] A. B. Pandav, A. V. Gosavi, D. N. Lanjewar, and R. V. Jagadale, "Gingival plasma cell granuloma," *Journal of Dental Research*, vol. 9, no. 6, pp. 816–820, 2012.

[32] S. V. Rajkumar and S. Kumar, "Multiple myeloma: diagnosis and treatment," *Mayo Clinic Proceedings*, vol. 91, no. 1, pp. 101–119, 2016.

[33] L. W. Solomon, R. O. Wein, I. Rosenwald, and N. Laver, "Plasma cell mucositis of the oral cavity: report of a case and review of the literature," *Oral Surgery, Oral Medicine, Oral Pathology, Oral Radiology, and Endodontics*, vol. 106, no. 6, pp. 853–860, 2008.

31

A Splint-to-CT Data Registration Strategy for Maxillary Navigation Surgery

Shinsuke Yamamoto,[1] **Shigeo Hara**,[2] **and Toshihiko Takenobu**[1]

[1]*Department of Oral and Maxillofacial Surgery, Kobe City Medical Center General Hospital, Kobe, Hyogo 650-0047, Japan*
[2]*Department of Pathology, Kobe City Medical Center General Hospital, Kobe, Hyogo 650-0047, Japan*

Correspondence should be addressed to Shinsuke Yamamoto; s.yamamoto@kcho.jp

Academic Editor: Jamil Awad Shibli

Computer-assisted navigation plays an important role in modern craniomaxillofacial surgery. Although headpins and skull posts are widely used for the fixation of the reference frame, they require the use of invasive procedures. Headbands are easily displaced intraoperatively, thus reducing the accuracy of the surgical outcome. This study reported the utility of a novel splint integrated with a reference frame and registration markers for maxillary navigation surgery. A maxillary splint with a 10 cm resin handle was fabricated before surgery, to fix the reference frame to the splint. The splint was set after the incorporation of fiducial gutta-percha markers into both the splint and resin handle for marker-based pair-point registration. A computed tomography (CT) scan was acquired for preoperative CT-based planning. A marker-based pair-point registration procedure can be completed easily and noninvasively using this custom-made integrated splint, and maxillary navigation surgery can be performed with high accuracy. This method also provides maximum convenience for the surgeon, as the splint does not require reregistration, and can be removed temporarily when required. The splint-to-CT data registration strategy has potential applicability not only for maxillary surgery but also for otolaryngologic surgery, neurosurgery, and surgical repair after craniofacial trauma.

1. Introduction

Computer-assisted navigation has been used in a wide range of craniomaxillofacial surgeries, including facial deformity correction, facial trauma management, temporomandibular joint arthroplasty, tumor resection, removal of foreign bodies, and dental implantation [1–9]. Precise registration is important in navigation surgery, as it has direct repercussions on the precision of all subsequent navigation tasks [4, 5].

Several methods have been developed to improve registration accuracy during craniomaxillofacial surgery. The combination of headpins, skull posts, or headbands with positioning screws implanted into the maxillary alveolar bone has been recently used for marker-based registration [3, 4, 8]. However, the use of headpins and skull posts is invasive; headbands, on the other hand, can be easily displaced intraoperatively, thus reducing the accuracy of registration. The splint was integrated with the reference frame and registration markers to overcome the issues associated with maxillary navigation surgery. This system is noninvasive, and more accurate than that involving the use of a headband, since the reference frame can be mounted more rigidly and closer to the surgical field. The aim of the present case report was to evaluate the feasibility of a novel custom-made integrated splint for maxillary navigation surgery.

2. Case Report

A 70-year-old Japanese man with a medical history of fibrous dysplasia of the craniofacial bones was referred to the oral and maxillofacial surgery department of a general hospital in March 2019 with chief complaints of swelling and pain in the left buccal region. The patient provided informed consent prior to treatment commencement, and the study

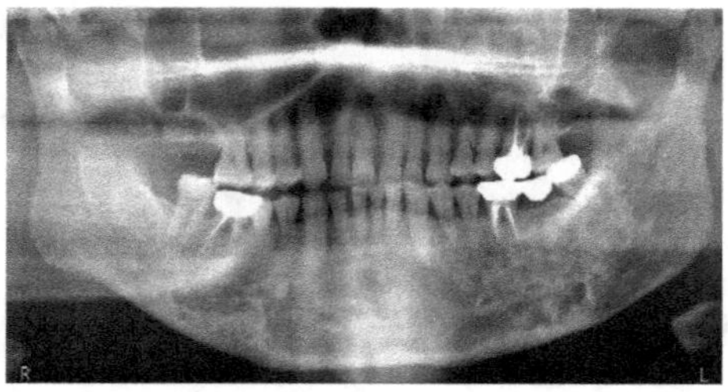

Figure 1: A panoramic radiograph obtained during the initial visit.

protocol was approved by the appropriate institutional ethics committee.

The patient had hypertension and was taking antihypertensive drugs. Clinical examination at the initial visit revealed facial asymmetry, mild swelling, and redness and tenderness over the left buccal region. No paresthesia was documented over the left buccal region. The left maxillary first molar was tender to percussion, and mild swelling and redness were observed on the buccal gingiva.

The panoramic radiograph revealed a "ground-glass" appearance in the left maxillary sinus and left mandibular body and ramus; a periapical radiolucency was observed with the left maxillary first premolar and first molar (Figure 1). Computed tomography (CT) revealed severe bone hyperplasia and "ground-glass" appearance with the left maxilla, mandible, and sphenoid bone, along with an osteolytic lesion extending from the root apex of the left maxillary first molar to the inferior aspect of the left infraorbital foramen and canal in the "ground-glass" lesion (Figure 2). Bone scintigraphy revealed the accumulation of technetium medronic acid in the right skull base, cervical spine, left maxilla, and left mandible (Figure 3).

The radiograph shows "ground-glass" appearance at the left maxillary sinus, mandibular body, and ramus. A periapical radiolucency is seen at the left maxillary first premolar and first molar.

Ampicillin/sulbactam was prescribed for 7 days. A clinical diagnosis of left maxillary infection caused by a periapical lesion of the left maxillary first molar in a fibrous dysplasia lesion was established. The left maxillary first premolar and first molar were extracted, and the osteolytic lesion was curetted (while preserving the infraorbital neurovascular bundle) using a navigation system and novel navigation splint (described below) in October 2019. The patient declined correction for facial asymmetry via bone reduction. Fibrous dysplasia with granulation tissue was observed on pathological examination of the surgical specimen (Figure 4). Ampicillin/sulbactam was prescribed for 7 days postoperatively, and the patient was discharged from the hospital 4 days after surgery. The patient's 1-year postoperative course was uneventful.

3. Navigation Technique

A maxillary splint was fabricated, which extended from the right maxillary first molar to the left maxillary second molar, prior to surgery. The splint was composed of 3 mm thick Erkoloc-Pro plates (Erkodent, Pfalzgrafenweiler, Germany),

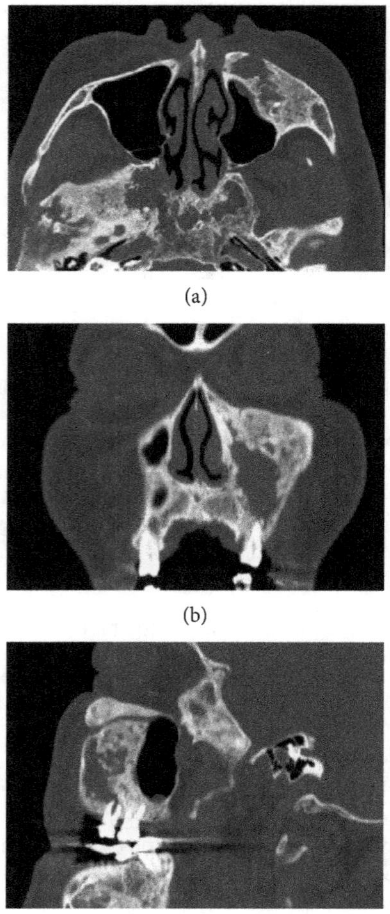

(a)

(b)

(c)

Figure 2: Computed tomography (CT) image obtained at the initial visit. CT shows bone hyperplasia and "ground-glass" appearance at the left maxilla, mandible, and sphenoidal bone, along with an osteolytic lesion extending from the root apex of the left maxillary first molar to the inferior aspect of the left infraorbital foramen and canal in the "ground-glass" lesion. Axial (a), coronal (b), and sagittal (c) CT views.

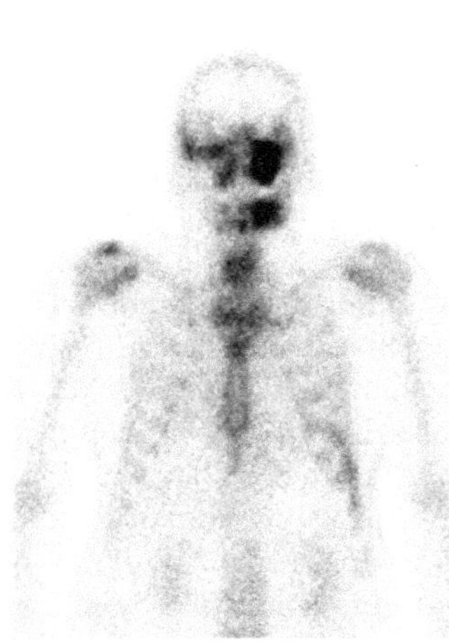

Figure 3: Bone scintigraphy findings obtained during the initial visit. Bone scintigraphy shows an accumulation of technetium medronic acid in the right skull base, cervical spine, left maxilla, and left mandible.

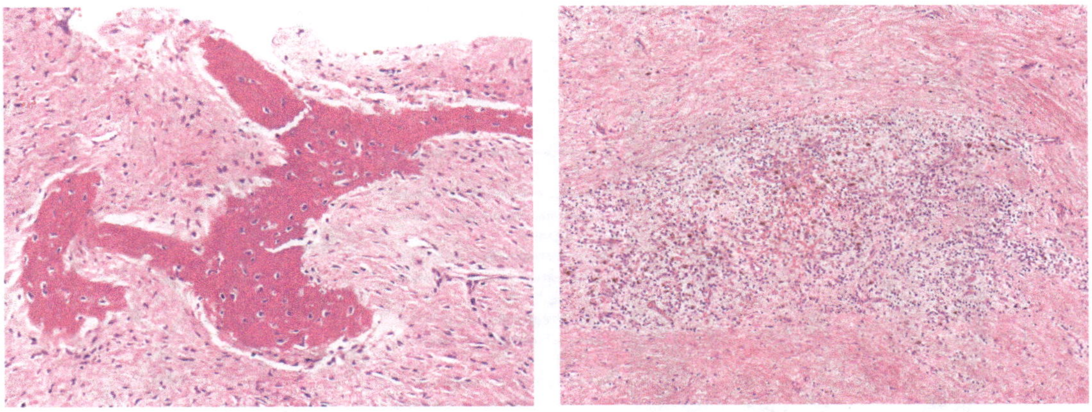

(a) (b)

FIGURE 4: Surgical specimen. (a) A characteristic pattern of disconnected, bizarrely contoured dysplastic trabeculae enmeshed in primitive mesenchymal cells (hematoxylin and eosin, ×200). (b) Granulation tissue can be observed in the mesenchymal stroma (hematoxylin and eosin, ×100).

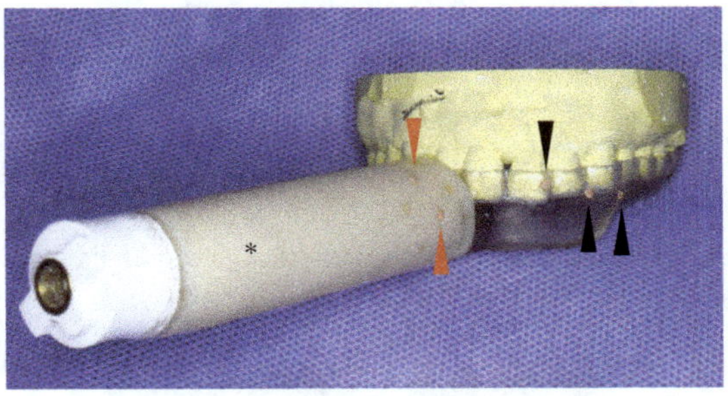

FIGURE 5: A custom-made splint. The 10 cm resin handle (with a connector), which was used to fix the reference frame (∗) and the gutta-percha markers are placed in asymmetric positions into both the splint (black arrowheads) and resin handle (red arrowheads) for marker-based pair-point registration.

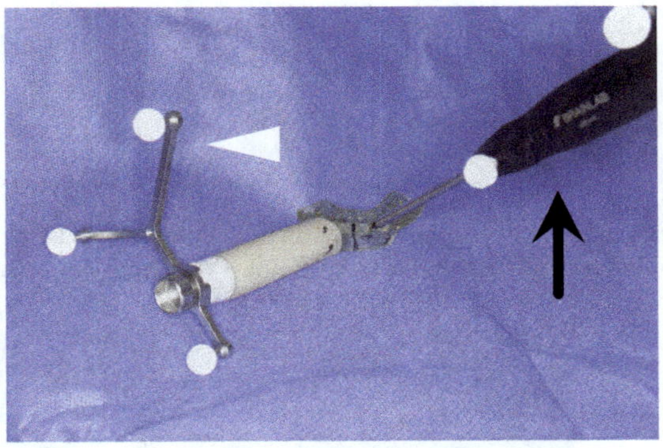

FIGURE 6: Marker-based pair-point registration using the custom-made splint, which is integrated with the reference frame and registration markers. The reference frame (white arrowhead) is fixed to the connector of the splint. The numbered landmarks (the 11 gutta-percha markers) are indicated within the optical tracking range of the navigation system and registered point-by-point in succession, using the pointer (black arrow).

and the resin extended to a point 1 cm below the incisal edges of the anterior teeth (Figure 5). A 10 cm resin handle with a connector, which was a reference star connector obtained from a reference headband (Brainlab AG, Feldkirchen, Germany), was used to fix the reference frame to the splint on the right side of the canine. The splint was set after the incorporation of 11 fiducial gutta-percha markers (each with a diameter of 1.5 mm) into the splint and resin handle for marker-based pair-point registration, and a CT scan was acquired [10]. Preoperative CT-based planning (iPlan CMF, Brainlab AG, Feldkirchen, Germany) entailed the determination of the region requiring curettage, as well as the registration and numbering of the 11 fiducial gutta-percha markers for the marker-based pair-point registration. The planning data were subsequently transferred to The Kick navigation system (Brainlab AG, Feldkirchen, Germany). The reference frame was fixed to the connector on the splint, and marker-based pair-point registration was performed, after the induction of general anesthesia and nasotracheal intubation. The practical procedure of the marker-based pair-point registration was as follows (splint-to-CT data registration): the numbered fiducial gutta-percha markers were indicated and registered point-by-point in succession within the optical tracking range of the navigation system, using the pointer (Figure 6). The splint was set on the maxillary dentition, and the presence of registration errors were determined with the pointer to assess the median positions of the maxillary central incisors and mesiobuccal line angles of the maxillary first molars on both sides. It took approximately 3 min to complete and confirm the marker-based pair-point registration before surgery; the mean fiducial registration error (FRE) was 0.68 ± 0.30 mm (Figure 7).

The splint was temporarily removed to facilitate extraction of the left maxillary premolar and first molar. A three-sided flap was subsequently elevated, and the splint was reinserted (Figure 8). The positions of the infraorbital foramen and canal were accurately identified in the surgical field using the pointer, which facilitated the removal of the osteolytic lesion (Figure 9). Both the splint and reference frame were stable, as the splint was rigidly fixed to the maxillary dentition, which prevented the risk of a navigation system error. Simple sutures were placed at the vertical incision, and

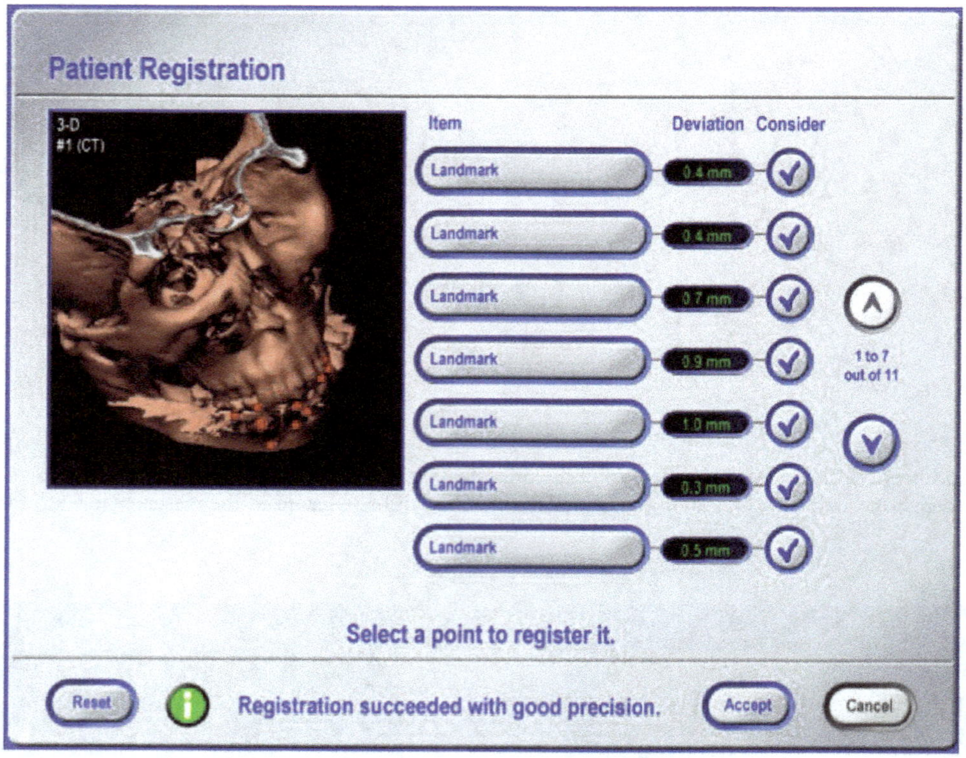

FIGURE 7: Screenshot of the navigation system during registration. The red points indicate the numbered landmarks (gutta-percha markers in the splint) for the marker-based pair-point registration. Deviations of each landmark are less than 1.0 mm.

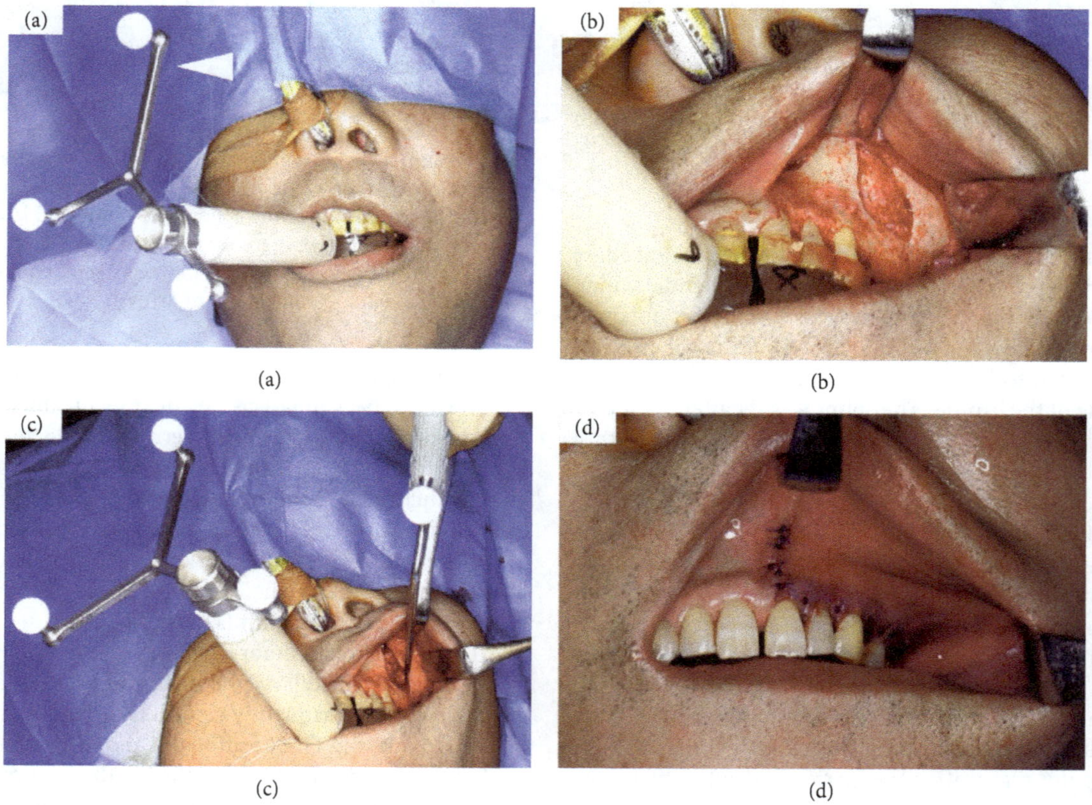

FIGURE 8: Intraoperative photographs. (a) The custom-made splint, which was integrated with the reference frame (white arrowhead), is set on the maxillary dentition. (b) The surgical field can be viewed clearly. (c) The positions of the osteolytic lesion are accurately identified in the surgical field using the pointer. (d) Placement of simple sutures at the vertical incision and horizontal mattress suture at the gingival margin.

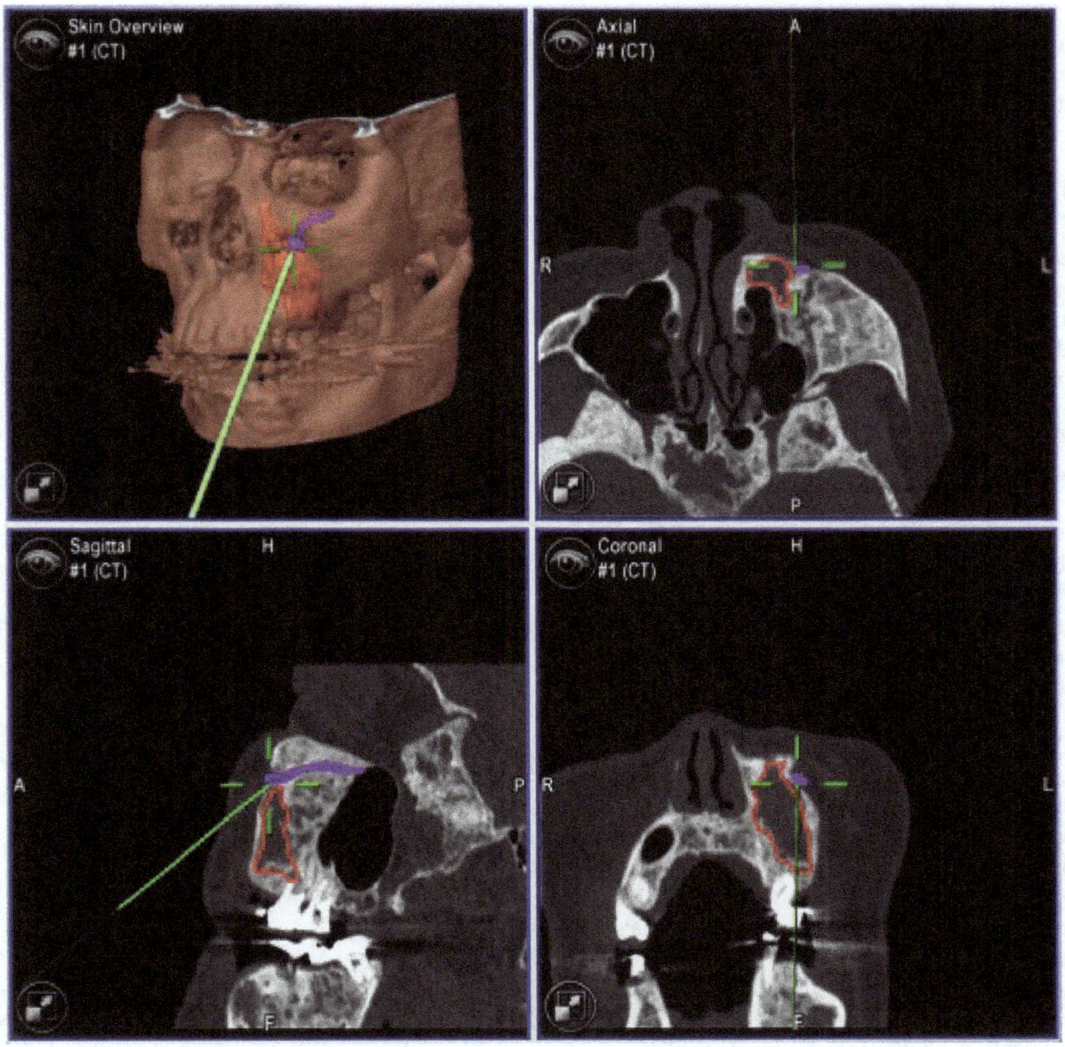

FIGURE 9: Intraoperative screenshot of the navigation system. The red line indicates the planned site for curettage. The contact of the pointer with the inferior border of the infraorbital foramen (purple line) is indicated.

horizontal mattress sutures were placed at the gingival margin after the splint was removed (Figure 8).

4. Discussion

The findings derived from this case have two crucial implications. First, the marker-based pair-point registration procedure can be completed easily and noninvasively using a maxillary splint integrated with the reference frame and registration markers, and the use of such a splint allows maxillary navigation surgery to be performed with high accuracy.

Fibrous dysplasia is a common benign skeletal lesion that may involve one bone (monostotic) or multiple bones (polyostotic), which can occur throughout the skeleton with a predilection for the long bones, ribs, and craniofacial bones [11, 12]. However, most lesions can be treated with clinical observation and patient education [11, 12]. In the present case, an infection originated from an apical lesion and spread to the region affected by fibrous dysplasia, which necessitated curettage of the infected lesion and extraction of the causative teeth. Furthermore, a method facilitating safe removal of the lesions was needed, owing to the severe hypertrophy and deformity of the left maxillary bone caused by fibrous dysplasia, and the contact of the osteolytic lesion with the infraorbital foramen and canal.

Headbands, skull posts, or headpins are generally used in craniomaxillofacial navigation surgery [3, 4, 6, 8, 13]. The reference frame is first fixed to the patient's head with a headband, skull post, or headpin, which is followed by marker-free or marker-based registration. However, the use of headpins and skull posts is invasive, and a headband can easily be displaced intraoperatively. Furthermore, it is known that surgical precision decreases linearly with the distance from the reference markers [5, 7, 8]. The splint was integrated with the reference frame and registration markers to overcome the above-mentioned issues associated with maxillary navigation surgery. This system is noninvasive and more accurate than the use of a headband, since the reference frame can be mounted more rigidly and closer to the surgical field. Furthermore, as 11 fiducial gutta-percha markers were incorporated within the splint in asymmetric positions, marker-based pair-point registration could be performed in the patient's absence. The resin handle was also used for marker incorporation as the maxillary splint did not have adequate space to accommodate each of the 11 fiducial gutta-percha markers. The low mean FRE for splint registration (0.68 ± 0.30 mm) suggested that a widely spaced three-dimensional arrangement of the 11 fiducial gutta-percha markers contributed to the increase in the accuracy of the splint-to-CT data registration. This splint-to-CT data registration strategy is extremely precise and rapid; approximately 3 min were required to complete and confirm the marker-based pair-point registration before surgery, and there was no evidence of instability in the splint and reference frame that could have induced a navigation system error. It was also possible to preserve the infraorbital neurovascular bundle with this approach.

Second, this novel method provides maximum convenience for the surgeon, as the splint does not require reregistration, and can be temporarily removed when required. During craniomaxillofacial surgery, surgeons often change the patient's head position slightly to secure the surgical field; this is not possible when using a headpin. Any change in head positioning may result in the displacement of the headband, thus necessitating reregistration [14]. In contrast, the use of a splint allows changes in head positioning without displacing the reference frame; furthermore, the splint can be temporarily removed when it obstructs the surgical field, and reregistration is not required.

In the present case, the patient declined to undergo bone reduction for the correction of facial asymmetry caused by fibrous dysplasia. However, it would have been technically possible to perform this procedure by using the splint and navigation system to capture the mirror images of the opposite, unaffected side of the facial skeleton.

A limitation of oral splints is that their use is not feasible in patients who are edentulous or have few remaining teeth. Nevertheless, provided that a sufficient number of teeth are present to ensure the stable positioning of the splint, the results of this case report suggest that the splint-to-CT data registration strategy may be used not only in maxillary surgery, but also in otolaryngologic surgery, neurosurgery, and surgical repair after craniofacial trauma (especially zygomatic fracture and orbital floor fracture). Further studies with larger sample sizes are required to compare the effectiveness and reliability of this technique with conventional approaches.

5. Conclusion

A marker-based pair-point registration procedure can be completed easily and noninvasively, and maxillary navigation surgery can be performed with high accuracy by incorporating a custom-made integrated splint. This method also provides maximum convenience for the surgeon, as the splint does not require reregistration, and can be temporarily removed when required.

Consent

The patient provided written informed consent for the use of their photographs in this publication.

Acknowledgments

The authors would like to thank T. Kawakami (Brainlab AG) for technical assistance with the navigation system, and K. Yoshida, S. Yao, and R. Mihara (Mihara Dental Laboratory) for providing technical assistance for the fabrication of the splint. This work was supported by JSPS KAKENHI, Grant Number JP20K18715.

References

[1] G. Schultes, V. Zimmermann, M. Feichtinger, A. Gaggl, and H. Karcher, "Removal of osteosynthesis material by minimally invasive surgery based on 3-dimensional computed tomography-guided navigation," *Journal of Oral and Maxillofacial Surgery*, vol. 61, pp. 401–405, 2003.

[2] R. Ewers, K. Schicho, G. Undt et al., "Basic research and 12 years of clinical experience in computer-assisted navigation technology: a review," *International Journal of Oral and Maxillofacial Surgery*, vol. 34, no. 1, pp. 1–8, 2005.

[3] H. Yu, G. Shen, X. Wang, and S. Zhang, "Navigation-guided reduction and orbital floor reconstruction in the treatment of zygomatic-orbital-maxillary complex fractures," *Journal of Oral and Maxillofacial Surgery*, vol. 68, no. 1, pp. 28–34, 2010.

[4] H. T. Lubbers, J. A. Obwegeser, F. Matthews, G. Eyrich, K. W. Gratz, and A. Kruse, "A simple and flexible concept for computer-navigated surgery of the mandible," *Journal of Oral and Maxillofacial Surgery*, vol. 69, pp. 924–930, 2011.

[5] C. Bettschart, A. Kruse, F. Matthews et al., "Point-to-point registration with mandibulo-maxillary splint in open and closed jaw position. Evaluation of registration accuracy for computer-aided surgery of the mandible," *Journal of Cranio-Maxillofacial Surgery*, vol. 40, no. 7, pp. 592–598, 2012.

[6] P. Li, Z. Li, W. Tian, and W. Tang, "A strategy for removal of foreign body in mandible with navigation system," *International Journal of Oral and Maxillofacial Surgery*, vol. 44, no. 7, pp. 885–888, 2015.

[7] S. Ohba, H. Yoshimura, K. Ishimaru, K. Awara, and K. Sano, "Application of a real-time three-dimensional navigation system to various oral and maxillofacial surgical procedures," *Odontology*, vol. 103, no. 3, pp. 360–366, 2015.

[8] Y. Opdenakker, G. Swennen, and J. Abeloos, "Application of a non-invasive reference headband and a surgical splint for intraoperative paediatric navigation," *International Journal of Oral and Maxillofacial Surgery*, vol. 46, no. 3, pp. 360–362, 2017.

[9] S. Yamamoto, N. Taniike, and T. Takenobu, "Application of an open position splint integrated with a reference frame and registration markers for mandibular navigation surgery," *International Journal of Oral and Maxillofacial Surgery*, vol. 49, pp. 686–690, 2020.

[10] P. Boeckx, H. Essig, H. Kokemuller, F. Tavassol, N. C. Gellrich, and G. R. J. Swennen, "Presentation and evaluation of a modified wax-bite dental splint for surgical navigation in craniomaxillofacial surgery," *Journal of Oral and Maxillofacial Surgery*, vol. 73, no. 11, pp. 2189–2195, 2015.

[11] M. M. Cohen Jr. and R. E. Howell, "Etiology of fibrous dysplasia and McCune-Albright syndrome," *International Journal of Oral and Maxillofacial Surgery*, vol. 28, no. 5, pp. 366–371, 1999.

[12] M. R. DiCaprio and W. F. Enneking, "Fibrous dysplasia pathophysiology, evaluation and treatment," *The Journal of Bone and Joint Surgery (American)*, vol. 87, pp. 1848–1864, 2005.

[13] O. Choudhri, S. A. Mindea, A. Feroze, E. Soudry, S. D. Chang, and J. V. Nayak, "Experience with intraoperative navigation and imaging during endoscopic transnasal spinal approaches to the foramen magnum and odontoid," *Neurosurgical Focus*, vol. 36, no. 3, p. E4, 2014.

[14] N. Casap, A. Wexler, and R. Eliashar, "Computerized navigation for surgery of the lower jaw: comparison of 2 navigation systems," *Journal of Oral and Maxillofacial Surgery*, vol. 66, no. 7, pp. 1467–1475, 2008.

32

Using the "One Shot" Concept for Immediate Loading Implant Protocol in Edentulous Patient Rehabilitation with a Fixed Prosthesis: A 6-Year Follow-Up

Philippe Bousquet,[1,2] **Delphine Carayon**,[3] **and Jean-Cedric Durand**[2,3]

[1]Department of Periodontology and Implantology, Faculty of Dentistry, University of Montpellier, Montpellier, France
[2]Laboratoire Bioingenierie et Nanosciences UR-UM104, University of Montpellier, Montpellier, France
[3]Department of Prosthetic Dentistry, Faculty of Dentistry, University of Montpellier, Montpellier, France

Correspondence should be addressed to Philippe Bousquet; dr.philippebousquet@free.fr

Academic Editor: Wen Lin Chai

Immediate-loaded implants with a fixed prosthesis are a viable option for the restoration of edentulous ridges. Several procedures now allow for the fabrication of immediate-loading provisional and definitive prostheses. However, this complex treatment is not accessible to all patients with budget restrictions. By using a unique master model with a single titanium framework prosthesis can simplify and shorten the treatment, as well as reduce costs. After surgical placement of implant fixtures, an interim prosthesis was fabricated using a laser-welded definitive titanium framework. The prosthesis was fitted intraorally following the immediate loading protocols. The master cast model used to fabricate interim prosthesis was conserved and subsequently used in modifying the final prosthesis. After the healing process and complete soft tissue stability, an impression was made to register the clearance between the gingiva and resin. The light silicone material was directly injected under the prosthesis screwed in the mouth. In the master cast model, the stone was eliminated between the implants and a new plaster was poured to modify the crest profile with the posthealing new shape. With this modified model, it is possible to rehabilitate the denture to the new gingival anatomy in 3 to 4 hours and, if necessary, the tooth rearrangement. This "one shot" concept combines the single definitive titanium welded framework and limited laboratory work with a unique master model thereby decreasing the cost and the time of treatment.

1. Introduction

Complete edentulism is a serious public health concern that has not decreased over time despite advances in dentistry [1]. Rehabilitation with implant-supported total prosthesis offers a greater quality of life benefits than conventional total prostheses, the latter presenting with less functional stability [2]. To reduce processing time and patient discomfort, immediately loaded implants with a fixed prosthesis have been proposed [3, 4]. This technique has been well-documented rehabilitation of edentulous patients and has become a viable option due to its high survival rate [5–7]. In a short period of time, from several hours to 2 days [8, 9], a provisional restoration is made, screwed on the implants, and then used by the patient for the duration of the osseointegration period. It is very important that the temporary prosthesis avoids compressing the swollen soft tissues and not hamper the soft-tissue healing [10]. During the initial healing, a soft-tissue recession occurs. After osseointegration from 3 to 6 months, a complete-arch conventional impression registering the implant position and the surrounding tissue anatomy must be made to prepare the final master models for the definitive restoration. All these steps for the rehabilitation of edentulous patients increase the cost of treatment. A definitive metal-framework prosthesis directly positioned, twenty-four hours after implant placement, has been proposed to reduce the cost of treatment [11, 12]. This allows the exclusion of an interim prosthesis. Another technique can be the intraoral welding to manufacture the definitive restoration in a short time [13, 14].

However, at the end of complete healing reconstruction, after the implant surgery, the soft tissue level may potentially become an important space between the prosthesis and tissue [10]. The resulting consequences include the disturbance of speech, discomfort during or after mastication, and air escape between the prosthesis and tissue. In many cases, patients require new impressions and a new laboratory protocol for the fabrication of the final prosthesis, or at least for the relining of the restoration, all of which lead to additional expenses.

Such treatment is not readily accessible to all patients with budget restrictions. The simplified technique "one shot" concept described herein a clinical case and allows the transformation of a single prosthesis, which can be used as a temporary prosthesis with the criteria necessary for immediate loading, to a definitive prosthesis adapted to the tissue after healing.

2. Case Presentation

A 68-year-old man visited our clinic presenting with maxillary and mandibular complete dentures; the chief complaint was the instability of his mandibular denture. He did not smoke and showed no significant risk factors and no contraindications to surgery. Optional treatment was presented which included the two implant-supported overdentures and 4 to 6 dental implants with screw-retained fixed prosthesis. The patient agreed to be treated with an immediately loaded implant screw-retained fixed prosthesis and provided written informed consent.

2.1. Surgical and Prosthetic Protocols. Before surgery, impressions of the maxilla and mandible were made using irreversible hydrocolloid impression material (Alginoplast®, Kulzer Mitsui Chemicals Groups, Hanau, Germany) and diagnostic laboratory casts were poured with type III stones. The vertical dimension was established using facial reference marks, and the casts were mounted in a semiadaptable articulator (Artex® Amann Girrbach AG, Koblach, Austria) with a facebow transfer. The diagnostic setup for the final restoration was made. The mandibular tooth arrangement was duplicated in clear acrylic resin for the fabrication of a radiology guide. The number and position of implants were chosen on the computed tomography, in prosthetically favored positions, to reduce the cantilever length.

The preliminary step included implant surgery and an interim prosthesis. In this case, 6 implants were inserted with an insertion torque of more than 45 Ncm (Tapered Screw-Vent®, Zimmer Biomet, Palm Beach Gardens, FL, USA). Abutments (tapered abutment TAC; Zimmer Biomet, Palm Beach Gardens, FL, USA) were tightened to 30 Ncm for the immediate loading protocol with a torque wrench.

Flap adaptation and suturing were performed. Analgesics were administered for pain control. Impression transfer copings (Tapered Abutment Direct Transfer, Zimmer Biomet, Palm Beach Gardens, FL, USA) were screwed on each implant abutment (Figure 1). A pickup open-tray impression was made with medium-bodied consistency polyether (Impregum™ Penta Soft, 3M Espe, Saint Paul, MN, USA) at the same time as the splitting impression transfer with resin (Luxabite®, DMG, Hamburg, Germany). After polymerization, the open tray was removed by loosening the transfer screws. Abutment analogs (Tapered Abutment Replica, Zimmer Biomet, Palm Beach Gardens, FL, USA) were tightened on impression transfer copings. The master cast was prepared and mounted on the articulator with the opposing cast using a bite record.

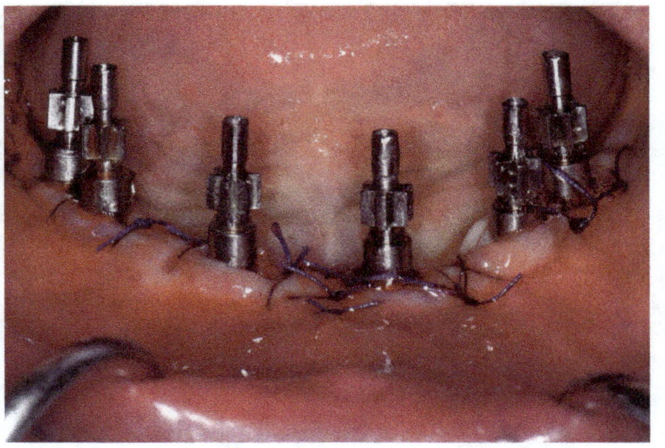

FIGURE 1: Impression transfer copings immediately after surgery.

2.2. Laboratory Work. A definitive metal framework was obtained immediately after surgery, using titanium milled cylinders (Titanium Bar Coping 5 mm TTC5, Zimmer Biomet, Palm Beach Gardens, FL, USA) and segments of cylindrical 3.5 mm titanium rods, which were adapted and inserted between the cylinders screwed on the abutment replicas in the master cast (Figure 2(a)). The titanium implant framework was performed using laser welding, with two distal cantilever extensions (Figure 2(b)). For welded frameworks, a high-strength joint is required. The tungsten inert gas welding with efficient argon shielding is important to increase the cantilever resistance [15]. The passive fit of the framework was evaluated by radiographic examination and was clinically ensured using the screw test. The framework was sandblasted to improve the mechanical bond, and a pink opaquer layer was applied (Gingiva opaquer pink Nexco, Ivoclar Vivadent® AG, Schaan, Liechtenstein). Acrylic teeth were arranged in accordance with the setup, and the prosthesis was tried on for aesthetic evaluation and occlusion control. Relatively flat cusps were ensured for the occlusal pattern, contact on the cantilever was eliminated, and occlusion was shortened to the second premolar [16] (Figure 2(c)). This reinforced interim prosthesis was performed in less than 12 hours and delivered to the patient (Figure 3).

2.3. Posthealing Prosthetic Transformation. Models on the articulator were preserved for the final transformation. After 3 months of osseointegration, the clearance between the gingiva and prosthesis was evaluated to edit the final prosthesis (Figure 4(a)). In the master cast model, the height of the stone between the implant analogs was reduced (Figure 4(b)). The interim restoration was unscrewed, and implants were checked with the prosthesis removed. To record the gingival recession and modify the denture in a

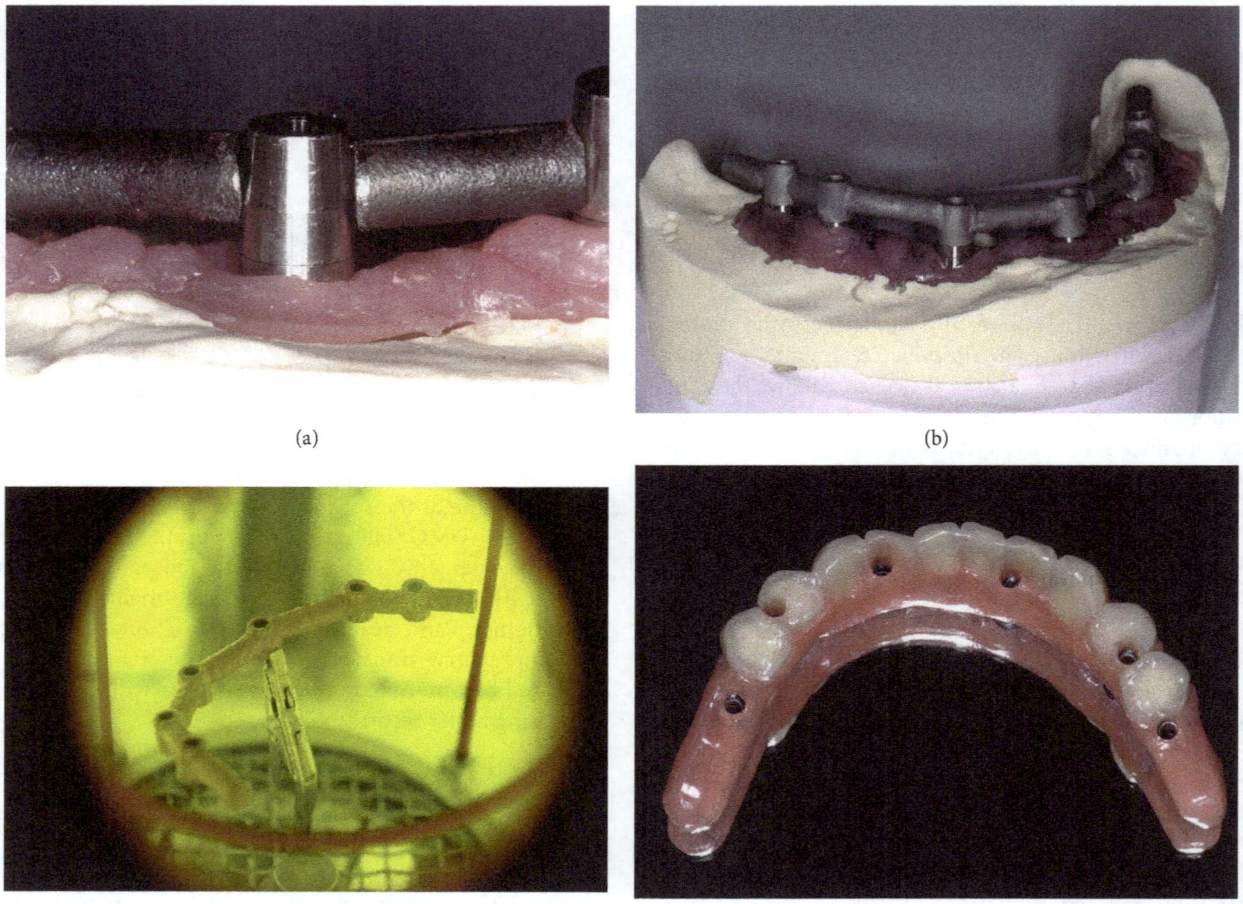

(a) (b) (c) (d)

Figure 2: Definitive titanium implant framework fabricated using a laser-welding technique. (a) Segments of titanium rod adapted and inserted into the space between the titanium milled cylinders. (b) Definitive framework. (c) Pink opaquer layer was applied to increase prosthetic resistance under occlusal forces. (d) Interim prosthesis with acrylic teeth after finishing. Occlusion was shortened to the second premolar.

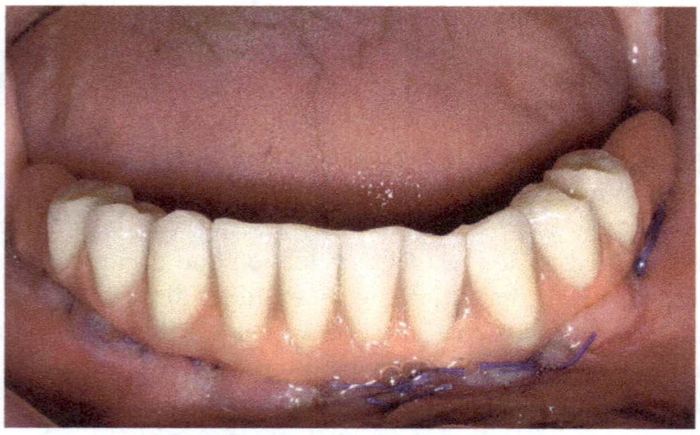

Figure 3: Interim prosthesis immediately after installation.

short time, a tray adhesive for use with silicone (universal adhesive, Kulzer Mitsui Chemicals Groups, Hanau, Germany) was applied to the gingival portion of the restoration. The prosthesis was screwed back on the patient's implants. An impression was made with silicone light-bodied material directly injected under the prosthesis while it is firmly screwed intraorally to fill the space underneath. Silicone must cover the buccal and lingual parts of the prosthesis to isolate the potential undercuts (Figure 5(a)). Simultaneously, the occlusion was also recorded (Luxabite®, DMG, Hamburg, Germany).

The model was encased with wax and silicone, and a new plaster was poured into the space between the light silicone and the master cast model (reduced to modify the crest profile according to the new anatomy; Figures 5 and 6). The final prosthesis was adapted to the new crest, and first molars were added on the cantilevers. Regarding occlusion, in case of group guide or bibalanced occlusion, the acrylic teeth can be repositioned or replaced when necessary. Before the addition of chemopolymerizable resin (PERform Inkovac, Coltene/Whaledent AG, Altstätten, Switzerland), the denture was ground and the master model was prepared (wax-up and varnish). Pressure firing was conducted according to the manufacturer's recommendations. These laboratory steps were completed by grinding off excess resin and working on the shapes (embrasures and profiles) prior to polishing. In order to limit the risk of fracture or damage to the connection areas, a muffle technique was avoided in this case.

2.4. Results. A new prosthesis was delivered 4 hours after the impression. This work was conducted in a relatively short

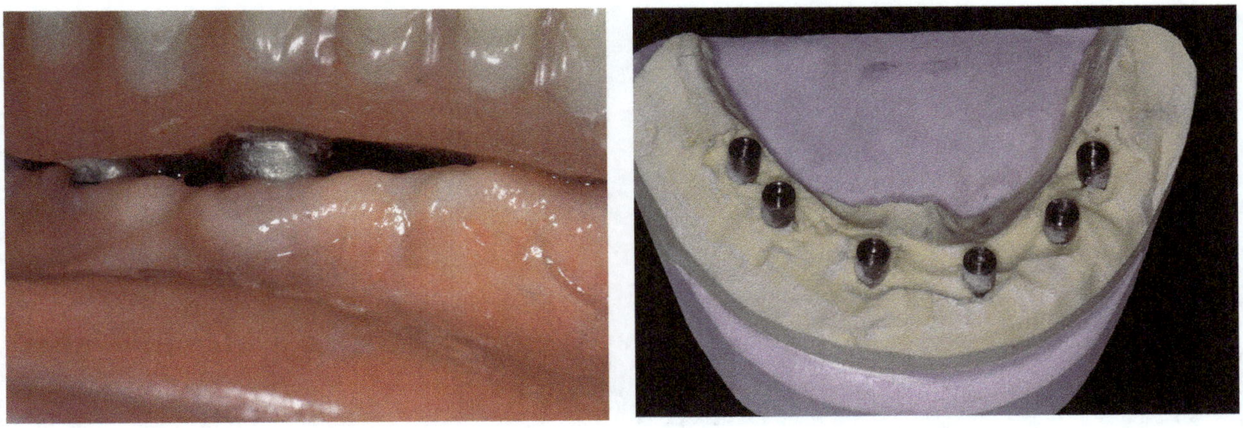

(a) (b)

FIGURE 4: Preparation after osseointegration and gingival recession. (a) After healing, clearance between the alveolar crest and the denture. (b) Stone was eliminated between the implant abutment analogs on the master cast model.

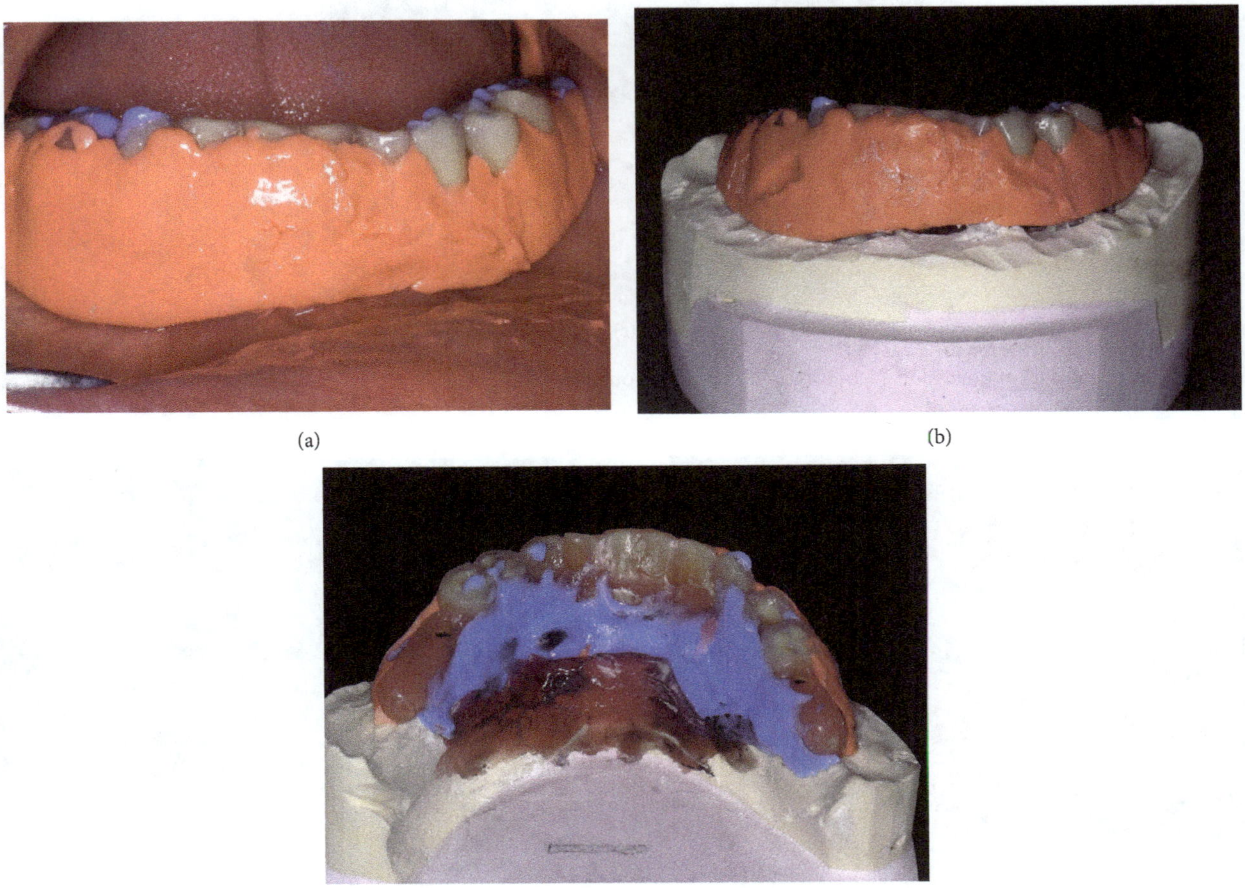

(a) (b) (c)

FIGURE 5: Posthealing prosthetic transformation. (a) Silicone impression material was injected under the prosthesis to fill the space, and occlusion was registered. (b) After the preparation of the model, the complex prosthesis and silicone are screwed onto the master cast model. (c) The restoration was boxed in the lingual area on the modified cast model.

period of time and the treatment cost was lower. The function after 6 years was stable (Figures 7 and 8). After 3 years of function, prosthetic complications occurred due to fractures of the complete antagonist prosthesis. This problem was solved by reinforcement with a palatal metal frame.

3. Discussion

The use of a temporary prosthesis for full arch rehabilitation is important for the patient's comfort and to respect the immediate loading criteria. Conversion prosthesis [17] has

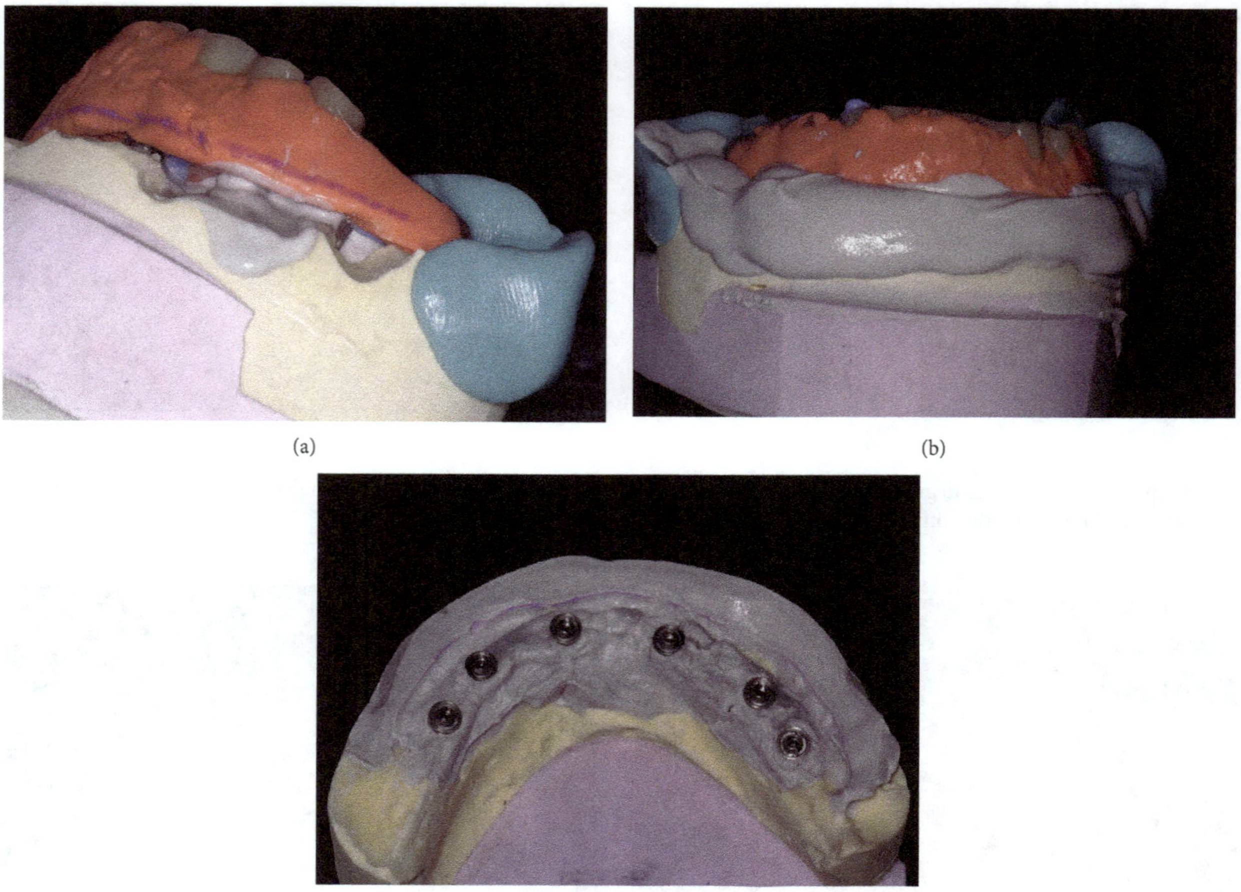

(a) (b) (c)

Figure 6: Master cast model modification. (a, b) New dental stone is poured into the space conserved on the buccal side. (c) Master cast model with the new crest anatomy.

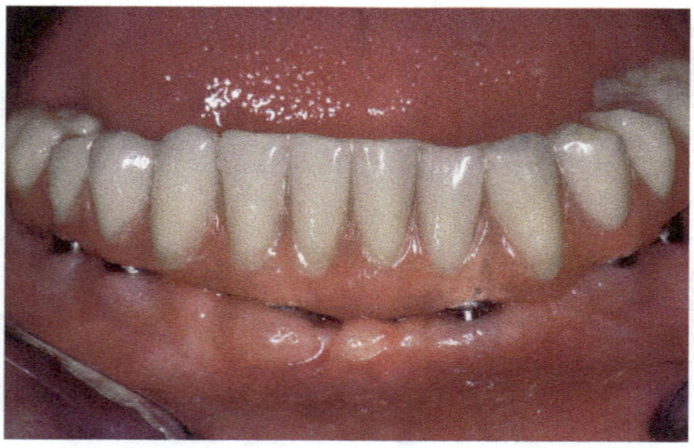

Figure 7: Final prosthesis. The molars and cantilevers were in occlusion, and a new adaptation to the crest was performed. The peri-implant tissues appeared healthy, indicating good oral hygiene level maintenance.

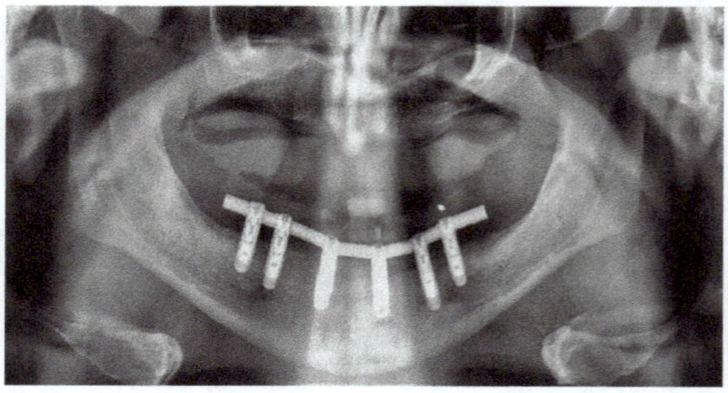

Figure 8: Radiographic panoramic control. After 6 years, bone level was stable.

been described as a technique for converting a transitional removable denture to a fixed provisional implant-supported prosthesis. This technique decreases the laboratory cost but increases the time of chair work. The precision of the prosthesis adaptation is often less than that of laboratory work. Moreover, it is difficult to incorporate metal renfort. Other authors have reported the feasibility of definitive all-acrylic resin prosthesis [18], but several studies have shown a better transmission of force and lack of micromovements on strengthened acrylic prosthesis [19, 20]. The micromovements of the implants during healing should not be more than 100 μm [21].

The use of a definitive restoration, directly positioned after implant placement, in place of the provisional prosthesis, can be used to achieve the same work in a shorter period of time [11, 12]. However, in all these techniques, after osseointegration and complete healing of the soft tissue, space appears between the gingiva and prosthesis. Moreover, the tooth arrangement, particularly on the cantilever, and the occlusion require improvement.

In this "one shot" simplified technique, the definitive framework is immediately built on the master cast model, thereby conserving it. The passive fit of the interim prosthesis was controlled on the implants, which validates the master model. The use of laser welding on milled cylinders allows for, in time compatible with immediate loading, manufacturing a framework with the same precision fit than the CAD-CAM titanium framework and yields a more accurate fit than the frameworks produced with the lost-wax technique [22]. Moreover, the possibility of using a titanium framework decreases the corrosion and metal leaching in comparison to a chrome-cobalt alloy [23, 24].

For the posthealing prosthetic transformation, occlusion and vertical dimensions were established on the articulator during the first step, using a facebow. These parameters after interim prosthesis function can be changed, but in most cases in our experience, the modifications are not common. During the gingival recession, the occlusion is controlled and the master cast model can be remounted in the semiadaptable articulator if necessary. This technique can be used for relining prosthetics after a long period of use if excessive spaces appear troublesome, but it is important to conserve the master cast model. This work can also be done in a short time, and the treatment cost is lower.

This technique requires suitable equipment and experience in laser welding laboratory work [15]. This clinical case was free from complications during service; the only problem was with the complete antagonist denture, but this has been previously described in the literature [25]. Fracture of titanium framework at the posterior cantilever can occur and will require a new welding and localized refection of the resin. The most frequently observed problems are cosmetic, with teeth fracture or resin veneer fracture. The bonding between metal and composite is an important point for prosthetic resistance under occlusal forces.

4. Conclusion

From the patient's point of view, the financial aspect of implant treatment is important. "One shot" concept, which combines a definitive framework with recession impression after healing, allows for a single prosthesis, which can be used as a temporary prosthesis with the necessary criteria for immediate loading. Adaptation to the tissue after the healing phase is important for patient comfort and can be achieved in a short time. The definitive restoration meets the specifications of the implant-supported screw-retained total prosthesis. This prosthetic simplification reduces the cost and is accessible to a large number of patients. Further studies with larger samples are required to better evaluate this promising low-cost patient treatment option.

Consent

The patient agreed to be treated and provided written informed consent.

Acknowledgments

The authors thank the dental laboratory technicians Hélène Mitjana and Hugues Doat for performing all laboratory steps involved in this clinical case.

References

[1] N. J. Kassebaum, A. G. C. Smith, E. Bernabé et al., "Global, regional, and national prevalence, incidence, and disability-adjusted life years for oral conditions for 195 countries, 1990-2015: a systematic analysis for the global burden of diseases, injuries, and risk factors," *Journal of Dental Research*, vol. 96, no. 4, pp. 380–387, 2017.

[2] M. V. Saintrain and E. H. de Souza, "Impact of tooth loss on the quality of life," *Gerodontology*, vol. 29, no. 2, pp. e632–e636, 2012.

[3] D. P. Tarnow, S. Emtiaz, and A. Classi, "Immediate loading of threaded implants at stage 1 surgery in edentulous arches: ten consecutive case reports with 1- to 5-year data," *The International Journal of Oral & Maxillofacial Implants*, vol. 12, no. 3, pp. 319–324, 1997.

[4] P. A. Schnitman, P. S. Wöhrle, J. E. Rubenstein, J. D. DaSilva, and N. H. Wang, "Ten-year results for Brånemark implants immediately loaded with fixed prostheses at implant placement," *The International Journal of Oral & Maxillofacial Implants*, vol. 12, no. 4, pp. 495–503, 1997.

[5] S. A. Alfadda, "A randomized controlled clinical trial of edentulous patients treated with immediately loaded implant-supported mandibular fixed prostheses," *Clinical Implant Dentistry and Related Research*, vol. 16, no. 6, pp. 806–816, 2014.

[6] A. Jokstad and H. Alkumru, "Immediate function on the day of surgery compared with a delayed implant loading process in the mandible: a randomized clinical trial over 5 years," *Clinical Oral Implants Research*, vol. 25, no. 12, pp. 1325–1335, 2014.

[7] P. Papaspyridakos, C. J. Chen, S. K. Chuang, and H. P. Weber, "Implant loading protocols for edentulous patients with fixed prostheses: a systematic review and meta-analysis," *The International Journal of Oral & Maxillofacial Implants*, vol. 29, pp. 256–270, 2014.

[8] M. Chiapasco, "Early and immediate restoration and loading of implants in completely edentulous patients," *The International Journal of Oral & Maxillofacial Implants*, vol. 19, pp. 76–91, 2004.

[9] G. O. Gallucci, D. Morton, and H. P. Weber, "Loading protocols for dental implants in edentulous patients," *The International Journal of Oral & Maxillofacial Implants*, vol. 24, pp. 132–146, 2009.

[10] H. De Bruyn, S. Raes, P. O. Ostman, and J. Cosyn, "Immediate loading in partially and completely edentulous jaws: a review of the literature with clinical guidelines," *Periodontology 2000*, vol. 66, no. 1, pp. 153–187, 2014.

[11] B. Yilmaz, T. B. Ozcelik, and E. McGlumphy, "Using the "final-on-four" concept to deliver an immediate metal-resin implant-fixed complete dental prosthesis," *The Journal of Prosthetic Dentistry*, vol. 114, no. 2, pp. 161–166, 2015.

[12] A. G. Paleari, C. D. Presoto, J. A. Vasconcelos et al., "An alternative technique for fabrication of frameworks in an immediate loading implant fixed mandibular prosthesis," *Case Reports in Dentistry*, vol. 2015, Article ID 102189, 4 pages, 2015.

[13] M. Degidi, D. Nardi, and A. Piattelli, "A six-year follow-up of full-arch immediate restorations fabricated with an intraoral welding technique," *Implant Dentistry*, vol. 22, no. 3, pp. 224–231, 2013.

[14] D. Bacchiocchi and A. Guida, "The Ball Welding Bar: A New Solution for the Immediate Loading of Screw- Retained, Mandibular Fixed Full Arch Prostheses," *International Journal of Dentistry*, vol. 2017, Article ID 2679085, 9 pages, 2017.

[15] C. N. Hart and P. R. Wilson, "Evaluation of welded titanium joints used with cantilevered implant-supported prostheses," *The Journal of Prosthetic Dentistry*, vol. 96, no. 1, pp. 25–32, 2006.

[16] J. Chow, E. Hui, J. Liu et al., "The Hong Kong Bridge Protocol. Immediate loading of mandibular Brånemark fixtures using a fixed provisional prosthesis: preliminary results," *Clinical Implant Dentistry and Related Research*, vol. 3, no. 3, pp. 166–174, 2001.

[17] T. J. Balshi and G. J. Wolfinger, "Conversion prosthesis: a transitional fixed implant-supported prosthesis for an edentulous arch a technical note," *The International Journal of Oral & Maxillofacial Implants*, vol. 11, no. 1, pp. 106–111, 1996.

[18] R. Crespi, R. Vinci, P. Capparé, G. E. Romanos, and E. Gherlone, "A clinical study of edentulous patients rehabilitated according to the "all on four" immediate function protocol," *The International Journal of Oral & Maxillofacial Implants*, vol. 27, no. 2, pp. 428–434, 2012.

[19] S. Holst, H. Geiselhoeringer, M. Wichmann, and A. I. Holst, "The effect of provisional restoration type on micromovement of implants," *The Journal of Prosthetic Dentistry*, vol. 100, no. 3, pp. 173–182, 2008.

[20] T. Ogawa, S. Dhaliwal, I. Naert et al., "Impact of implant number, distribution and prosthesis material on loading on implants supporting fixed prostheses," *Journal of Oral Rehabilitation*, vol. 37, no. 7, pp. 525–531, 2010.

[21] J. B. Brunski, "In vivo bone response to biomechanical loading at the bone/dental-implant interface," *Advances in Dental Research*, vol. 13, no. 1, pp. 99–119, 1999.

[22] J. Abduo, K. Lyons, V. Bennani, N. Waddell, and M. Swain, "Fit of screw-retained fixed implant frameworks fabricated by different methods: a systematic review," *The International Journal of Prosthodontics*, vol. 24, no. 3, pp. 207–220, 2011.

[23] L. Hjalmarsson, "On cobalt-chrome frameworks in implant dentistry," *Swedish Dental Journal Supplement*, vol. 201, pp. 3–83, 2009.

[24] N. Eliaz, "Corrosion of metallic biomaterials: a review," *Materials*, vol. 12, no. 3, p. 407, 2019.

[25] A. Ortorp and T. Jemt, "Early laser-welded titanium frameworks supported by implants in the edentulous mandible: a 15-year comparative follow-up study," *Clinical Implant Dentistry and Related Research*, vol. 11, no. 4, pp. 311–322, 2009.

33

Delayed Healing of Tooth Extraction Sockets with Ramucirumab use

Yosuke Iijima ,[1] Miki Yamada,[1] Shunsuke Hino,[1] Motohiko Sano,[2] Takahiro Kaneko,[1] and Norio Horie[1]

[1]*Department of Oral and Maxillofacial Surgery, Saitama Medical Center, Saitama Medical University, Saitama, Japan*
[2]*Division of Applied Pharmaceutical Education and Research Hoshi University, Tokyo, Japan*

Correspondence should be addressed to Yosuke Iijima; yoiijima@saitama-med.ac.jp

Academic Editor: Darko Macan

Objective. An angiogenesis inhibitor can cause medication-related osteonecrosis of the jaw (MRONJ). To our knowledge, there has been no report that an angiogenesis inhibitor causes delayed healing of tooth extraction socket. Here, we describe a case of delayed healing of tooth extraction sockets associated with an angiogenesis inhibitor, ramucirumab, which showed characteristics similar to MRONJ. *Materials and Methods.* A 76-year-old male patient, who was diagnosed with gastric cancer with liver metastasis, received tooth extraction twice during continuous chemotherapy comprising paclitaxel and ramucirumab. *Results.* The first extraction was performed 30 days after ramucirumab discontinuation without complication. The second extraction was conducted without ramucirumab discontinuation. Although tooth socket healing was finally achieved, it took about 150 days. *Discussion.* This case was considered to be delayed healing of dry sockets rather than MRONJ due to ramucirumab. Dentists and oral surgeons need to be aware that angiogenesis inhibitors can cause not only MRONJ but also dry sockets after tooth extraction.

1. Introduction

Many new cancer chemotherapeutic agents have been recently developed and administered. Among chemotherapeutic agents, angiogenesis inhibitors reduce or slow cancer progression by blocking the nutritional supply that the tumor requires. Ramucirumab, which was relatively newly approved by the United States Food and Drug Administration, binds to the extracellular domain of vascular endothelial growth factor-2 (VEGF-2) with high affinity and selectivity and blocks the binding of multiple VEGF ligands (VEGF-A, VEGF-C, and VEGF-D) to VEGFR-2 [1, 2]. Clinically, angiogenesis inhibitors are used alone or in combination with other chemotherapeutic agents. Ramucirumab has been used in second-line treatment of cancers such as gastric cancer, nonsmall cell lung cancer, and colorectal cancer [2].

Chemotherapeutic agents cause various adverse events, and major adverse events of angiogenesis inhibitors are hypertension, vomiting, neutropenia, and anemia [3]. Angiogenesis inhibitors can also interfere with wound healing, which is caused by blocking of vasodilation, increased vascular permeability and angiogenesis, and complication of wound healing was found in 0.5% of patients treated with ramucirumab [2, 4].

Medication-related osteonecrosis of the jaw (MRONJ) has been identified as a common oral adverse event of chemotherapy [5]. MRONJ is principally caused by bone-modifying agents (BMAs) including bisphosphonates and denosumab, which inhibit bone resorption, and MRONJ also occurs upon taking angiogenesis inhibitors without the use of BMAs [5, 6]. Invasive dental surgery, such as tooth extraction, is the predisposing factor of MRONJ.

To date, there has been no report of delayed healing of a tooth extraction socket complicated by MRONJ during ramucirumab use. In this article, the authors report on two tooth extractions in a patient treated with ramucirumab. The first tooth extractions occurred 30 days after ramucirumab discontinuation and the sockets healed well. The second extractions were performed without ramucirumab cessation and severe contact pain of the socket quickly developed.

Although healing was finally possible, it took about 150 days for the socket to heal completely. From a comprehensive perspective, these findings suggested that the second extraction sockets might be caused by delayed dry socket healing (alveolar otitis) rather than MRONJ.

2. Case Report

In July 2018, a 76-year-old man was referred to the oral surgery clinic from the gastroenterology and hepatology clinic for dental caries treatment. In August 2016, the patient was diagnosed with gastric cancer with multiple liver metastases and lymph node metastases. The patient began chemotherapy comprising cisplatin and tegafur/gimeracil/oteracil. In February 2017, the lymph node metastases had shrunk and the patient underwent surgery for gastric cancer. Subsequently, beginning in June 2017, he started chemotherapy comprising paclitaxel (100 mg) and ramucirumab (310 mg) as second-line treatment. Paclitaxel was given weekly, and ramucirumab was given every 2 weeks. The patient was also prescribed concomitant antihypertensive and diuretic medications. In July 2018, there was no evidence of recurrence of liver metastasis by positron emission tomography. Furthermore, the patient desired to treat dental caries and stop chemotherapy; thus, chemotherapy was discontinued. Thirty days after the last dose of ramucirumab, the right maxillary central incisor, right maxillary second premolar, left maxillary first and second molars, and left mandibular lateral incisor were extracted (Figure 1). The postextraction course was uneventful with good healing of tooth extraction sockets. In November 2018, computed tomography showed recurrence of liver metastasis and the patient restarted chemotherapy with paclitaxel and ramucirumab (same dose as before). In January 2019, the patient experienced repeat pericoronitis in the right mandibular third molar and eating difficulties. Thus, the right mandibular third molar and right mandibular first molars and second premolar, which were difficult to treat conservatively, were extracted in March 2019 without ramucirumab discontinuation after discussion between the patient and the chemotherapy team. The extractions were performed 8 days after ramucirumab administration, taking into consideration the half-life of ramucirumab (8 days) and the timing of the next administration of ramucirumab. The third molar, which was an impacted tooth, was extracted with elevation of the mucoperiosteal flap and bone removal. After the tooth extractions, the patient received amoxicillin (750 mg) for 7 days, and acetaminophen (400 mg) was given as an analgesic. Seven days after the extractions, the patient felt strong contact pain in the sockets. He had no other symptoms that suggested the spread of inflammation. Dry sockets were strongly suggested, and the analgesic was continued. Paclitaxel and ramucirumab were restarted according to the chemotherapy regimen. Twenty-three days after the extractions, the patient stated that he was still in severe pain but the pain was better than before (Figure 2(a)). Subsequently, paclitaxel and ramucirumab were continued. Twenty-five days after the extractions, the lower denture was extended to cover the extraction socket to decrease the contact pain. Forty-seven days after the extractions, the pain was moderately diminished, but soft tissue did not completely cover the extraction sockets. Sixty-one days after the extractions, the pain was considerably diminished, and soft tissue mostly covered the extraction sockets of the first molar and second premolar, but not that of the third molar (Figure 2(b)). This was probably because the third molar extraction was more invasive with bone removal. Seventy-five days after the extractions, the socket of the third molar was slightly covered with soft tissue (Figure 2(c)). One hundred and three days after the extractions, the socket of the third molar was still not completely covered with soft tissue. One hundred and seventeen days after the extractions, the socket of the third molar was partially covered with soft tissue. There was almost no contact pain. By comparison, the extraction sockets of the first molar and second premolar were completely covered with soft tissue (Figure 2(d)). One hundred and thirty days after the extractions, the extraction socket of the third molar was almost completed covered with soft tissue with almost no pain (Figure 2(e)). On the same day, the final doses of paclitaxel and ramucirumab were given because the patient's liver metastasis subsequently progressed. Third-line treatment with nivolumab (240 mg) was started 158 days after the tooth extractions, and the patient reported no pain in the sockets at this time. One hundred and eighty-four days after tooth extractions, the patient continued to receive nivolumab, and complication of the socket such as bone exposure was not observed.

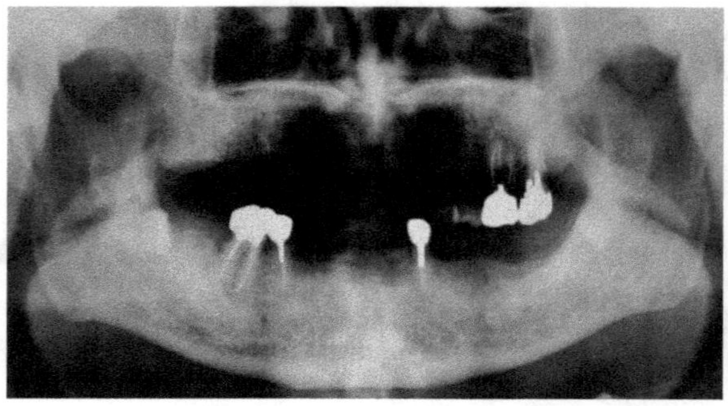

FIGURE 1: Photoradiograph showing the patient's teeth before the first extractions.

3. Discussion

Dental treatment of patients during chemotherapy, especially surgical intervention, is recommended prior to chemotherapy and, when absolutely necessary, during chemotherapy intervals. However, chemotherapy is seldom needed once, commonly requiring repeated administrations with a long duration, and the interval between chemotherapy cycles may be too short for adequate dental treatment. Furthermore, depending on the patient's condition, it may be necessary to provide dental treatment without considering chemotherapy withdrawal and interval periods.

MRONJ is defined as the presence of exposed bone or bone that can be probed through an intraoral or extraoral fistula in the maxillofacial region, which is present for more than 8 weeks and without a history of radiation therapy to the jaws [5]. In this case, delayed healing of the second

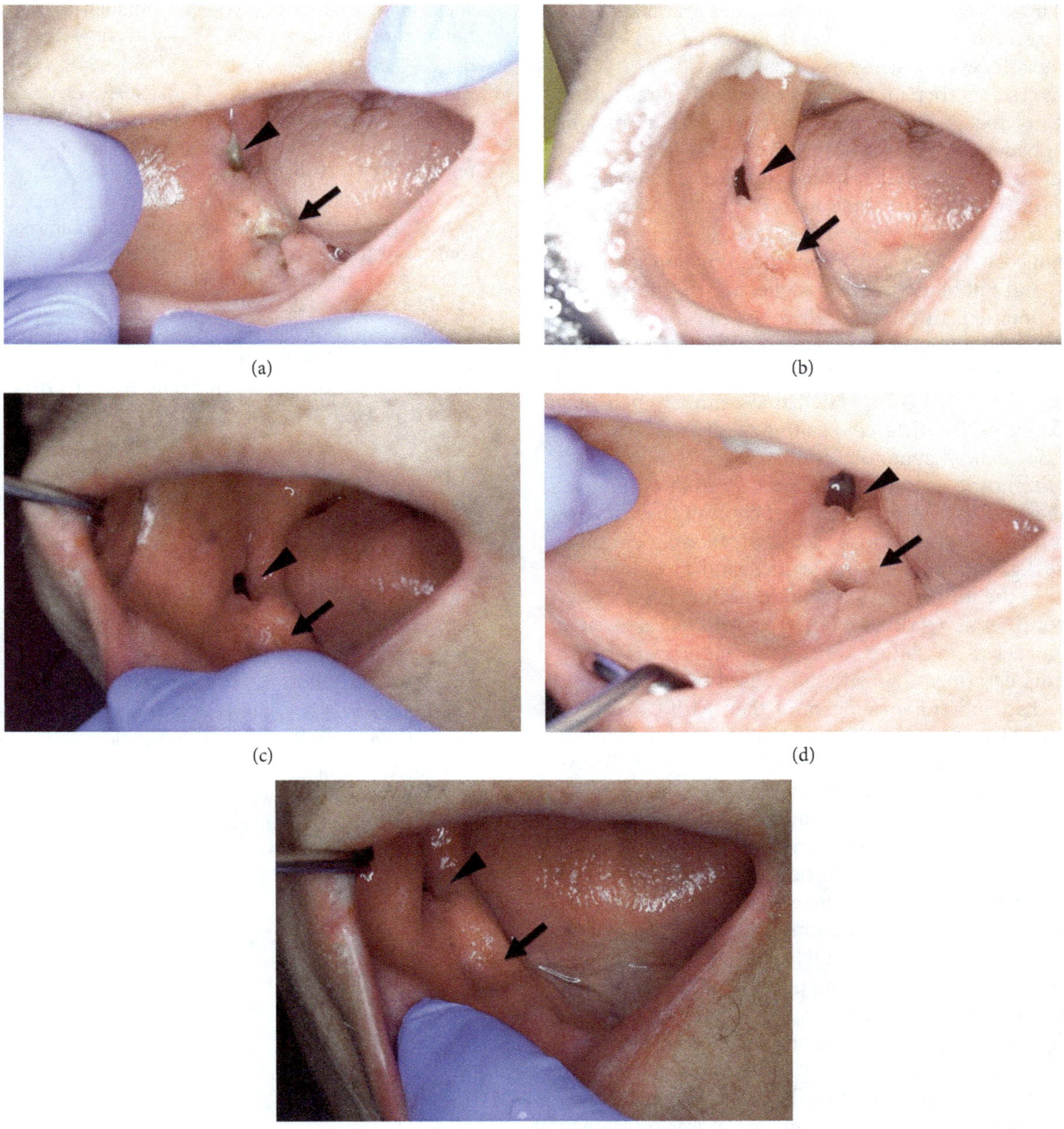

Figure 2: Photographs showing the healing process of the sockets. (a) Bone exposure was noted 23 days after the extractions in each socket (arrow, sockets of the first molar and second premolar; arrowhead, socket of the third molar). (b) Sixty-one days after the extractions, sockets of the first molar and second premolar were mostly covered with soft tissue (arrow), whereas the socket of the third molar was not covered (arrowhead). (c) Seventy-five days after the extractions, sockets of the first molar and second premolar were almost completely covered with soft tissue (arrow), but the socket of the third molar was only slightly covered (arrowhead). (d) One hundred and seventeen days after extractions, sockets of the first molar and second premolar were completely covered with soft tissue (arrow). However, the socket of the third molar was only partially covered (arrowhead). (e). One hundred and thirty days after extraction, the socket of the third molar was almost completely covered with soft tissue (arrowhead).

extraction socket occurred with bone exposure of more than 8 weeks, and the patient had no history of radiation therapy to the jaws or metastatic disease to the jaws. Based on these findings, the patient would typically be considered to have stage 2 MRONJ. However, the authors were concerned that this case differed from the typical MRONJ clinical course.

As with MRONJ, dry socket is a common complication after tooth extraction, wherein the socket is not covered with soft tissue. Fibrinolysis of blood clots has been considered the main cause of dry socket. Although the mechanism is unclear, bacterial involvement has been suggested [7]. The socket is partly covered or totally devoid of blood clots with exposed, rough, painful bone. Considering the action of angiogenesis inhibitors, it is quite possible that these agents cause dry sockets. Dry sockets are characterized by severe and persistent pain, which lasts till the exposed (and nonvital) bone is either eventually covered by granulation tissue or is separated from the underlying bone and sequestrated. This process can take more than 4 weeks.

In this case, severe pain occurred soon after extraction. In a case of dry socket, it is usually sharp pain. There may be local lymphadenitis, and a few untreated cases of dry socket may progress to infection that spreads through the bone marrow (osteomyelitis) [8]. Pain is improved by covering the wound, as in this case. However, in MRONJ, severe pain rarely occurs immediately after extraction, inflammation gradually increases, and antibiotic therapy is effective to improve the patient's condition. In this case, there was no pus discharge from the extraction sockets, and the extraction sockets healed without continuous antibiotic therapy, although it took a long time. These results suggested that ramucirumab may cause relatively long-delayed healing of dry sockets, and patients may exhibit symptoms similar to MRONJ or meet MRONJ diagnostic criteria. In comparison to bevacizumab, which binds to VEGF-A and is the first clinically used angiogenesis inhibitor, ramucirumab blocks the binding of multiple VEGF ligands. This difference in ligand blocking may be related to the formation of a delayed healing dry socket.

Pimolbutr et al. reported 35 cases of MRONJ associated with angiogenesis inhibitors other than ramucirumab [6]. The authors described that MRONJ caused by angiogenesis inhibitors had superior healing rates than MRONJ caused by BMAs. Thus, there might be a qualitative difference in bone modification effects between MRONJ caused by BMAs and MRONJ caused by angiogenesis inhibitors.

If delayed socket healing is caused by a common dry socket rather than MRONJ, then treatment for a dry socket is necessary. Good oral hygiene is necessary not only to keep the socket clean but also to prevent adverse events associated with concomitant use of chemotherapeutic agents. Good oral hygiene is also essential for MRONJ treatment. In addition, analgesics are effective to manage postoperative pain in dry socket. Antibiotics may reduce infection when used as surgical prophylaxis, but postoperative administration is not recommended [8, 9]. Irrigation with warm saline to remove the debris, chlorhexidine mouthwash, and dressings to cover the exposed bone are effective. In this case, it was possible to alleviate the patient's oral pain by extending the denture to cover the extraction sockets.

In conclusion, this case was considered to be delayed dry socket healing rather than MRONJ caused by ramucirumab. If a patient has a dry socket, the dry socket treatment is necessary. Dentists and oral surgeons need to be aware that angiogenesis inhibitors can cause not only MRONJ but also dry sockets after tooth extractions that are very slow to heal.

References

[1] M. Janning and S. Loges, "Anti-angiogenics: their value in lung cancer therapy," *Oncology research and treatment*, vol. 41, no. 4, pp. 172–180, 2017.

[2] J. Tabernero, T. Yoshino, A. L. Cohn et al., "Ramucirumab versus placebo in combination with second-line FOLFIRI in patients with metastatic colorectal carcinoma that progressed during or after first-line therapy with bevacizumab, oxaliplatin, and a fluoropyrimidine (RAISE): a randomised, double-blind, multicentre, phase 3 study," *The Lancet Oncology*, vol. 16, no. 5, pp. 499–508, 2015.

[3] Z. G. Bai and Z. T. Zhang, "A systematic review and meta-analysis on the effect of angiogenesis blockade for the treatment of gastric cancer," *Oncotargets and Therapy*, vol. Volume 11, pp. 7077–7087, 2018.

[4] D. Arnold, C. S. Fuchs, J. Tabernero et al., "Meta-analysis of individual patient safety data from six randomized, placebo-controlled trials with the antiangiogenic VEGFR2-binding monoclonal antibody ramucirumab," *Annals of Oncology*, vol. 28, no. 12, pp. 2932–2942, 2017.

[5] S. L. Ruggiero, T. B. Dodson, J. Fantasia et al., "American Association of Oral and Maxillofacial Surgeons position paper on medication-related osteonecrosis of the jaw–2014 update," *Journal of Oral and Maxillofacial Surgery*, vol. 72, no. 10, pp. 1938–1956, 2014.

[6] K. Pimolbutr, S. Porter, and S. Fedele, "Osteonecrosis of the jaw associated with antiangiogenics in Antiresorptive-Naïve patient: a comprehensive review of the literature," *BioMed Research International*, vol. 2018, Article ID 8071579, 14 pages, 2018.

[7] L. H. Shen, E. Xiao, E. B. Wang, H. Zheng, and Y. Zhang, "High-throughput sequencing analysis of microbial profiles in the dry socket," *Journal of Oral and Maxillofacial Surgery*, vol. 77, no. 8, pp. 1548–1556, 2019.

[8] J. Pedlar and W. Frame, "Oral and Maxillofacial Surgery," in *4 - Extraction of teeth*, Elsevier Ltd, 2nd edition, 2007.

[9] H. Cho, A. J. Lynham, and E. Hsu, "Postoperative interventions to reduce inflammatory complications after third molar surgery: review of the current evidence," *Australian Dental Journal*, vol. 62, no. 4, pp. 412–419, 2017.

Rehabilitation of Edentulous Jaws with Full-Arch Fixed Implant-Supported Prostheses: An Approach with Short and Ultrashort Implants and Metal-Free Materials

Riccardo Aiuto,[1] Christian Barbieri,[1] Daniele Garcovich,[2] Mario Dioguardi,[3] Mattia Redaelli,[4] and Luca De Micheli[5]

[1]*Department of Biomedical, Surgical, and Dental Science, University of Milan, Italy*
[2]*Universidad Europea de Valencia, Spain*
[3]*Department of Clinical and Experimental Medicine, University of Foggia, Italy*
[4]*Private Practice, Albavilla, Como, Italy*
[5]*Department of Periodontology, Italian Stomatological Institute, Milan, Italy*

Correspondence should be addressed to Riccardo Aiuto; riccardo.aiuto@unimi.it

Academic Editor: Konstantinos Michalakis

Introduction. Short implants represent a valid alternative to bone regeneration techniques. In addition, metal-free prosthetic materials have several advantages for predictable rehabilitation. This case report is aimed at illustrating the advantages of fixed implant-prosthetic rehabilitation on short and ultrashort implants and metal-free prosthetic materials. *Case report.* A 66-year-old male patient with bone atrophy was treated with temporary denture placement performed based on a rapid protocol. Once the tissues after extractions matured and aesthetic/function was studied, short implants were prosthetically placed, and a fiber-reinforced composite (FRC) bar was digitally designed for a double full-arch fixed rehabilitation. The 2-year follow-up showed the absence of peri-implantitis signs and a stable occlusal relationship of prostheses. *Discussion and conclusions.* The FRC material has excellent aesthetic properties and is low cost with a simplified and fast workflow owing to digital dentistry methods. Further studies are still needed to confirm the effectiveness of long-term therapy; however, the combination of new minimally invasive surgery and prosthetic advances seems to be very promising.

1. Introduction

Complete edentulism is a serious problem that affects many individuals, with different incidence and prevalence rates worldwide. Owing to advances in dentistry, the situation has improved; however, there is an increase in incidence in the elderly population. The loss of teeth without replacement with dentures implies severe loss of oral functioning [1]. Therefore, despite the progress in prevention, diagnosis, and treatment, dentists are facing the challenge of rehabilitation of patients with edentulism daily.

Sivaramakrishnan and Sridharan in their meta-analysis confirmed that oral implantology can improve the quality of life of patients with total prosthesis through the realization of implant-supported rehabilitations [2]. Total oral rehabilitation is a complex therapeutic procedure because it includes many aspects, such as the patient's emotional sphere and general health status; however, clinical difficulties are represented, for example, by atrophy of the jaw bone or limitation imposed by the presence of the inferior alveolar nerve (IAN) if endosseous implants are planned [3]. Thus, oral surgery is becoming less invasive to limit the risks and prevent excessive discomfort of the patient, who prefers to avoid bone grafts and prevent intra- and postoperative morbidity in terms of pain, swelling, bleeding, or extended operative time [4]. With a view to minimally invasive implant surgery, short implants or ultrashort implants (<6 mm in length) are a valid alternative. In a systematic review of RTCs, Amine et al. showed promising results in terms of bone loss in these types of implants that are increasingly used [5].

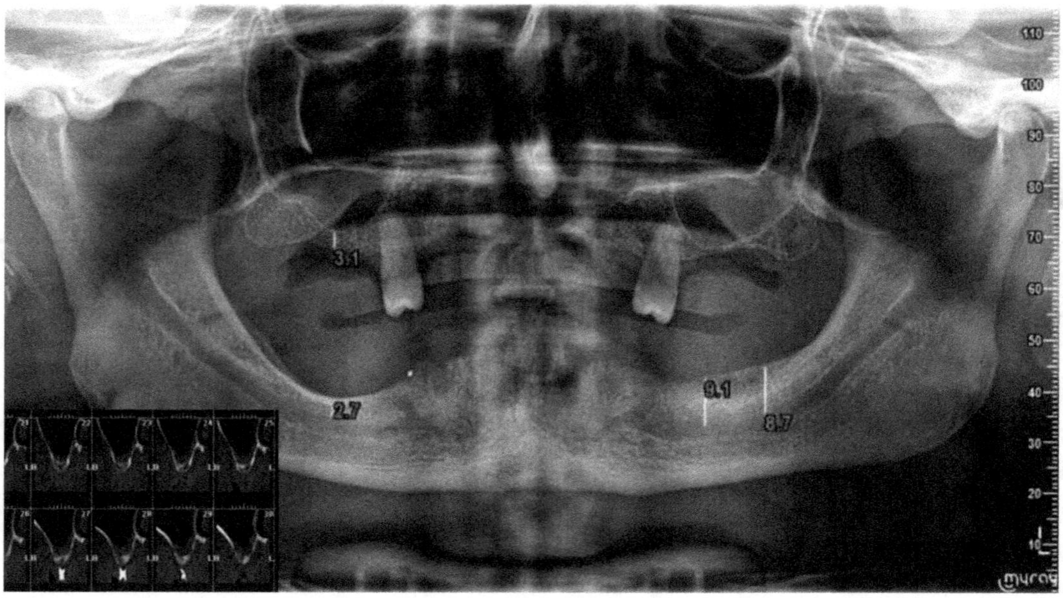

Figure 1: Preoperative orthopantomography and CBCT.

In addition to the surgical phase, the design of the prosthesis also plays an important role. In the past years, the interest in prosthetic dentistry has focused on composite materials, and many studies have been conducted to evaluate the performance of fixed partial dentures made of composite materials. The advantages of these composite materials over traditional metal-ceramic systems include improved aesthetics, excellent biomechanical behavior, and possibility of repair or modifying denture chairside [6]. Zaparolli et al. have recently analyzed different bar materials and manufacturing techniques, proving that fiber-reinforced composite (FRC) materials have achieved excellent functional-aesthetic and biotolerability results [7].

This case report is aimed at illustrating the advantages of fixed implant-prosthetic rehabilitation on short implants and metal-free prosthetic materials.

2. Case Report

A 66-year-old man, with hypertension and a history of smoking, consulted us at an Italian center qualified for short dental implants. The patient had previously undergone extractions of the lower teeth and is totally edentulous, apart from the two upper second premolars. The patient had severe atrophy (Cawood and Howell classes IV and V) [8] of the jaw bones (Figure 1) and is currently wearing an incongruous mobile prosthesis. The patient requested to undergo fixed-prosthetic implant rehabilitation. In agreement with the patient, the treatment plan included extraction of remaining teeth (with 2° mobility, as described by Miller) [9], creation of two temporary upper and lower total prostheses, and finalization of the case with the prosthetically guided insertion of short implants and manufacturing of a fixed prosthesis with an FRC bar.

Four weeks after the planned extractions, the realization of total prosthesis followed a simplified protocol that started with alginate impressions (standard stainless steel trays) and detection of the craniomandibular relationships with JIG BTHB (the articulator Condylator® was then used). In the second appointment, the tooth assembly test and phonetic and aesthetic tests were performed (Figure 2). In the next visit, the prosthesis was terminated.

Implant surgery was performed after the maturation of the tissues, approximately 3 months after the extractions. For prosthetically guided surgery, duplicates of the prosthesis were used: in the first phase, a check was made thanks to a cone beam which showed a radiopaque material positioned inside the prosthesis; subsequently, the duplicate was drilled and used as a surgical guide. Surgical interventions involved local anesthesia with Optocain® (mepivacaine 1 : 100.000), full-thickness flap, and use of a surgical template built with the duplication of the new prostheses for implant-guided positioning. The following short implants (Bicon LLC, Boston, MA, USA) were inserted in another appointment a month later: 4.5 × 6 mm and 4.5 × 5 mm in zones 16 and 26, respectively, with transcrestal sinus lift without biomaterials and 4 × 8 mm in zone 13 and 4 × 6 mm in zone 24. In a second appointment, a few weeks later with the same modality, the lower implants were inserted in the intraforaminal region: two implants 3 × 8 mm in the areas 34 and 42 and two implants 3.5 × 8 in areas 32 and 43. The suturing material used was 4-0 Silk. The implant in zone 26 was removed after a few weeks for an osseointegration failure. Four months after the first surgical stage, the implants were uncovered, and healing abutments were placed. After 15 days of healing, the abutments were removed, and related transfers with their copings were connected and splinted to the fixtures. An implant-level transfer impression was recorded in the silicone material. The bite was recorded with articulation wax. For the realization of the prosthesis's FRC bar with Trinia® on implants, it is essential to use a partially digital workflow: not being a traditional cast bar, the design takes place

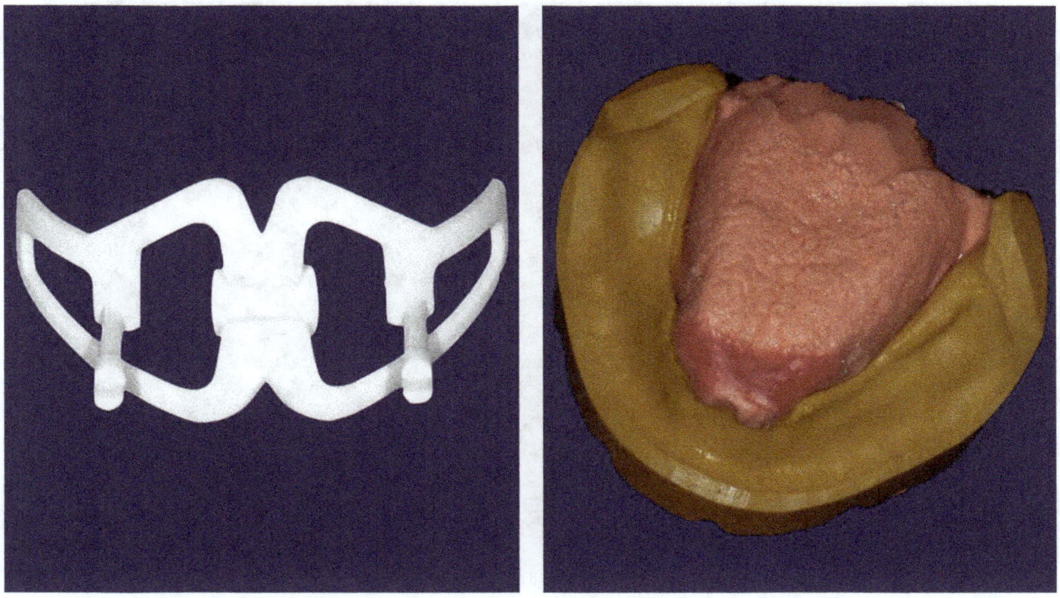

FIGURE 2: JIG BTHB device and tongue position in the model.

thanks to a software. Trinia® CAD/CAM discs and blocks are composed of a multidirectional interlacing of fiberglass and resin in several layers. In performing this procedure, the laboratory model was digitally scanned after proving its accuracy with a light-cured resin bar for intraoral confirmation. The fiber-resin bar was digitally designed (exocad) on a computer (Figure 3). The project was performed using a milling machine operating on five axes (Roland DWX-50). The construction of the prosthesis on the bar reflected the parameters of the temporary prosthesis. The fitting of the framework was checked thanks to a radiopaque light cured resin bar for an intraoral and radiograph confirmation, and the Morse taper connection was activated. Temporary cementation of the framework was achieved (Temp-Bond, Kerr). The occlusion was evaluated and adjusted (Figures 4 and 5). The clinical protocol initially included checks every 4 months, then every 6 months. The following checks were performed: clinical examination, peri-implant probing, plaque and bleeding score, and radiographs.

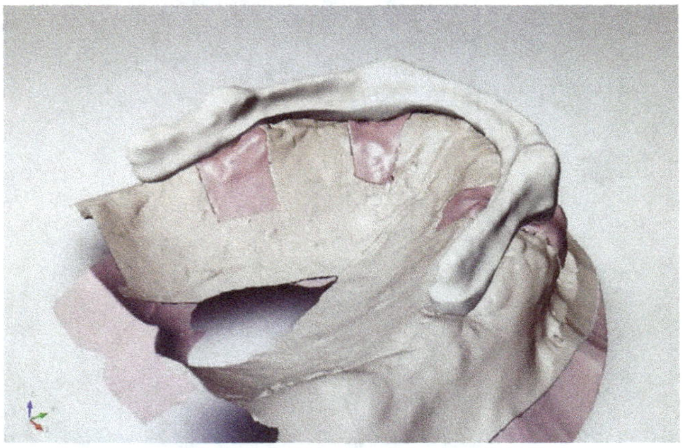

FIGURE 3: Trinia® bar CAD.

3. Discussion

The necessary occlusal adjustments were minimal, and the patient was immediately comfortable with the new rehabilitation. He was able to chew and speak correctly, and social life and consequently psychological well-being improved. The patient was also extremely satisfied with the aesthetics achieved.

Regarding the prosthetic aspect, there are important cantilevers in the distal areas of quadrants 2, 3, and 4, none of which exceeded 21 mm. As for the surgical aspect, the implant in zone 26 was lost due to lack of osseointegration before loading, but the 2-year radiographic follow-up showed the absence of signs of bone resorption around the implants (Figure 6). The fixture was characterized by a conometric connection with the abutments, both made from Ti-6Al-4V alloy, and a calcium phosphate-based treatment. A critical point for a potential microbial colonization and peri-implantitis is the connection between the implant and the prosthetic abutment [10]. The locking taper design of the implant allows a valid seal against bacteria [11].

The therapy's success was also confirmed by the absence of other clinical problems and stable and balanced occlusal relationship. In fact, the patient no longer had those discomforts that he had with the previous incongruous dentures. The patient was provided with home oral hygiene rules; in any case, he regularly returns to the clinic for periodic checks and professional oral hygiene sessions.

Complex implant-prosthetic rehabilitation, such as that described here, requires special attention from different points of view to ensure long-term clinical success. The first aspect to consider is the diagnosis and requests of the patient, who in this case preferred a fixed prosthesis. To complete the diagnosis, radiographs are fundamental: in this case of severe atrophy, in addition to orthopantomography, three-dimensional imaging techniques were also performed, which are fundamental for a correct preoperative evaluation [12].

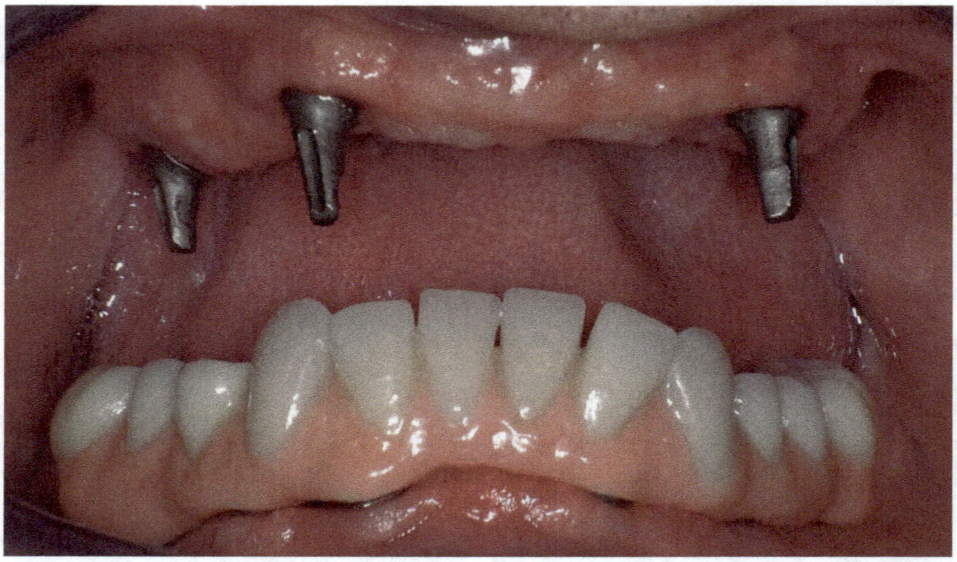

(a)

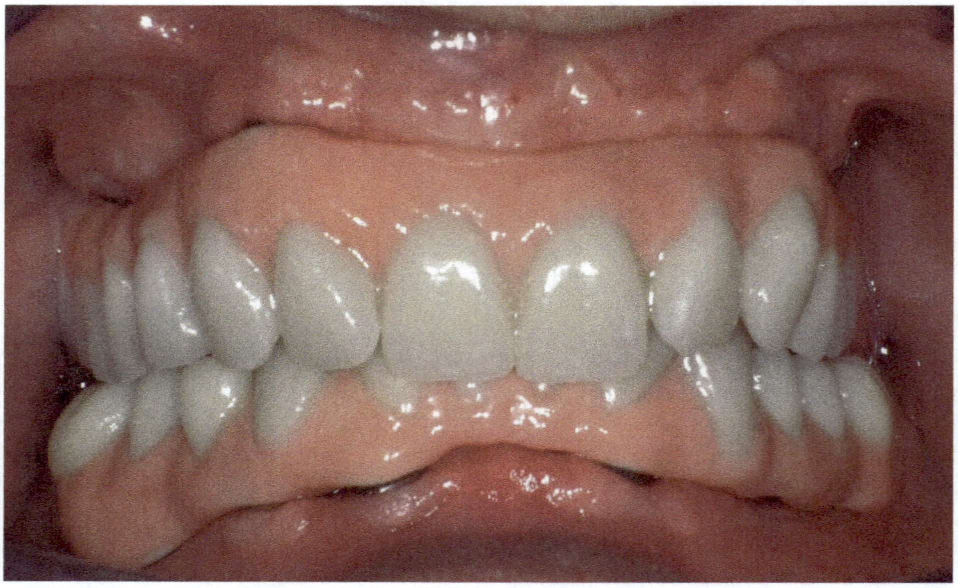

(b)

FIGURE 4: Implant abutments and full-arch fixed implant-supported prosthesis.

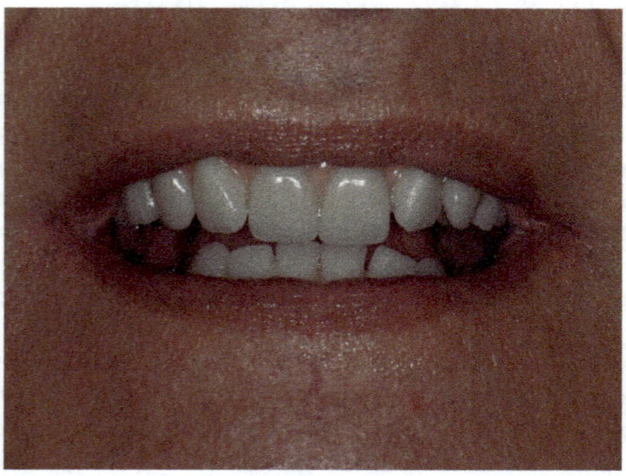

FIGURE 5: Final smile aesthetic results.

However, it was greatly important to start from a correct design of the removable temporary prosthesis. This is to not only satisfy the aesthetic requests of the patient but also create a prosthesis respecting the neutral zone for perfect adaptation and therefore avoid dangerous forces or uncomfortable situations of poor retention. Owing to the JIG BTHB device, it was possible to perform the procedure quickly, recording the craniomandibular relationship and tongue position of the patient. In 1976, Beresin and Schiesser described the neutral zone, affirming that the soft tissues that form the internal and external boundaries of the denture space exert forces that greatly influence the stability of the dentures [13]. Therefore, the aim was to locate that area in the edentulous mouth where the teeth should be positioned so that the forces exerted by muscles will stabilize rather than unseat the denture.

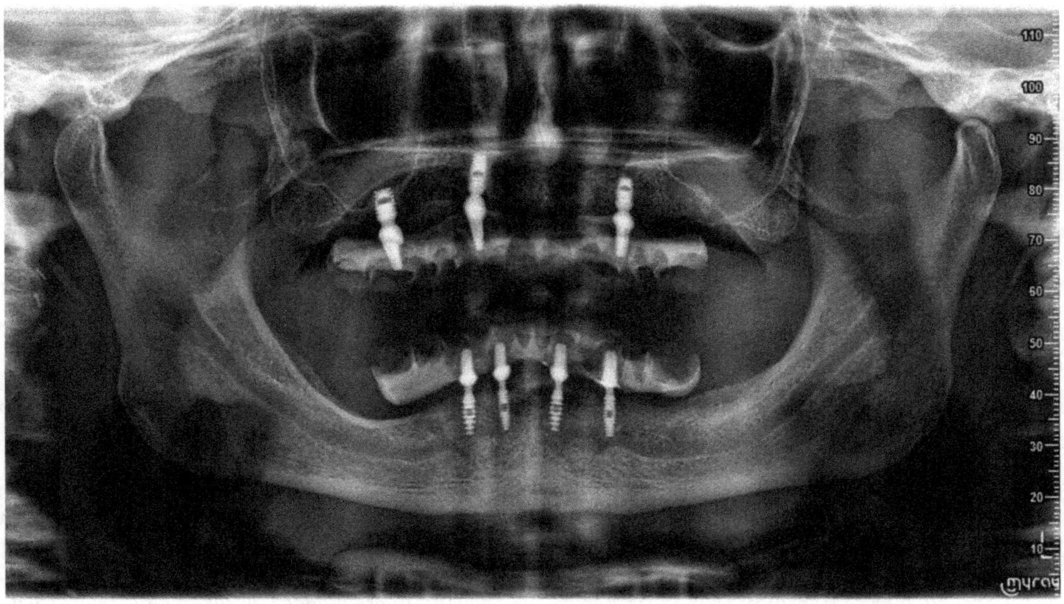

FIGURE 6: Postoperative orthopantomography at the 2-year follow-up.

A recent consensus statement also considers the importance of a balanced occlusion in an All-On-4 protocol [14]. Therefore, correct positioning of the teeth allowed the patient to not only accept the occlusal scheme but also correctly position the implants and avoid forces that cause stress on both the prosthetic and implant components. The desire for a predictable prosthesis, particularly for fixed partial dentures, led to the development of the concept of "prosthetically guided implantology." This concept establishes the correct implant position during the diagnostic stage according to planned definitive restoration. The importance of this approach was analyzed by Tallarico and Meloni in a recent multicenter study [15].

Additionally, in this case, the use of short implants in the native bone limits the indication for tilted implants. As claimed by Scarano et al. in their study [16], the protocol with short implants avoids more invasive tissue regeneration interventions, and it can be a solution in cases of limited bone height, but it has also some limitations. In fact, an immediate load was not performed. In any case, several authors question the immediate load because, in order to immediately load an implant, primary stability is required, with a bone compression that often may cause reabsorption and replacement of nonfunctional, avascular bone [17]. This patient already had a denture and anamnesis that allowed the clinical choice for a low-risk treatment-oriented procedure.

Therefore, despite the failure of an implant, the initial prosthetic project was completed without problems. The initial program included four dental implants in maxilla, but after the loss of one of these, the patient did not want to undergo other operation for implant replacement. The choice to continue even without an implant was also dictated by the fact that occlusal contacts had been carefully studied, and a high-performance metal-free material was used.

After the analog impression, with specially splinted transfers to ensure excellent precision [18], the bar for the fixed prosthesis was designed using digital methods and is made of FRC. This material allows better distribution of occlusal loads, an advantage that contributes to the maintenance of the peri-implant bone: the implant-supported FRC not only eliminates excessive stresses in the bone-implant interface but also maintains normal physiological loading of the surrounding bone [19]. The reason for this is the lower material's flexural modulus that permits the absorption of energy from the masticatory cycle. Despite this characteristic, the performance in terms of resistance is comparable to that of other materials generally used for these purposes.

Finally, there is a biocompatibility issue. The FRC material was also found as an optimized alternative to similar materials used for the reconstruction of craniofacial bone defects [20]. Compared to metal alloys, it prevents corrosion that represents a concrete risk; for example, cobalt and nickel can be released into the oral cavity in other types of prosthesis [6]. Therefore, the advantages are multiple: the FRC material has excellent aesthetic properties and low cost with a simplified and fast workflow, owing to digital dentistry methods. Although the results are very encouraging, further studies are still needed to confirm the effectiveness of long-term therapy.

4. Conclusions

Rehabilitation of a patient with complete edentulism still represents a great challenge for dentists. Owing to scientific and technological advances, it is possible to implement protocols that allow less invasive implant surgery and prosthesis that correctly responds to rehabilitation needs, while respecting biology. This combination translates, for the surgical phase, into the use of short implants to reduce operative risks, limit patient discomfort, and more easily manage situations of bone atrophy that is often present in these cases. However, in the prosthetic phase, which starts from the fundamentals of the mobile prosthesis, it indicates the use of more high-performance materials, such as metal-free FRC materials, which reduce the number of implants and have great advantages in terms of durability, biotolerability, aesthetics, and treatment costs. All are facilitated by a partially digital workflow, as evidenced by the clinical case presented.

Acknowledgments

The authors would like to express their gratitude to Mr. Roberto Mariconti for his insightful contribution.

References

[1] P. E. Petersen, D. Kandelman, S. Arpin, and H. Ogawa, "Global oral health of older people–call for public health action," *Community Dental Health*, vol. 27, Supplement 2, pp. 257–268, 2020.

[2] G. Sivaramakrishnan and K. Sridharan, "Comparison of implant supported mandibular overdentures and conventional dentures on quality of life: a systematic review and meta-analysis of randomized controlled studies," *Australian Dental Journal*, vol. 61, no. 4, pp. 482–488, 2016.

[3] A. C. Pimentel, M. A. Sanches, G. C. Ramalho, C. V. Roman-Torres, M. R. Manzi, and W. R. Sendyk, "Lateralization technique and inferior alveolar nerve transposition," *Case Reports in Dentistry*, vol. 2016, Article ID 4802637, 10 pages, 2016.

[4] B. Pommer, G. Mailath-Pokorny, R. Haas, D. Busenlechner, R. Fürhauser, and G. Watzek, "Patients' preferences towards minimally invasive treatment alternatives for implant rehabilitation of edentulous jaws," *European Journal of Oral Implantology*, vol. 7, Supplement 2, pp. S91–S109, 2014.

[5] M. Amine, Y. Guelzim, S. Benfaida, A. Bennani, and A. Andoh, "Short implants (5–8 mm) vs. long implants in augmented bone and their impact on peri-implant bone in maxilla and/or mandible: systematic review," *Journal of Stomatology, Oral and Maxillofacial Surger*, vol. 120, no. 2, pp. 133–142, 2019.

[6] A. Passaretti, G. Petroni, G. Miracolo, V. Savoia, A. Perpetuini, and A. Cicconetti, "Metal free, full arch, fixed prosthesis for edentulous mandible rehabilitation on four implants," *Journal of Prosthodontic Research*, vol. 62, no. 2, pp. 264–267, 2018.

[7] D. Zaparolli, R. F. Peixoto, D. Pupim, A. P. Macedo, M. B. Toniollo, and M. da Glória Chiarello de Mattos, "Photoelastic analysis of mandibular full-arch implant-supported fixed dentures made with different bar materials and manufacturing techniques," *Materials Science and Engineering: C*, vol. 81, pp. 144–147, 2017.

[8] J. I. Cawood and R. A. Howell, "A classification of the edentulous jaws," *International Journal of Oral and Maxillofacial Surgery*, vol. 17, no. 4, pp. 232–236, 1988.

[9] S. C. Miller, *Textbook of Periodontia*, Blakiston Co, Philadelphia, PA, USA, 1950.

[10] F. Carinci, D. Lauritano, C. A. Bignozzi et al., "A new strategy against peri-implantitis: antibacterial internal coating," *International Journal of Molecular Sciences*, vol. 20, no. 16, article 3897, 2019.

[11] S. Dibart, M. Warbington, M. F. Su, and Z. Skobe, "In vitro evaluation of the implant-abutment bacterial seal: the locking taper system," *The International Journal of Oral & Maxillofacial Implants*, vol. 20, no. 5, pp. 732–737, 2005.

[12] S. Arora, A. K. Lamba, F. Faraz, S. Tandon, and A. Ahad, "Role of cone beam computed tomography in rehabilitation of a traumatised deficient maxillary alveolar ridge using symphyseal block graft placement," *Case Reports in Dentistry*, vol. 2013, Article ID 748405, 6 pages, 2013.

[13] V. E. Beresin and F. J. Schiesser, "The neutral zone in complete dentures," *The Journal of Prosthetic Dentistry*, vol. 36, no. 4, pp. 356–367, 1976.

[14] M. Peñarrocha-Diago, M. Peñarrocha-Diago, R. Zaragozí-Alonso, D. Soto-Peñaloza, and On Behalf Of The Ticare Consensus M, "Consensus statements and clinical recommendations on treatment indications, surgical procedures, prosthetic protocols and complications following All-On-4 standard treatment. 9th Mozo-Grau Ticare Conference in Quintanilla, Spain," *Journal of Clinical and Experimental Dentistry*, vol. 9, no. 5, pp. e712–e715, 2017.

[15] M. Tallarico and S. Meloni, "Retrospective analysis on survival rate, template-related complications, and prevalence of peri-implantitis of 694 anodized implants placed using computer-guided surgery: results between 1 and 10 years of follow-up," *The International Journal of Oral & Maxillofacial Implants*, vol. 32, no. 5, pp. 1162–1171, 2017.

[16] A. Scarano, C. Mortellaro, M. Brucoli, A. G. Lucchina, B. Assenza, and F. Lorusso, "Short implants: analysis of 69 implants loaded in mandible compared with longer implants," *The Journal of Craniofacial Surgery*, vol. 29, no. 8, pp. 2272–2276, 2018.

[17] G. Leonard, P. Coelho, I. Polyzois, L. Stassen, and N. Claffey, "A study of the bone healing kinetics of plateau versus screw root design titanium dental implants," *Clinical Oral Implants Research*, vol. 20, no. 3, pp. 232–239, 2009.

[18] A. Pozzi, M. Tallarico, F. Mangani, and A. Barlattani, "Different implant impression techniques for edentulous patients treated with CAD/CAM complete-arch prostheses: a randomised controlled trial reporting data at 3 year post-loading," *European Journal of Oral Implantology*, vol. 6, no. 4, pp. 325–340, 2013.

[19] E. Erkmen, G. Meriç, A. Kurt, Y. Tunç, and A. Eser, "Biomechanical comparison of implant retained fixed partial dentures with fiber reinforced composite versus conventional metal frameworks: a 3D FEA study," *Journal of the Mechanical Behavior of Biomedical Materials*, vol. 4, no. 1, pp. 107–116, 2011.

[20] M. A. Lazar, H. Rotaru, I. Bâldea et al., "Evaluation of the biocompatibility of new fiber-reinforced composite materials for craniofacial bone reconstruction," *The Journal of Craniofacial Surgery*, vol. 27, no. 7, pp. 1694–1699, 2016.

35

Implications and Considerations of Dental Materials in MRI: A Case Report and Literature Review

Brenton J. Wilson[1] **Phoebe E. O'hare**[1] **and John Zacariah**[2]

[1]*James Cook University, Cairns, Australia*
[2]*Oral Health Services Northern Territory, Australia*

Correspondence should be addressed to Brenton J. Wilson; brenton.wilson@my.jcu.edu.au

Academic Editor: Wen Lin Chai

Magnetic resonance imaging (MRI) has an increasing role as a diagnostic imaging modality. Dental materials have important implications on the use of MRI as a diagnostic imaging modality. A case of a dislodged crown while in an MRI machine prompted a review of the literature for the implications and considerations of dental materials with magnetic resonance technology. An understanding of the basic physics involved in magnetic resonance is required to appreciate the relevance of dental materials in an MRI scanner. This case report supported by a literature review recommends assessing a patient's crown retention prior to and after MRI scanning.

1. Introduction

Magnetic resonance imaging (MRI) has an increasing role as a diagnostic imaging modality in Australia. In 2015, there were 41 MRI scans performed per 1000 population [1]. Although MRI technology currently has limited uses in dentistry, such as evaluation of temporomandibular joint anatomy, dental patients are increasingly exposed to MRI for medical indications. There are a number of reasons why MRI technology is becoming more frequently utilised internationally, including increased accessibility, the absence of ionizing radiation, and superior soft tissue resolution compared to other imaging modalities [2].

Dental materials have important implications on the use of MRI as a diagnostic imaging modality. A case of a dislodged crown while in an MRI machine prompted a review of the literature for the implications and considerations of dental materials with magnetic resonance technology, with particular relevance to the Australian setting. These implications can be divided into radiofrequency-driven heating, magnetically induced displacement forces, and image artefact [3]. An understanding of the basic physics involved in magnetic resonance is required to appreciate the relevance of dental materials in an MRI scanner.

2. Case Study

A 74-year-old lady presented to a public dental clinic in the Northern Territory with a dislodged crown from tooth 11. She was undergoing an MRI as part of her workup for a brain tumour. As the machine started up, she felt the crown "pull" on her tooth and dislodge into her mouth. There was no documentation of the metallic composition of this porcelain fused metal crown, which was constructed and cemented in Indonesia approximately 8 years ago. She has had no issues with the crown until this MRI. She presented to the dental clinic within 4 hours of dislodgement.

On examination, the crown preparation was in good condition, except for a small area of marginal caries on the distal. The patient opted to have the caries excavated and restored with a glass ionomer cement (GIC) and the crown recemented with a resin-reinforced luting GIC. Given the need for ongoing MRI scans as part of her brain tumour monitoring and consequent risk of recurrent dislodgement, it was

Table 1: Dental materials and impact on MR image artefact.

Classification	Clinical significance	Materials
Compatible	No image artefact or distortion	Glass ionomers, resin, gutta percha, zirconium dioxide, some composites
Compatible I	Limited image artefact or distortion localised to imaging site	Amalgam, gold alloy, gold ceramic crowns, titanium, some composites
Noncompatible	Significant image distortions, even when imaging site distant from material	Stainless steel, cobalt-chrome

recommended that she have an alternative restoration considered in the future. Signed informed consent was sought from this patient to present her case.

3. Discussion

The temporal relationship between the crown dislodging and commencement of the MRI mechanism is indicative as the probable cause of the dislodgement. Other causes of fixed prosthodontic retention loss include adhesive or cohesive failure of cement, excessive crown taper, short clinical crown length, or recurrent caries [4]. These factors may contribute but would be significantly coincidental given the timing of retention failure with the diagnostic scan. In our review of literature, we identified only one other similar case in a published letter to the editor, where a patient felt the MRI "nearly pulled his crown out" [5]. In this case, the cast core and crown were found to be made with 82% nickel content. Potential reasons for the scarcity of published literature are the relatively recent introduction of MRI to Australia in 1998 in addition to the change in profile of dental materials globally in recent times.

MRI technology relies on a strong uniform magnetic field that results in uniform alignment of protons within its field. A magnetic vector along the axis of the MRI scanner is consequently generated, and radiofrequency waves are then directed towards these protons. The returning waveforms are detected by radiofrequency receptors and converted into images reflecting the different tissue compositions [2]. The strength of the magnetic field can have a "projectile effect," by pulling ferromagnetic materials. Due to this strong magnetic field, stringent safety mechanisms are practised in Australia to prevent harm and injury. The Royal Australian and New Zealand College of Radiologists MRI safety guidelines require patients to be screened for potentially hazardous items before entering the magnetic field zone. Metal objects are removed by the patient prior, and any medical implantable devices need to be checked for their compatibility with magnetic resonance [6]. The three commonest ferromagnetic metals are iron, nickel, and cobalt.

3.1. Dental Materials. There is a wide array of materials used in dentistry, many left in the mouth long-term, such as implants and dental crowns. Ferromagnetic metals are commonplace in orthodontic brackets and wires, dentures, and crowns. The most common issue with dental materials is their susceptibility to creating artefacts and distortions in MRI. These have been divided by Tymofiyeva et al. into compatible, compatible I, and noncompatible based on the resultant distortion of the image (Table 1) [7].

With regard to displacement of the crown in this case, there are two potential methods of displacement. The first is that radiofrequency energy is absorbed, resulting in heating, compromising the adhesion of the crown to the tooth structure. Hasegawa et al. investigated the temperature increase of fixed prosthodontic appliances in MRI scanners and found an increase of <2°C, which would have negligible effect on the luting cement.

The second factor is the magnetically induced displacing forces created by the MRI machine. Ferromagnetic components of the patient's crown may have created enough displacing forces to overcome the already compromised retentive force of the luting cement on the crown [8]. For this reason, Chockattu et al. recommend that ferromagnetic containing dental prostheses are checked for retention prior to and after the MRI scan [3].

3.2. The Australian Context. Of potential relevance in this case is the Indonesian origin of the patient's crown. The material used in the crown is unclear, and the patient did not allow permission for this to be removed for testing. Medical and dental tourism is an increasing trend around the world, whereby patients seek lower-cost medical and dental care overseas in countries such as Indonesia [9]. In many countries, the dental industry, including the use of dental materials, is subject to approval by the Therapeutic Goods Administration (TGA). Dental materials require testing certificates for approval by TGA and consequently do not require an implantable card and considered safe for MRI. Other implantable materials such as cardiac defibrillators and cochlear implants that do not meet MR requirements necessitate the patient to be given a card highlighting that the material is MR conditional or MR unsafe, depending on the field condition of the MRI [10].

3.3. Conclusions/Recommendations. With the increasing use of MRI technology, dentists should be aware that dental materials affect MR images and MR technology affects dental materials. The most significant impact is the effect on image quality. Recommendations from the literature are based predominately on scientific ex vivo studies on the effect of MR on materials as well as small retrospective studies on image quality. With regard to improving image quality, removable dentures and orthodontic wires should be removed where possible prior to scanning, particularly when the head and neck region is being imaged. This case report highlights a case where a crown has dislodged at the commencement of

MRI scanning and the potential mechanisms of this. In terms of displacement and heating, the literature is limited to ex vivo studies of dental materials and appliances placed in MRI scanners. These studies have found limited risk of dental materials causing damaging heating or significant displacement in the magnetic field. This case report, however, supports the Chockattu et al. recommendation of assessing a patient's crown retention prior to and after MRI scanning.

References

[1] Commonwealth of Australia, "Community Affairs References Committee. Availability and accessibility of diagnostic imaging equipment in AustraliaCanberra," 2018, March 2020 https://www.aph.gov.au/Parliamentary_Business/Committees/Senate/Community_Affairs/Diagnosticimaging/Report/c03.

[2] P. Allisy-Robert and J. Williams, "Magnetic resonance imaging," in *Farr's Physics for Medical Imaging 2nd Edition*, pp. 169–195, Edinburgh: Elsevier Health Sciences, 2008.

[3] S. J. Chockattu, D. B. Suryakant, and S. Thakur, "Unwanted effects due to interactions between dental materials and magnetic resonance imaging: a review of the literature," *Restorative Dentistry & Endodontics*, vol. 43, no. 4, 2018.

[4] S. D. Heintze, "Crown pull-off test (crown retention test) to evaluate the bonding effectiveness of luting agents," *Dental Materials Journal*, vol. 26, no. 3, pp. 193–206, 2010.

[5] D. Sinkiewicz, "MRI scan hazard," *British Dental Journal*, vol. 214, no. 8, p. 376, 2013.

[6] "Royal Australian and New Zealand College of Radiologists. MRI safety guidelines. Sydney," 2017, March 2020 https://www.ranzcr.com/college/document-library/ranzcr-mri-safety-guidelines.

[7] O. Tymofiyeva, S. Vaegler, K. Rottner et al., "Influence of dental materials on dental MRI," *Dentomaxillofacial Radiology*, vol. 42, no. 6, article 20120271, 2013.

[8] M. Hasegawa, K. Miyata, Y. Abe, and T. Ishigami, "Radiofrequency heating of metallic dental devices during 3.0 T MRI," *Dentomaxillofacial Radiology*, vol. 42, no. 5, p. 20120234, 2013.

[9] P. Leggat and U. Kedjarune, "Dental health, 'dental tourism' and travellers," *Travel Medicine and Infectious Disease*, vol. 7, no. 3, pp. 123-124, 2009.

[10] Therapeutic Goods Administration, "Medical device patient information leaflets and implant cards: requirements for new and on-market implantable medical devices," March https://www.tga.gov.au/publication/medical-device-patient-cards-and-leaflets.

36

A Retrospective Case Report on the Longevity of a Reimplanted Closed-Apex Avulsed Canine

Julian Leow and Robin Amanullah

Eastman Dental Hospital, 256 Grays Inn Rd, London WC1X 8LD, UK

Correspondence should be addressed to Robin Amanullah; robinamanullah@hotmail.com

Academic Editor: Daniel Torres-Lagares

For an avulsed tooth with closed apices, it is recommended that the tooth undergoes elective root canal treatment. We however present in this case report a 73-year-old Afro-Caribbean lady, with an asymptomatic, untreated, self-replanted lower left canine which suffered an avulsion 45 years ago. The patient reported no loss of function. This case illustrates the potentially positive outcome of a replanted, non-root-treated, avulsed closed-apex tooth while highlighting the significance of patient-related factors.

1. Introduction

Dental avulsion is described when a tooth has been completely displaced from its socket—which severs the periodontal ligament and the neurovascular connection. It constitutes 0.5%-3% of dental trauma injuries [1]. Treatment guidelines depend on the development of the root apices (open or closed) and the amount of extra oral dry time (< or > than 60 minutes) [2]. Ideally, the tooth should be reimplanted immediately. An extraoral dry period of more than 60 minutes is associated with poor prognosis due to drying of the periodontal ligament (PDL) and pulpal cells, which are key proponents to the prognosis of the tooth. Extensive PDL necrosis is likely to cause ankylosis and in growing patients will cause infraposition of the tooth.

For an avulsed tooth with closed apices, it is recommended that if replanted, the tooth undergoes elective root canal treatment [1–5]. The tooth is normally splinted with a flexible splint for up to 2 weeks instead of a rigid splint to prevent ankylosis. Antibiotics such as doxycycline are normally prescribed. Oral hygiene and dietary advice such as soft foods for 2 weeks are usually recommended [6]. Patients are then followed up regularly. Some contraindications for replanting avulsed teeth include a patient who is immunocompromised, deciduous teeth and severe cardiac defects, unrestorable decay, severe uncontrolled diabetes, and severe mental disability. Long-standing, widely regarded guidelines have been available for dealing with dental trauma cases, and there are numerous studies on the outcome of avulsed teeth [1, 3–9]. There is however a scarcity of studies which describe the outcome of replanted closed-apex permanent teeth which have not undergone root canal treatment (RCT)—such as abscess formation, discoloration, and tooth loss. Most studies report performing root canal treatment on replanted closed-apex teeth [8]. This case report is a retrospective patient recall of the lower left canine (LL3) avulsion experienced 45 years ago, which was self-replanted into the socket and untreated.

2. Case Report

A 73-year-old Afro-Caribbean lady attended the dental practice in 2018 complaining of sensitivity when brushing the upper left side. She was fit and well and did not smoke or drink any alcohol. Her dental history revealed that she experienced avulsion of the LL3 due to trauma in 1973. The tooth however remained within the oral cavity and was instinctively repositioned by the patient into the socket. She attended her dentist the following day who decided against any further treatment (i.e., no RCT and no splinting).

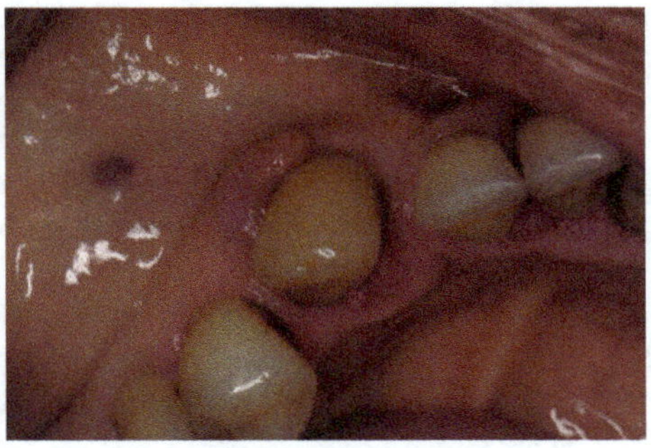

Figure 1: Occlusal view of LL3 before treatment.

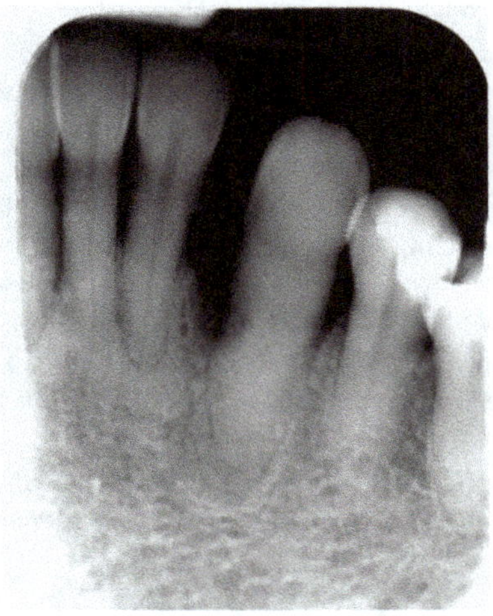

Figure 2: Long-cone periapical radiograph of the LL3 showing loss of about 50% bony support, obliteration of the root canal, radiolucency on the mesial surface of the root, and sclerosing osteitis periapically. No signs of caries intraorally. The LL2, LL1, and LR1 show 50-70% bone loss and bony sclerosis apically which could indicate late-stage periapical cemento-osseous dysplasia.

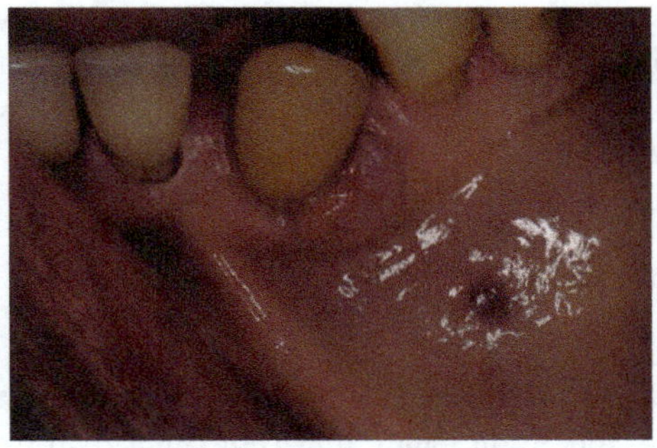

Figure 3: Buccal view of LL3 before treatment.

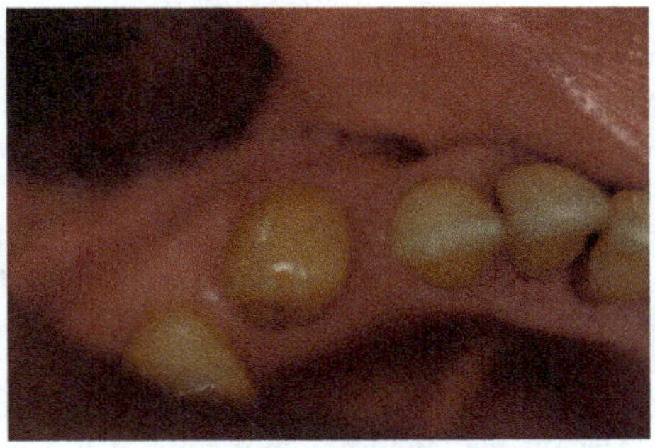

Figure 4: Occlusal view of LL3 after treatment.

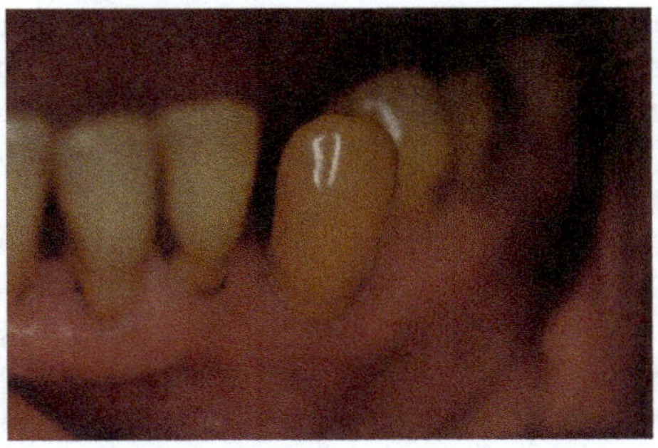

Figure 5: Buccal view of LL3 after treatment.

Following on from this first review of the tooth, there have been no reported symptoms relating to limited function or otherwise.

Both extraoral and intraoral medicine-related observations were unremarkable. After a basic periodontal examination screening, a 6-point pocket chart and appropriate radiographs were taken. The patient was diagnosed with generalised severe chronic periodontitis and UL4 cavity and was thus scheduled for nonsurgical root surface debridement and restoration of UL4. Despite the LL3 being out of the line of the arch form and displaying grade 2 mobility, the patient reported no symptoms from the tooth such as loss of function or pain. Furthermore, the LL3 was notably discolored (Figure 1) and bleeding on all sites with deep pockets. The tooth was unresponsive to the electric pulp test, which may be due to either a necrotic or obliterated pulp in the absence of periapical radiolucency. A periapical radiograph (Figure 2) of the LL3 showed reduced bony support, complete obliteration of its canal, and radiolucency involving the mesial aspect of the tooth at the midroot level. Expected outcomes of replantation of a tooth include ankylosis or external root resorption [2]. The patient was not concerned about the aesthetics.

At the following appointment, the LL3 presented with an exophytic, nonpedunculated red swelling in the buccodistal gingiva which was 10 mm in diameter (Figures 1 and 3). The LL3 was unrestored and was free from coronal caries. It was not tender to vertical percussion. Due to the long history of symptomless and issueless use of the tooth, the patient stated from the start that she was opposed to have it extracted. A provisional diagnosis of lateral periodontal abscess with secondary external root resorption was made. The treatment provided was oral hygiene advice and nonsurgical root surface debridement.

Future advanced treatment options were discussed with several specialist periodontal colleagues, and the treatment proposed was open surgical access for root surface debridement and appropriate restorative intervention on the radiolucent lesion seen radiographically, with or without local periodontal regeneration.

At her review appointment 2 weeks later, the swelling had resolved and she was happy with the outcome of the treatment. The patient was symptom free (Figures 4 and 5) and reported returning to eating as normal. The patient was given the option stated above; however, she decided to monitor the tooth. A 3-month recall for reassessment was planned; however, the patient never returned.

3. Discussion

International Association of Dental Traumatology (IADT), American Association of Endodontists (AAE), and other guidelines and studies state that root canal treatment must be commenced 7-14 days after replantation of a closed-apex tooth as "revascularisation is not expected" and inflammatory root resorption is a risk [2, 3, 7]. Further risks include abscess formation and ankylosis.

This case illustrates the positive outcome of replantation of a closed-apex tooth without further treatment. This is demonstrated via the LL3's symptom-free 45-year survival postavulsion with no reported loss of function (i.e., mastication). This is likely due to a combination of factors including nil extraoral time, nil dry time, immediate replantation [2, 9], and patient factors.

Although the outcome of this case does not meet the IADT criteria [2] for favourable outcome, it is a functional tooth which the patient was able to use for 45 years.

This case demonstrates how clinical outcomes may fall outside those "expected" as documented in the literature. For this patient, the 45 years and the ongoing function of this tooth are regarded as a positive outcome. Multifactorial reasons for this would include individual patient factors such as adaptation to less than ideal conditions of teeth, tolerance, and host response. Taking into consideration the long-term positive outcome of this tooth, its response to treatment, and this particular patient's factors, the prognosis of this tooth is deemed good. A possible reason for the absence of ankylosis is the retention of the tooth in the oral cavity after avulsion and immediate reimplantation which are favourable factors for the viability of the periodontal ligament cells.

Clearly, there is a limitation in that this highlights a single tooth-single case scenario, but a remarkable one at that. Reliance upon a patient history may carry bias, but given the clinical presentation of a 45-year-old avulsed tooth and associated symptoms, which also responded positively to the treatment, it is certainly notable in the least.

4. Conclusion and Clinical Implications

This case illustrates the potential long-term survivability and useful function of replanted, non-root-treated, avulsed closed-apex teeth and shows the importance of patient factors as well. A study collecting data on patients with closed-apex teeth who decline root canal treatment postavulsion would be able to further support this case report in justifying the "leave" option in select patients.

References

[1] A. Zürcher and A. Filippi, "Management of avulsed teeth," in *Management of Dental Emergencies in Children and Adolescents*, vol. 16, p. 177, Wiley-Blackwell, 2019.

[2] L. Andersson, J. O. Andreasen, P. Day et al., "International Association of Dental Traumatology guidelines for the management of traumatic dental injuries: 2. Avulsion of permanent teeth," *Dental Traumatology*, vol. 28, no. 2, pp. 88–96, 2012.

[3] A. Sigurdsson, *Colleagues for excellence-the treatment of traumatic dental injuries*, American Association of Endodontists, 2014.

[4] R. Krug, K. Kremeier, and G. Krastl, "Long-term retention of avulsed maxillary permanent incisors replanted after prolonged non-physiological storage," *Dental Traumatology*, vol. 35, no. 2, pp. 147–152, 2019.

[5] E. Özlek, B. Ak, and E. Akkol, "Five-year follow-up of a delayed reimplanted avulsed tooth: case report," *Eastern Journal of Medicine*, vol. 23, no. 4, pp. 350–354, 2018.

[6] E. Bendoraitiene, S. Zemgulyte, and M. Borisovaite, "Reasonable outcome of avulsed permanent upper incisor after seven years follow-up period: a case report," *Journal of Oral & Maxillofacial Research*, vol. 8, no. 4, article e6, 2017.

[7] C. J. Stewart, R. O. Elledge, M. J. Kinirons, and R. R. Welbury, "Factors affecting the timing of pulp extirpation in a sample of 66 replanted avulsed teeth in children and adolescents," *Dental Traumatology*, vol. 24, no. 6, pp. 625–627, 2008.

[8] V. Chappuis and T. Von Arx, "Replantation of 45 avulsed permanent teeth: a 1-year follow-up study," *Dental Traumatology*, vol. 21, no. 5, pp. 289–296, 2005.

[9] M. Trope, "Clinical management of the avulsed tooth: present strategies and future directions," *Dental Traumatology*, vol. 18, no. 1, pp. 1–11, 2002.

37

Complete Denture Fabrication using Digitally Fabricated Copy Dentures for a Patient with Moderate Dementia

Korehide Arai,[1] **Yuto Tanaka**,[1] **Shinsuke Matsuda,**[2] **Tomohiko Okamura,**[1] **Kazufumi Iwayama,**[1] **and Yoshiaki Ono**[1]

[1]*Department of Special Care Dentistry, Osaka Dental University Hospital, Osaka, Japan*
[2]*Matsuda Oral Appliance, Osaka, Japan*

Correspondence should be addressed to Yuto Tanaka; yutotanaka.0106@gmail.com

Academic Editor: Rui Amaral Mendes

A 91-year-old woman was referred to our hospital with a chief complaint of unsatisfactory fit and pain associated with her complete dentures. She had moderate dementia with difficulty in communication (Mini-Mental State Examination, 16; Barthel Index, 15). The closed impressions and jaw record were taken with the digitally fabricated copy dentures as follows. First, the tissue conditioner was used to correct the poor fit of the old dentures, following which minor occlusal alterations were made. Second, the copy dentures that copied the morphology of the corrected old dentures using three-dimensional (3D) scanner were fabricated with a 3D printer. The new dentures were then fabricated using conventional methods as follows. The impressions were cast and articulated, and the dentures were subsequently processed. This case report documented the following results. First, the acceptance of new dentures appeared to be easier since the new dentures copied the morphology of the familiar dentures digitally. Moreover, the 3D data of the dentures could be used for immediate denture fabrication in case of fracture or loss of the dentures. Second, only two visits were required for taking an impression and delivering the complete dentures. In addition, her old dentures were brought to our dental office by the patient's family after the patient's dinner; immediately after copying the dentures' morphology, the dentures were returned to the patient's family, thus avoiding any disturbance to the patient's eating routine. These reduced the burden on the patient and her family.

1. Introduction

Some elderly patients requiring complete denture fabrication are medically frail or are homebound with major limitations in mobility [1]. While some individuals can independently access the dental office, others are institutionalized or require long-term care at home; these individuals might require a dentist to provide care at their place of residence. These facts emphasize the need to reduce the number of visits to dental clinics for fabrication of complete dentures [2]. On the other hand, it is difficult to ensure the safety of dental treatment for these patients. In particular, treatment requiring low-viscosity materials place a heavy burden on the patients with impaired oropharyngeal function [3]. Therefore, in such nondexterous patients, denture modification is preferred over a new denture fabrication. However, temporary denture modifications, such as tissue conditioning with acrylic-based tissue conditioner, lead to several problems, including bond failures to the denture base, accumulation of oral microorganisms, poor tear strength, and hardness changes.

In contrast, digital dental technologies, with the aim of highly safe dental treatment and efficiency, have significantly improved in the last decade [4]. For example, based on the results of an integrative review, no significant difference was found regarding the marginal discrepancy of single-unit ceramic restorations fabricated following digital and conventional impressions [5]. Therefore, in this case report, new dentures were manufactured by incorporating digital dental technology with conventional methods to reduce the burden on edentulous patients with severe dementia and to improve overall safety.

2. Case Presentation

The patient was 91 years of age and a female. As the chief complaint, the patient expressed unsatisfactory fit and pain associated with use of the complete dentures. The patient's family desired new dentures for her, as her dentures appeared to fit loosely, and she was unable to eat properly.

For the degree of care, the patient exhibited difficulty in communicating (Mini-Mental State Examination, 16; Barthel Index, 15). Her medical history is as follows: The patient developed symptoms of Alzheimer's-type dementia five years prior, following which she has been under the care of her family. In addition to taking an acetylcholinesterase inhibitor to treat the dementia, the patient had been prescribed antihypertensive and antihyperuricemic drugs.

The patient has a height of 150.0 cm and weight of 47.0 kg.

A home-visit dentist manufactured the complete dentures for the upper and lower jaws two years prior. The following year, she complained of pain in the left alveolar ridge of the mandible and requested a home visit for dental treatment; however, her symptoms and food intake did not improve. She was referred to our hospital for the fabrication of new dentures. Figure 1 shows the oral findings (Figures 1(a) and 1(b)) and the old dentures (Figures 1(c)–1(f)). An ulcer was noted in the left alveolar ridge of the mandible, with severe bilateral ridge resorption (Figure 1(b)).

3. Procedure

(1) First clinical stage: the minimum amount of tissue conditioner required (Tissue Conditioner II, Shofu, Inc., Kyoto, Japan) was used to correct the poor fit of the old dentures and to record dynamic impressions of the dentures, following which minor occlusal alterations were undertaken. One week later, a follow-up teleconsultation of the patient revealed disappearance of pain in the mucosa of the jaw ridge during meals and an increase in the food intake. We asked the patient's family (her son) to bring her upper and lower dentures to our hospital to record optical impressions for the upper and lower dentures using an optical scanner (Neway; Open Tech 3D s.r.l., Rezzato, Brescia, Italy) (Figures 2(a) and 2(b)); the dentures were returned to the patient immediately

(2) First laboratory stage: the scanned data were converted into standard tessellation language (STL) data and exported to a three-dimensional (3D) printer interface software (Composer; Asiga, Sydney, Australia) (Figure 2(c)), and then a 3D printer (Asiga MAX UV; Asiga) using dental photocurable resin (Freeprint Tray UV; Detax, Ettlingen, Germany) which fabricated the copy denture at 100 μm/layer. After washing the copy dentures with isopropyl alcohol, final polymerization was performed using a dental polymerization apparatus (Asiga Flash; Asiga). The copy dentures were polished with a dental carbide cutting tool (H251GSQ-060; Komet, Lemgo, Germany) (Figures 2(d)–2(g)). 3D scanning of each of the upper and lower dentures according to the software's instructions and saving of the STL data were completed in 10 min. An additional 1 min was required for transfer of the STL data to a composer. The time required for setting the support bars in the composer was 5 min; printing, 75 min; washing, 6 mins; final polymerization, 30 min; and polishing, 10 min. The total laboratory work required approximately 2.5 h

(3) Second clinical stage: the copy dentures were slightly adjusted to ensure the correct occlusal contact. A closed mouth impression was recorded using the minimum required amount of a light-body wash impression (Fusion II Extra Wash Type, GC Corp. Tokyo. Japan) in the copy dentures for both the maxillary and mandibular bases inside the patient's mouth. While taking the impressions, the patient was asked to sit upright and close her mouth. The jaw record was obtained at the same time

(4) Second laboratory stage: the impressions were cast and articulated, the morphology of the polishing surface of the copy dentures were converted into wax rims utilizing plaster masks, and teeth were set on those rims. After deflasking, the dentures were checked using the articulator for processing errors and subsequently polished (Figure 3).

(5) Third clinical stage: we visited the patient's home and delivered the completed dentures following an intraoral check. The fit and occlusion of the dentures were good

(6) Fourth clinical stage: telephonic follow-up was performed twice every other week, and there was no complaint of pain during meals; an increase in food intake and a decrease in the duration of meals were noted. The procedures followed in this case are shown in Figure 4. Only two visits were required for taking the impression and delivering the complete dentures. In addition, the patient's dentures were sent to the dental office after her dinner and returned to her the next morning, thus avoiding disturbance of the patient's normal eating routine

4. Discussion

Recording oral impressions in elderly individuals requiring long-term home care is often challenging. Although dentists have tried various measures, such as the use of impression materials with low fluidity and a short curing time, the risk of accidental ingestion and aspiration during impression taking has been reported in elderly patients [2]. On the other hand, intraoral scanners have significantly improved with the aim of providing highly safe and effective dental treatment over the last decade. For example, a previous study examined the patient's comfort and stress levels while taking

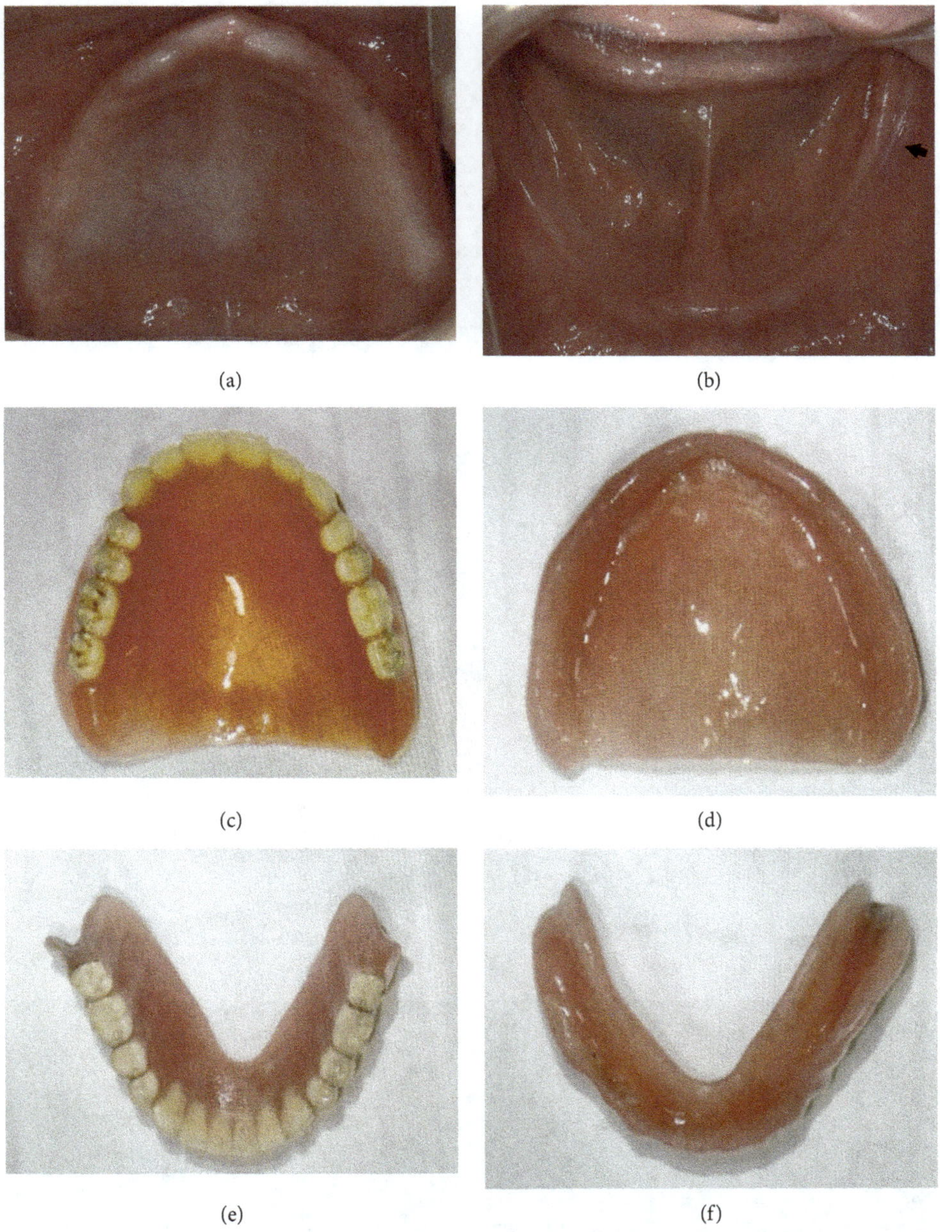

Figure 1: Intraoral findings ((a) upper jaw, (b) lower jaw) and a familiar denture used by the patient ((c) occlusal surface of upper denture, (d) mucosal surface of upper denture, (e) occlusal surface of lower denture, and (f) mucosal surface of lower denture). The arrowhead indicates an ulcer in the left alveolar ridge of the lower jaw.

oral impressions digitally and conventionally in patients with gag reflex or breathing difficulty; the study revealed that the intraoral scanner scored better than the conventional method [6]. Another previous study found no significant difference in the accuracy between dental prostheses manufactured using an alginate impression and those made using an intraoral scanner [5]. However, certain challenges remain with the use of intraoral scanners. It is impossible to record an impression of areas that are outside the scanning range, such as undercuts of ridges and deep grooves. The accuracy of the impression is also affected by moisture, including salivary contamination [7–11]. Moreover, a digital jaw relation record can be obtained in edentulous patients [12]. However, the success or failure of the scan is seemingly dependent on the operator's technique. Therefore, at present, it is practical to incorporate digital dental technology into the manufacturing process of the conventional method for improvement of safety and efficiency of the dental treatment, rather than using a digital workflow for all the processes. In the present case, for a patient with dementia with difficulty communicating, incorporating digital dental technology into the manufacturing process of the conventional method enabled us to provide high-quality complete dentures safely because of the following reasons.

First, acceptance of new dentures in this case appeared relatively simple owing to the use of dentures that copied the morphology of a familiar denture that the patient had been using for a long time. In contrast, previous studies

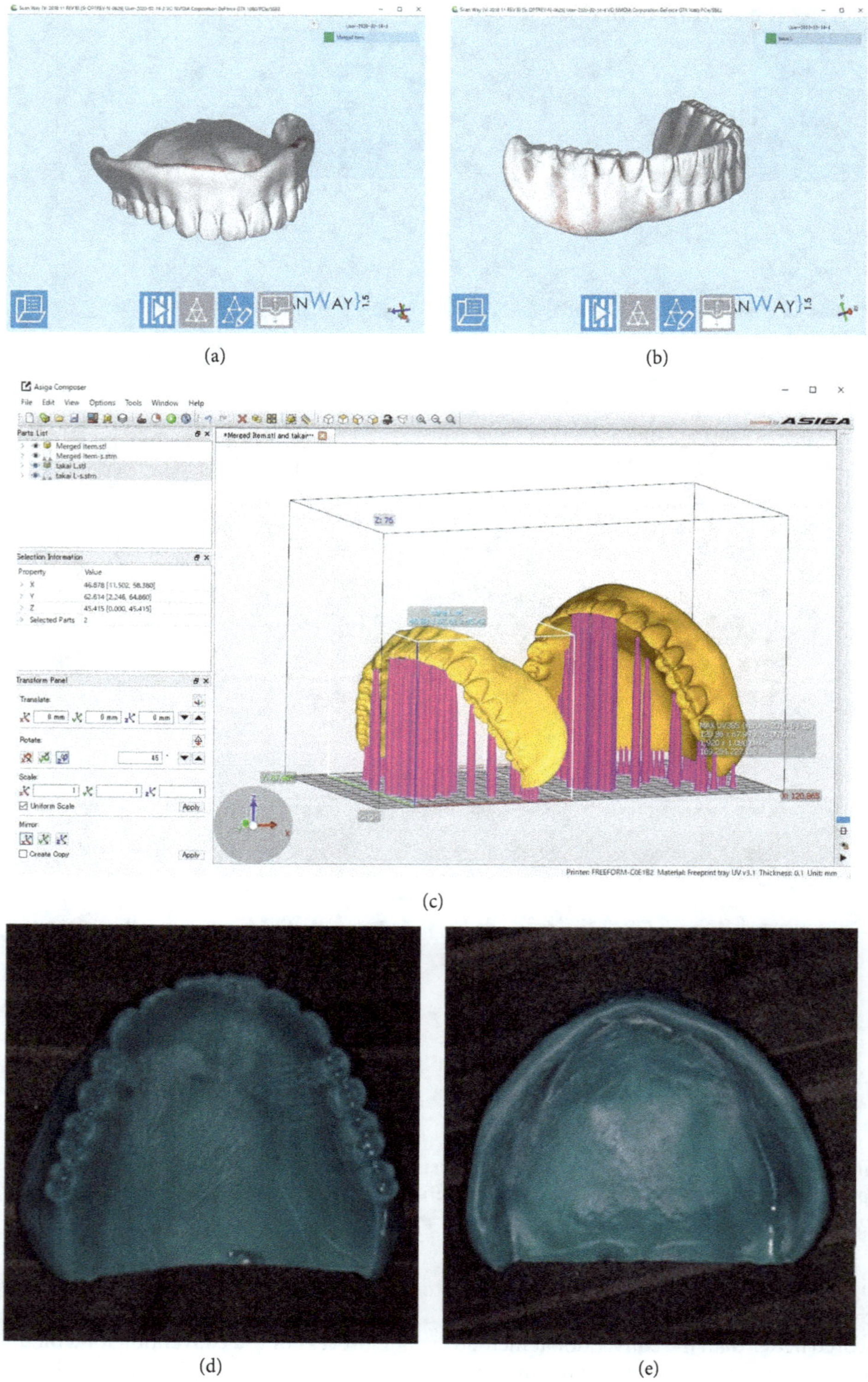

Figure 2: Continued.

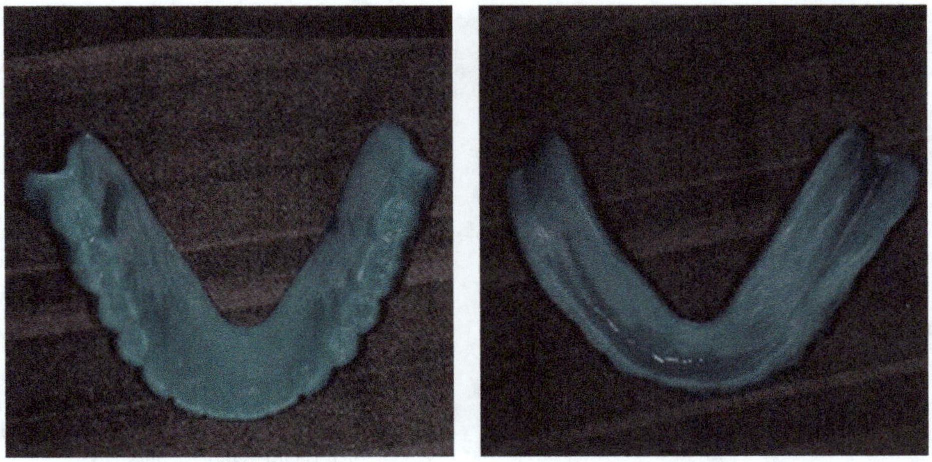

(f) (g)

FIGURE 2: Optical impressions recorded for the upper (a) and lower (b) dentures with an optical scanner. The scanned data were converted into standard tessellation language (STL) data and exported to a three-dimensional (3D) printer interface software, after which the support bars were set (c). A 3D printer using dental photocurable resin fabricated the copy denture at 100 μm/layer ((d) occlusal surface of upper denture, (e) mucosal surface of upper denture, (f) occlusal surface of lower denture, and (g) mucosal surface of lower denture).

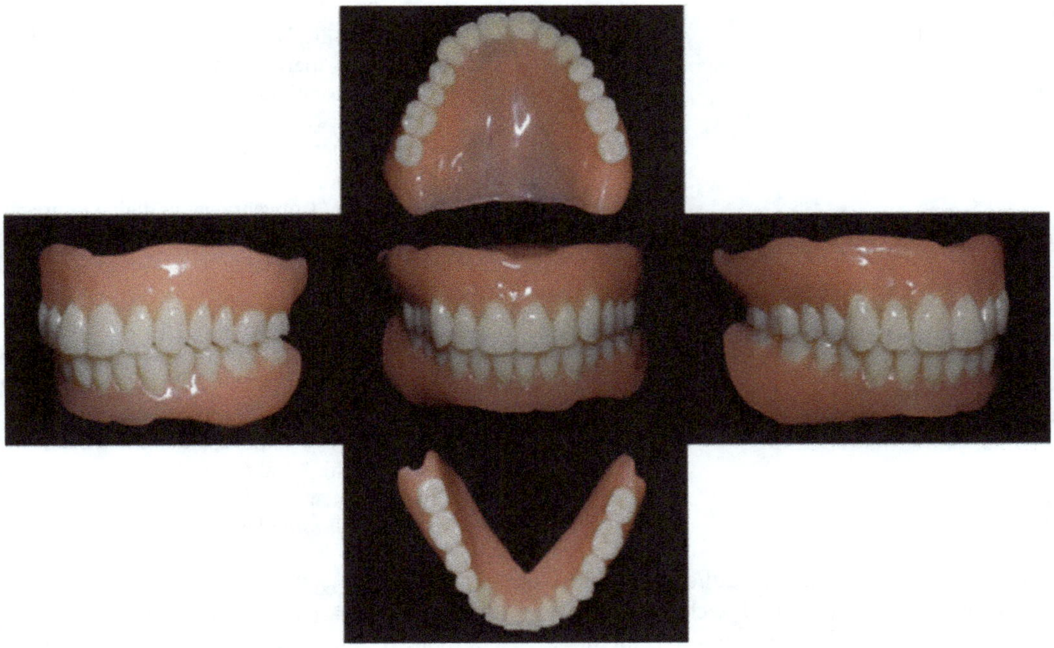

FIGURE 3: New dentures.

reported that older patients have difficulty accepting new dentures [13]. Dentists have been trying to determine a technique for transferring the morphology of familiar dentures to new dentures. For example, the neutral zone technique [14] uses impressions of the polishing surface of the denture followed by boxing using a silicone putty material to obtain the tongue and facial matrices. Similar to the method used in this case, the polished surface morphology can be transferred easily using optical scanning. Moreover, we could obtain 3D data of the familiar dentures in case the patient loses or breaks the dentures in the future; in such cases, the 3D data of the dentures could be used for new denture fabrication.

Second, only two visits were required for taking the impression and delivering the complete dentures, reducing the quantity of impression material used and frequency of impressions taken. Many such patients who require long-term care, especially those with moderate or severe dementia, refuse long-duration or highly invasive treatment [15]; therefore, selection of a simple and minimally invasive treatment for such patients is desirable.

Finally, the reduction in contact and time spent between patients and healthcare professionals owing to the use of digital dental technology could help reduce the risk of spread of the new coronavirus disease (COVID-19), which is currently present worldwide. According to public health authorities,

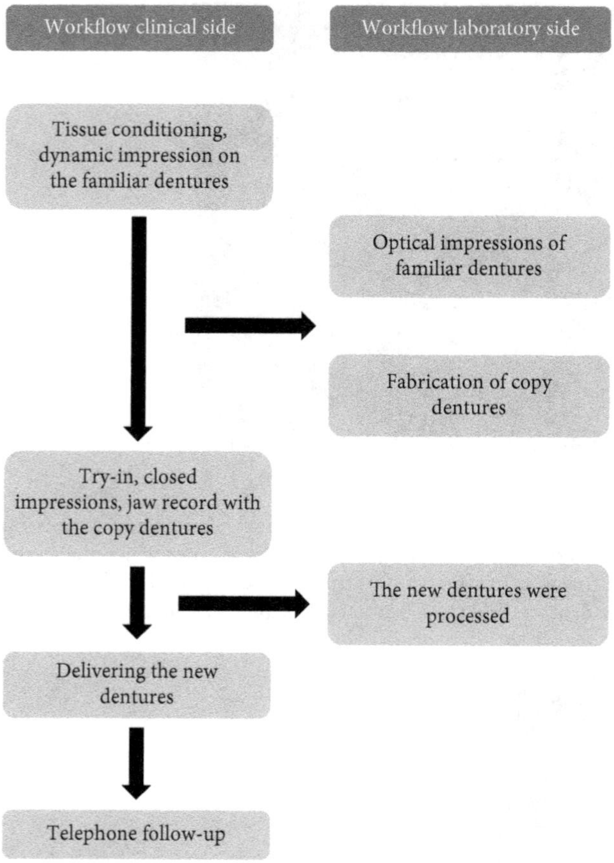

FIGURE 4: Flowchart of the combined workflow.

significant exposure is defined as a "face to face contact within 2 m with a patient with symptomatic COVID-19" in the range of a few minutes up to 30 min [16]. Therefore, conventional "face to face" dental treatment, which increases the risk of acquiring infection, should be minimized.

5. Conclusion

Our case of a patient with dementia with difficulty in communication, incorporating digital dental technology into the manufacturing process of the conventional method, enabled us to provide high-quality complete denture safely, due to the following reasons. First, acceptance of new dentures was enhanced by using dentures that copied the morphology of a familiar denture. Second, only two visits were required for recording the impression and delivering the complete dentures. Moreover, the patient's dentures were brought to the dental office by her son after her dinner and returned to her son immediately, thus avoiding any disturbance to her eating routines. These factors reduced the burden on the patient and her family.

Consent

Informed consent was voluntarily obtained from the patient and her family for publication of the photographs in this report.

Acknowledgments

The authors wish to thank Dr. Tatsuyuki Mori for his clinical advice.

References

[1] W. Q. Qiu, M. Dean, T. Liu et al., "Physical and mental health of homebound older adults: an overlooked population," *Journal of the American Geriatrics Society*, vol. 58, no. 12, pp. 2423–2428, 2010.

[2] H. Morita, A. Hashimoto, R. Inoue, S. Yoshimoto, M. Yoneda, and T. Hirofuji, "Successful Fitting of a Complete Maxillary Denture in a Patient with Severe Alzheimer's Disease Complicated by Oral Dyskinesia," *Case Reports in Dentistry*, vol. 2016, Article ID 4026480, 5 pages, 2016.

[3] E. Nicolas, C. Lassauzay, G. Pickering, J. Croze, and M. Hennequin, "Needs in screening cardiovascular parameters during dental care in the elderly," *Aging Clinical and Experimental Research*, vol. 20, no. 3, pp. 272–276, 2008.

[4] K. Suese, "Progress in digital dentistry: the practical use of intraoral scanners," *Dental Materials Journal*, vol. 39, no. 1, pp. 52–56, 2020.

[5] P. Tsirogiannis, D. R. Reissmann, and G. Heydecke, "Evaluation of the marginal fit of single-unit, complete-coverage ceramic restorations fabricated after digital and conventional impressions: a systematic review and meta-analysis," *The Journal of Prosthetic Dentistry*, vol. 116, no. 3, pp. 328–35.e2, 2016.

[6] A. Mangano, M. Beretta, G. Luongo, C. Mangano, and F. Mangano, "Conventional vs digital impressions: acceptability, treatment comfort and stress among young orthodontic patients," *The Open Dentistry Journal*, vol. 12, no. 1, pp. 118–124, 2018.

[7] M. Kurz, T. Attin, and A. Mehl, "Influence of material surface on the scanning error of a powder-free 3D measuring system," *Clinical Oral Investigations*, vol. 19, no. 8, pp. 2035–2043, 2015.

[8] T. Arakida, M. Kanazawa, M. Iwaki, T. Suzuki, and S. Minakuchi, "Evaluating the influence of ambient light on scanning trueness, precision, and time of intra oral scanner," *Journal of Prosthodontic Research*, vol. 62, no. 3, pp. 324–329, 2018.

[9] M. Revilla-León, P. Jiang, M. Sadeghpour et al., "Intraoral digital scans–Part 1: Influence of ambient scanning light conditions on the accuracy (trueness and precision) of different intraoral scanners," *The Journal of Prosthetic Dentistry*, vol. 124, no. 3, pp. 372–378, 2020.

[10] M. Revilla-León, P. Jiang, M. Sadeghpour et al., "Intraoral digital scans: Part 2–influence of ambient scanning light conditions on the mesh quality of different intraoral scanners," *The Journal of Prosthetic Dentistry*, vol. 124, no. 5, pp. 575–580, 2020.

[11] M. Revilla-León, S. G. Subramanian, M. Özcan, and V. R. Krishnamurthy, "Clinical study of the influence of ambient light scanning conditions on the accuracy (trueness and precision) of an intraoral scanner," *Journal of Prosthodontics*, vol. 29, no. 2, pp. 107–113, 2020.

[12] M. Kanazawa, M. Iwaki, T. Arakida, and S. Minakuchi, "Digital impression and jaw relation record for the fabrication of CAD/CAM custom tray," *Journal of Prosthodontic Research*, vol. 62, no. 4, pp. 509–513, 2018.

[13] B. Bergman and G. E. Carlsson, "Review of 54 complete denture wearers. Patients' opinions 1 year after treatment," *Acta Odontologica Scandinavica*, vol. 30, no. 4, pp. 399–414, 1972.

[14] K. Ikebe, I. Okuno, and T. Nokubi, "Effect of adding impression material to mandibular denture space in piezography," *Journal of Oral Rehabilitation*, vol. 33, no. 6, pp. 409–415, 2006.

[15] J. Fiske, H. Frenkel, J. Griffiths, V. Jones, British Society of Gerodontology, and British Society for Disability and Oral Health, "Guidelines for the development of local standards of oral health care for people with dementia," *Gerodontology*, vol. 23, Supplement 1, pp. 5–32, 2006.

[16] M. Klompas, C. A. Morris, J. Sinclair, M. Pearson, and E. S. Shenoy, "Universal masking in hospitals in the COVID-19 era," *The New England Journal of Medicine*, vol. 382, no. 21, article e63, 2020.

38

A Case Report of Dental Implants and Site Augmentation in a Patient with Erosive Lichen Planus

Abdulrahman Aseri

Department of Preventive Dental Sciences, Faculty of Dentistry, Najran University, Saudi Arabia

Correspondence should be addressed to Abdulrahman Aseri; aaaseri.p@gmail.com

Academic Editor: Paolo Giacomo Arduino

Lichen planus (LP) is an autoimmune inflammatory disease that affects oral mucosal tissue, leading to complications in patients treated with dental implant therapy. This case report discusses the clinical management of a patient diagnosed with an erosive type of LP. After disease management, the patient was treated with dental implants in the upper and lower jaws with augmentation procedures around the implants. All implants were loaded after a three-month period of healing. Slight bone loss was observed in the upper premolar area following an exaggerated soft tissue response to the augmentation procedure. Within one year of implant placement, no additional complications were encountered.

1. Introduction

Oral lichen planus is an inflammatory autoimmune mucocutaneous disease that affects the skin, oral mucosa, genitalia, scalp, and nails. It mainly affects people in their middle age with an estimated prevalence ranging from 0.1 to 2.2% of the population, with 3 : 2 female predilection. LP can be present orally in several forms; the most common forms are reticular and erosive LP [1–3].

Dental implant prostheses have been widely used to effectively replace missing teeth with a survival rate ranging from 93 to 95% [4]. Multiple factors can dictate dental implant success or failure, including systemic health, history of periodontal disease, quality, and quantity of hard and soft tissues [5]. Following a dental extraction, the alveolar ridge can undergo up to 50% dimensional changes within 12 months [6]. Even with ridge preservation techniques, the alveolar ridge cannot be preserved entirely [7, 8]. Additional hard and soft tissue augmentations around the implant can aid in maintaining stable alveolar bone and provide healthier peri-implant tissues [9].

LP in its erosive form can affect the quality of soft tissue. Few studies have looked at the effect of oral mucosal lesions, namely LP, on the success of dental implants [10, 11]. Furthermore, there is a scarcity of evidence investigating the effect of LP on soft tissue quality and tissue response to surgical implant therapy. These surgeries include guided bone regeneration around the alveolar ridge or simultaneously with implant placement. These surgical procedures require flap manipulation at the mucosal level to achieve tension-free primary closure [12]. This case report was aimed at assessing and discussing the surgical management of a patient with LP treated with dental implant therapy with implant site augmentation.

2. Materials and Methods

A 65-year-old female patient was referred to the periodontics clinic to evaluate extraction of the hopeless upper left second premolar and dental implants placement. Medical history showed high cholesterol and hypothyroidism under control of medication. Upon clinical examination, the patient had fair oral hygiene with a history of regular visits to the dental office for maintenance every six months. Erythematous and ulcerated mucosal tissue were observed on the buccal vestibule of the upper left and lower left quadrants (Figures 1 and 2). The patient reported sensitivity to citrus fruits and spices in these specific oral areas. A partially edentulous area was seen on radiographs at the upper left first premolar and lower right, as well as a retained root tip

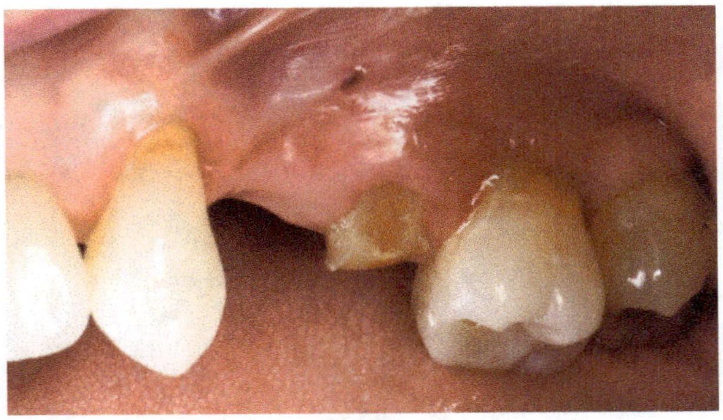

FIGURE 1: Desquamative erythematous lesion in the vestibular area upper left quadrant.

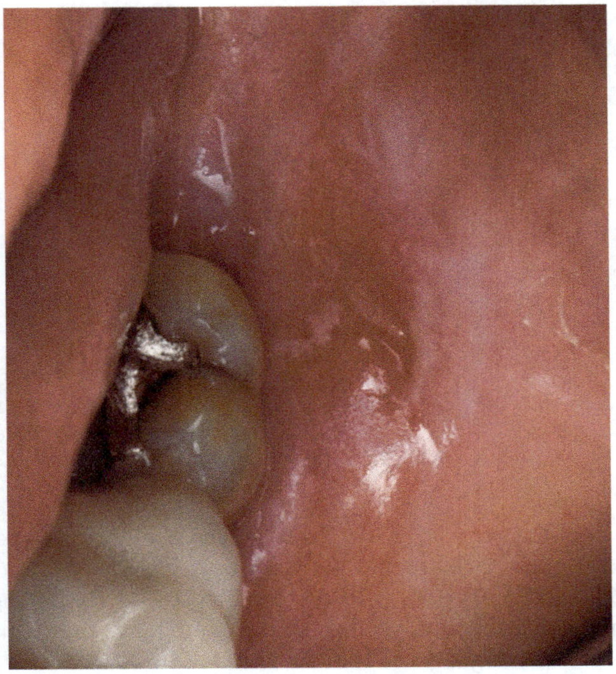

FIGURE 2: Lichenoid lesion related to tooth #37.

at the upper left second premolar. The patient was referred to an oral medicine specialist to manage the oral lesion. Two punch biopsies were taken from the upper left quadrant; the first biopsy was placed in formalin solution for H&E staining, and the second was submitted in Michel's solution for an immunofluorescence test. The diagnosis of erosive lichen planus was confirmed by a pathology report. After that, the patient began applying fluocinonide 0.05 percent gel three times a day. Meanwhile, dental procedures like scaling, polishing, and oral hygiene instructions were conducted carefully while monitoring the status of the soft tissue response to the corticosteroid therapy. Two months after systemic and local treatments, the patient presented with an improved soft tissue status and healthier-looking tissue (Figure 3). Clearance for dental implant therapy was obtained from the oral medicine specialist. A cone beam CT scan revealed adequate bone height and width to place an immediate implant at tooth #25 and implant placement at #24 with contoured bone augmentation. Before surgery,

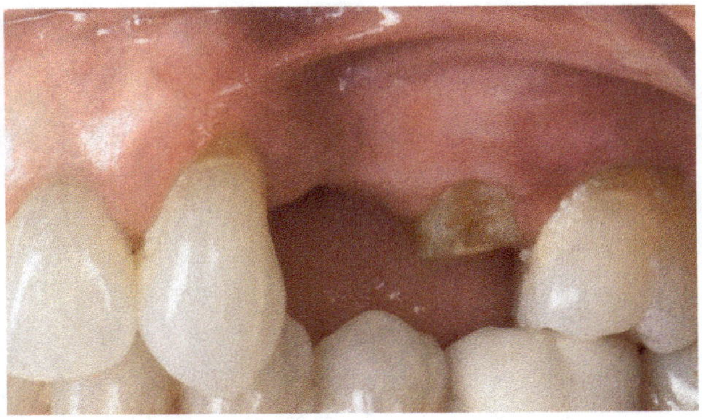

FIGURE 3: Improved soft tissue response to topical corticosteroid therapy two months after diagnosis.

verbal and written consent was obtained, and the patient was premeditated with 1 g of amoxicillin one hour before the surgery to minimize the risk of complications or implant failure [13]. Tooth #25 was then extracted as minimally traumatic as possible, followed by curettage to ensure that all granulomatous tissues were removed. The socket was then thoroughly irrigated with normal saline. The immediate implant (Biomet 3i), #25, was placed in the freshly extracted socket, and #24 was placed in the healed ridge with buccal ridge deficiency. The buccal gap at the extraction socket and the buccal concavity at the first premolar site were grafted with freeze-dried bone allograft (Oragraft, Lifenet Health) and covered with collagen membrane (Ossix plus, ColBar Life Sciences Ltd). A periosteal releasing incision was made deep into the buccal flap to achieve tension-free primary closure. The flap was sutured using 4-0 expanded polytetrafluoroethylene. The tissue was difficult to suture at this point, and tears at the buccal mucosa were noticed upon tightening the sutures (Figure 4). The patient was then given verbal and written postoperative instructions, and medication was prescribed 500 mg of amoxicillin and nonsteroidal anti-inflammatory drugs as an analgesic, ibuprofen 400 mg. The patient presented with an exaggerated response to the procedure eight days after implant placement, as sloughed tissue covered the surgical site. At this stage, it was decided to remove the sutures after irrigating with normal saline. Healing was within normal limits after four weeks, with no sign of inflammation except at the area of the second premolar, where slightly ulcerated tissues were still clinically evident. On eight weeks follow-up, healing appeared to be better with around 2×2 mm soft tissue exposure of cover screw at the site of the second premolar (Figure 5). The patient was then scheduled for a second-stage appointment. During that procedure, minimal flap manipulation was used to minimize further exaggerated tissue response. After the second-stage surgery, healing was uneventful. The tissue appeared firm, pink in color, and free of inflammation (Figure 6). The same procedure was performed for tooth #46, where the implant was placed in a healed ridge with adequate bone and soft tissue thickness. When compared to the other site, no abnormal tissue response was observed. Furthermore, no flare-ups were detected during the subsequent appointments, and the patient was referred to the

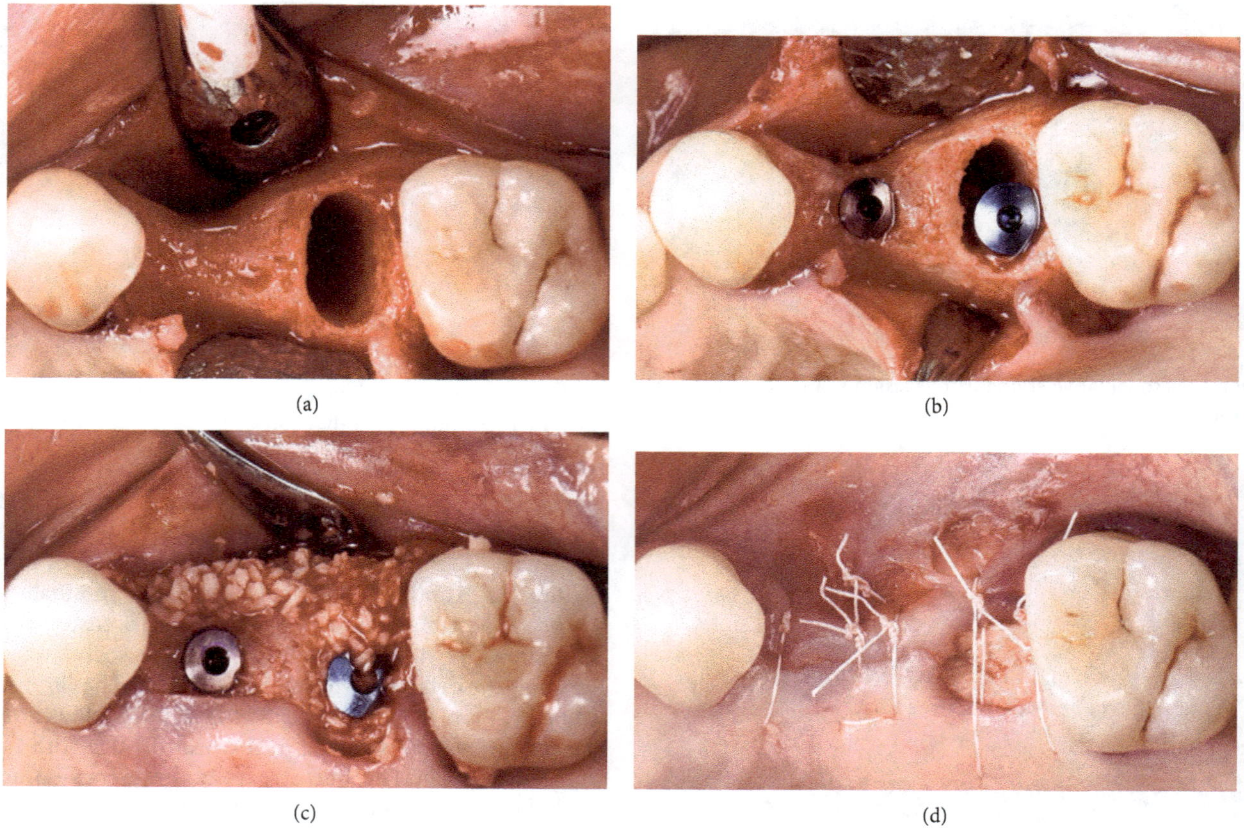

FIGURE 4: The sequence of the surgical management of the upper left quadrant. (a) After tooth extraction and ridge deficiency is noticed at the 1st premolar site. (b) Implant placement at #25 and 24. (c) Allograft bone material is used to fill the buccal gap at the extraction socket and augment the buccal ridge at #24. (d) Upon flap closure, a tissue tear was noticed at the mucosal area of the site.

restorative dentist for a final impression and crown fabrication.

3. Discussion

In this case of erosive LP, the patient was treated with dentoalveolar implant placement in the upper left and lower right quadrants with variable degrees of tissue response to the surgical therapy. Even though few studies have examined the success of implant placement in patients with LP, when the disease is appropriately managed by a specialist, it can be assumed that implant placement and site augmentation can be a viable approach to restoring missing dentition in such patients [11].

A total of fourteen patients who received 1-15 implants were investigated over a two-year period in a retrospective study to investigate whether oral LP affected the success of dental implant therapy. The study suggested that a well-treated LP does not appear to negatively impact the success of dental implants [14]. In a cross-sectional study evaluating clinical parameters of 16 patients diagnosed with LP who received dental implants loaded for at least a year, the clinical parameters were peri-implant mucositis, peri-implantitis, bone loss, pain, and bleeding. The study did not find any statistically significant difference in all these parameters when comparing dental implants placed in patients with LP and those without LP [15].

Several studies investigated the effect of soft tissue thickness on the stability and health of peri-implant bone [16, 17]. Linkevicius et al. in 2015 reported in a study evaluating implant placement with platform switching prosthetic design in two groups of thick and thin soft tissues. The study found that implants placed in thin soft tissue had more bone loss when compared to those placed in thick soft tissue after one year of loading [18]. One of the clinical challenges encountered with patients with LP is the risk of exaggerated oral tissue response to surgical therapy, which may have an impact on the quality and quantity of soft tissue. This was a clear finding in the patient in this case report where crestal bone loss was evident three months after placing the implant in the upper premolar site. This observation could be attributed to the soft tissue exposure that eventually affected the soft tissue thickness around the implant.

In a systematic review, Chrcanovic et al. reported a low failure rate of implants placed in patients with LP (2.7%). The study recommended that dental implant surgery be performed in the disease remission stage in a site with no desquamative gingivitis to avoid peri-implant soft tissue inflammation [11]. In the case presented in this report, surgery was postponed until better soft tissue quality was evident after disease management and adequate plaque control were achieved by the patient.

The most common types of LP are the reticular and erythematous erosive [1]. Many therapeutic approaches have

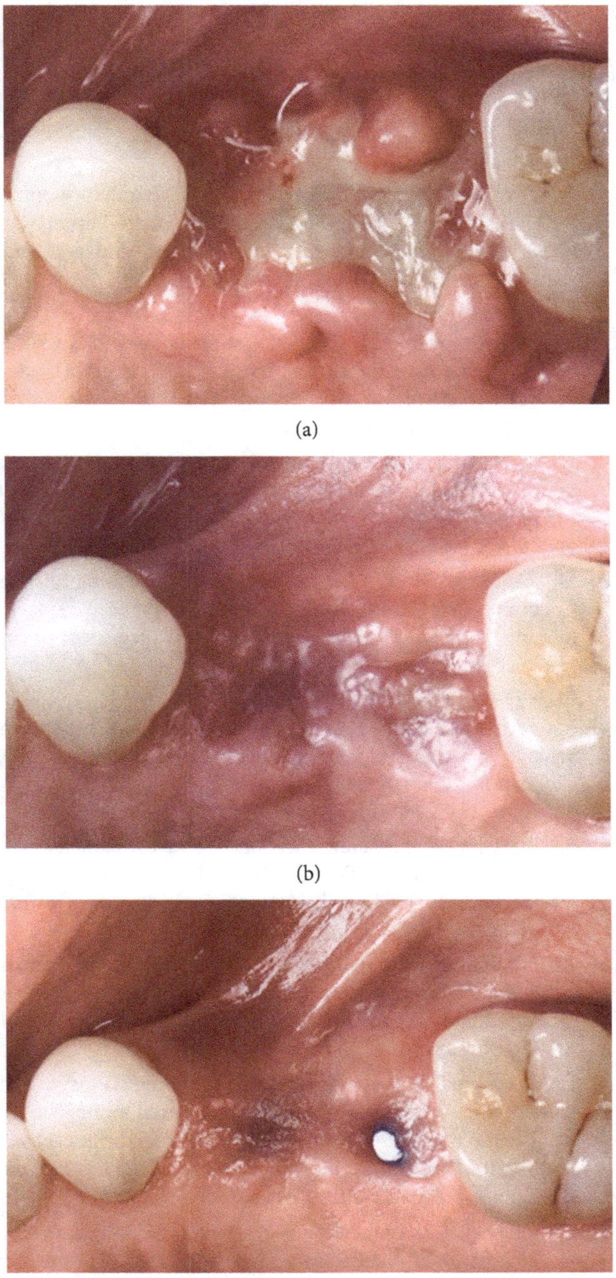

FIGURE 5: (a) Eight days of follow-up presented with exaggerated tissue response to the surgery. (b) Four weeks postoperative with better soft tissue response. (c) Eight weeks postoperative with thin, soft tissue covering the implants.

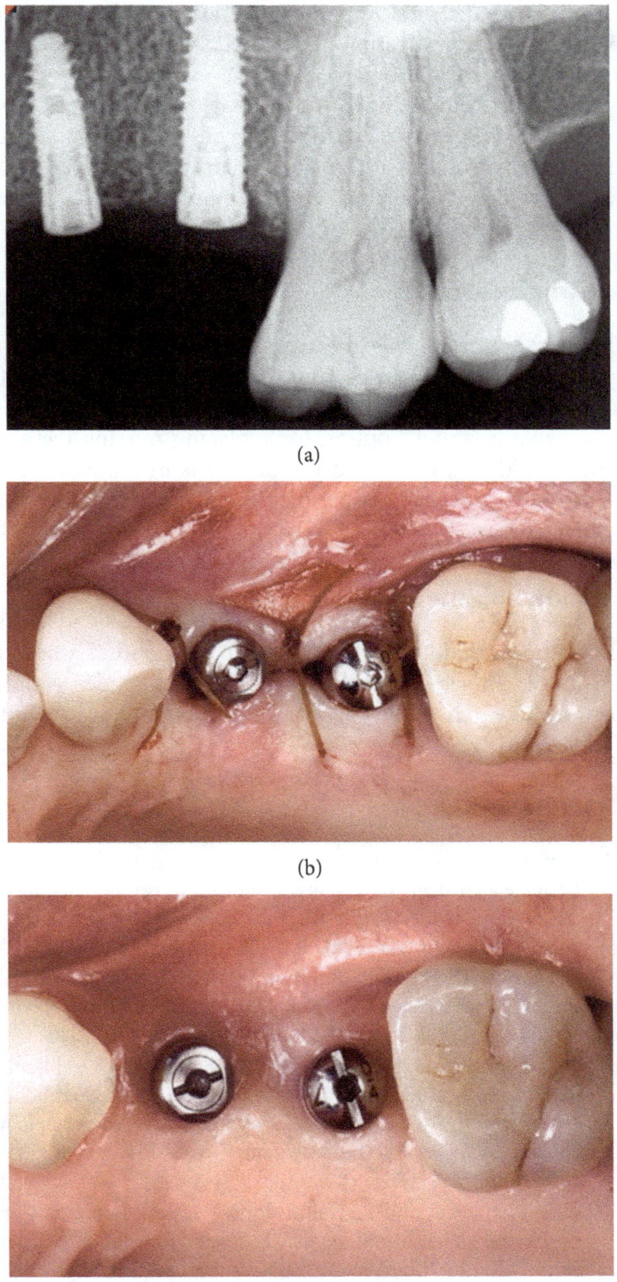

FIGURE 6: (a) At three months postimplant placement, the radiograph showed slight crestal bone loss. (b) Implants exposure with healing abutments. (c) Two weeks healing with better soft tissue healing and healthier-looking tissue.

been documented for the treatment of LP, like glucocorticoids, calcineurin derivatives, vitamins A and E, and laser therapy [19] [20]. Following a referral to an oral medicine specialist for disease management, a topical corticosteroid was recommended to ensure that the patient was asymptomatic and in no discomfort prior to any surgical intervention.

Good plaque control should be an essential part of disease management in patients diagnosed with LP to eliminate soft tissue inflammation triggering factors. These patients may experience sensitivity to regular plaque control regimens and some toothpaste, which may lead to suboptimal oral hygiene and negatively impact the patient's life [21] [22]. As a result, a structured plaque control regimen and products can reduce the severity of LP lesions while also enhancing the individuals' oral health-related quality of life [23].

López-Jornet et al. evaluated the quality of life of 3 groups of patients: implants with LP, LP patients with no implant, and implants with no LP. This study found a difference between the three groups in which the patients with LP and no implant experienced the worst quality of life compared to the other two groups. The author attributed that the presence of dental implant prosthesis may have a positive impact on mastication and esthetic whether the patient is diagnosed with LP or not [15].

Few studies in the literature evaluated the effect of LP on dental implant therapy. Future researches need to investigate the long-term impact of LP on the survival and success of dental implants, utilizing larger samples and a longer follow-up period.

4. Conclusion

This case report details the treatment of a female patient with erosive lichen planus who underwent dental implants and site augmentation surgery. Dental implant therapy can be a viable treatment option for replacing missing teeth in patients with LP, given that the disease is in remission and the surgical procedure is performed on a good quality soft tissue.

Acknowledgments

The author is thankful to the Deanship of Scientific Research at Najran University for funding this work under Najran Region Research Program Funding program grant code NU/NAR/MRC/11/9.

References

[1] I. van der Waal, "Oral Lichen Planus and Oral Lichenoid Lesions; a Critical Appraisal with Emphasis on the Diagnostic Aspects," *Oral Medicine, Oral Pathology and Oral Surgery*, vol. 14, no. 7, pp. E310–E314, 2009.

[2] C. Camisa, C. M. Allen, B. Bowen, and R. G. Olsen, "Indirect immunofluorescence of oral lichen planus," *Journal of Oral Pathology & Medicine*, vol. 15, no. 4, pp. 218–220, 1986.

[3] I. Al-Hashimi, M. Schifter, P. B. Lockhart et al., "Oral lichen planus and oral lichenoid lesions: diagnostic and therapeutic considerations," *Oral Surgery, Oral Medicine, Oral Pathology, Oral Radiology, and Endodontology*, vol. 103, pp. S25.e1–S25.12, 2007.

[4] B. E. Pjetursson and K. Heimisdottir, "Dental implants - are they better than natural teeth?," *European Journal of Oral Sciences*, vol. 126, Supplement 1, pp. 81–87, 2018.

[5] T. Berglundh, G. Armitage, M. G. Araujo et al., "Peri-implant diseases and conditions: consensus report of workgroup 4 of the 2017 world workshop on the classification of periodontal and peri-implant diseases and conditions," *Journal of Periodontology*, vol. 89, pp. S313–S318, 2018.

[6] L. Schropp, A. Wenzel, L. Kostopoulos, and T. Karring, "Bone healing and soft tissue contour changes following single-tooth extraction: a clinical and radiographic 12-month prospective study," *International Journal of Periodontics and Restorative Dentistry*, vol. 23, no. 4, pp. 313–323, 2003.

[7] M. Nevins, M. Camelo, S. De Paoli et al., "A study of the fate of the buccal wall of extraction sockets of teeth with prominent roots," *The International Journal of Periodontics & Restorative Dentistry*, vol. 26, no. 1, pp. 18–29, 2006.

[8] S. Fickl, A. Therese Kröger, T. Dietrich, and M. Kebschull, "Influence of soft tissue augmentation procedures around dental implants on marginal bone level changes-a systematic review," *Clinical Oral Implants Research*, vol. 32, Supplement 21, pp. 108–137, 2021.

[9] U. Grunder, S. Gracis, and M. Capelli, "Influence of the 3-D bone-to-implant relationship on esthetics," *The International Journal of Periodontics & Restorative Dentistry*, vol. 25, no. 2, pp. 113–119, 2005.

[10] A. Torrejon-Moya, C. Saka-Herran, K. Izquierdo-Gomez, A. Mari-Roig, A. Estrugo-Devesa, and J. Lopez-Lopez, "Oral lichen planus and dental implants: protocol and systematic review," *Journal of Clinical Medicine*, vol. 9, no. 12, p. 4127, 2020.

[11] B. R. Chrcanovic, A. F. Cruz, R. Trindade, and R. S. Gomez, "Dental implants in patients with oral lichen planus: a systematic review," *Medicina*, vol. 56, no. 2, p. 53, 2020.

[12] D. Buser, K. Dula, H. -P. Hirt, H. Berthold, and U. Belser, "Localized ridge augmentation using guided bone regeneration. I. Surgical procedure in the maxilla," *International Journal of Periodontics and Restorative Dentistry*, vol. 13, no. 1, pp. 28–45, 1993.

[13] M. Esposito, M. G. Grusovin, H. V. Worthington, and Cochrane Oral Health Group, "Interventions for replacing missing teeth: antibiotics at dental implant placement to prevent complications," *Cochrane Database of Systematic Reviews*, vol. 2013, no. 7, article CD004152, 2013.

[14] R. Czerninski, M. Eliezer, A. Wilensky, and A. Soskolne, "Oral lichen planus and dental implants–a retrospective study," *Clinical Implant Dentistry and Related Research*, vol. 15, no. 2, pp. 234–242, 2013.

[15] P. López-Jornet, F. Camacho-Alonso, and M. Sánchez-Siles, "Dental implants in patients with oral lichen planus: a cross-sectional study," *Clinical Implant Dentistry and Related Research*, vol. 16, no. 1, pp. 107–115, 2014.

[16] T. Berglundh, I. Abrahamsson, M. Welander, N. P. Lang, and J. Lindhe, "Morphogenesis of the peri-implant mucosa: an experimental study in dogs," *Clinical Oral Implants Research*, vol. 18, no. 1, pp. 1–8, 2007.

[17] T. Linkevicius, P. Apse, S. Grybauskas, and A. Puisys, "The influence of soft tissue thickness on crestal bone changes around implants: a 1-year prospective controlled clinical trial," *The International Journal of Oral & Maxillofacial Implants*, vol. 24, no. 4, pp. 712–719, 2009.

[18] T. Linkevicius, L. Linkeviciene, A. Puisys, E. Vindasiute, and M. Steigmann, "Influence of vertical soft tissue thickness on crestal bone changes around implants with platform switching: a comparative clinical study," *Clinical Implant Dentistry and Related Research*, vol. 17, no. 6, pp. 1228–1236, 2015.

[19] M. J. García-Pola, L. González-Álvarez, and J. M. Garcia-Martin, "Treatment of oral lichen planus. Systematic review and therapeutic guide," *Medicina Clínica (Barcelona)*, vol. 149, no. 8, pp. 351–362, 2017.

[20] C. Bacci, V. Vanzo, A. C. Frigo, E. Stellini, L. Sbricoli, and M. Valente, "Topical tocopherol for treatment of reticular oral lichen planus: a randomized, double-blind, crossover study," *Oral Diseases*, vol. 23, no. 1, pp. 62–68, 2017.

[21] M. Cabras, A. Gambino, R. Broccoletti, and P. G. Arduino, "Desquamative gingivitis: a systematic review of possible treatments," *Journal of Biological Regulators and Homeostatic Agents*, vol. 33, no. 2, pp. 637–642, 2019.

[22] K. Thongprasom, P. Luengvisut, A. Wongwatanakij, and C. Boonjatturus, "Clinical evaluation in treatment of oral

lichen planus with topical fluocinolone acetonide: a 2-year follow-up," *Journal of Oral Pathology & Medicine*, vol. 32, no. 6, pp. 315–322, 2003.

[23] S. J. Stone, P. A. Heasman, K. S. Staines, and G. I. McCracken, "The impact of structured plaque control for patients with gingival manifestations of oral lichen planus: a randomized controlled study," *Journal of Clinical Periodontology*, vol. 42, no. 4, pp. 356–362, 2015.

39

Complete and Fast Recovery from Idiopathic Facial Paralysis using Laser-Photobiomodulation

João Paulo Colesanti Tanganeli[1] **Simone Saldanha Ignácio de Oliveira,**[2] **Tamiris da Silva,**[3] **Kristianne Porta Santos Fernandes,**[4] **Lara Jansiski Motta**[4] **and Sandra Kalil Bussadori**[4]

[1]*Post-Doctoral Student Program in Biophotonics Applied to Health Sciences, University Nove de Julho, SP, Brazil*
[2]*PhD University of São Paulo, SP, Brazil*
[3]*Post-Graduate Program in Biophotonics Applied to Health Sciences, University Nove de Julho, SP, Brazil*
[4]*PhD Biophotonics Applied to Health Sciences, University Nove de Julho, SP, Brazil*

Correspondence should be addressed to João Paulo Colesanti Tanganeli; tanganeliodonto@hotmail.com

Academic Editor: Jose López-López

Idiopathic facial paralysis, also known as Bell's palsy, exerts a negative effect on the quality of life. Although the prognosis is good in the majority of cases, a significant percentage of affected individuals may have sequelae that can negatively affect their lives. The use of therapeutic measures as early as possible can improve the prognosis. This article describes the successful use of laser-photobiomodulation as a single therapy in a patient with Bell's palsy and confirms the possibility of using this therapeutic modality as a good choice, since it is a therapy that is painless, comfortable, and without systemic side effects. The findings demonstrate that the adequate use of laser-photobiomodulation can be an effective therapeutic option for patients with Bell's palsy, regardless of the age, shortening the recovery time obtained with conventional therapies and avoiding sequelae. Further studies are needed for the establishment of adequate protocols.

1. Introduction

Idiopathic facial paralysis, also known as Bell's palsy, is the most common form of facial paralysis, accounting for 60 to 75% of cases [1]. This condition affects the seventh cranial nerve and is characterized by acute, unilateral onset that compromises function and esthetics, exerting a considerable impact on the social, professional, and psychological aspects of the lives of affected individuals [2].

The etiology of this condition remains unclear [3–5]. However, some aspects are considered possible triggers, such as genetic factors, viral infection, autoimmune disease, diabetes mellitus, pregnancy, Lyme disease, emotional factors, and stress [2, 3, 5, 6]. Moreover, recent studies point to the reactivation of herpes simplex virus and/or herpes zoster (shingles) as possible triggers for the onset of paralysis [3, 5, 7].

The diagnosis can be obtained through clinical examination, but complementary exams can be useful, especially for the elucidation of the differential diagnosis in relation to certain diseases, such as Ramsay Hunt syndrome [3, 8], Lyme disease [9], and lymphoma [10].

The incidence of Bell's palsy is between 23 and 35 cases for every 100,000 people [2]. The most common age group for the onset of facial paralysis is between 30 and 50 years [2], but children can be affected, which is a situation that deserves an even more detailed investigation [11–13]. The initial symptoms include the appearance of an earache several days prior to the onset of the paralysis that requires analgesia [1]. The condition ranges from mild to complete paralysis of the affected side of the face [1, 3, 4].

Different treatments have been proposed to achieve rapid recovery without significant sequelae. Such treatments include

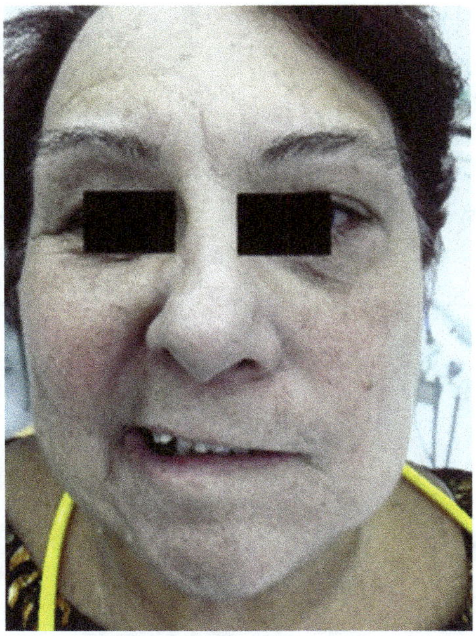

Figure 1: Patient with Bell's palsy—pretreatment.

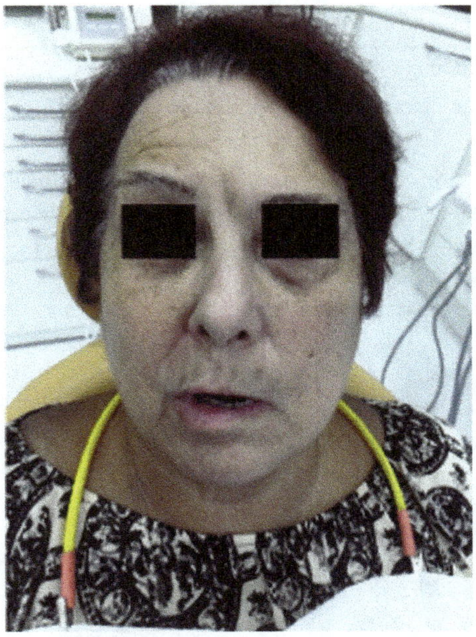

Figure 2: Patient with Bell's palsy—pretreatment.

botulinum toxin [14], acupuncture, kinesio taping [15], facial expression exercises [2, 3], corticoids, antiviral drugs, electrical stimulation [3], and laser-photobiomodulation (L-PBM) [2, 4, 12, 16].

The occurrence of Bell's palsy during pregnancy [17] requires integrated follow-up with the prenatal medical team. Individuals with diabetes can suffer unusual consequences, such as hearing loss [6, 18]. Permanent speech difficulties [19] and an association with temporomandibular disorders have also been described [16].

Some studies have been conducted to predict the prognosis and quantify the degree of impairment in Bell's palsy [5, 20]. Although the prognosis is good, with complete or adequate recovery in 70 to 85% of cases [1, 3], shortening the recovery time is a common concern for both affected individuals and the health professionals in charge of treating this condition. Indeed, the early institution of measures to accelerate the recovery process leads to better results [1–4, 16]. Laser-photobiomodulation administered with adequate protocols by trained professionals has proven to be a good option for accelerating the recovery process in both adults and children [2, 4, 12, 16].

2. Case Presentation

AMFC, a 71-year-old female patient, presented with a sudden onset of unilateral facial paralysis preceded by pain in the masticatory muscles (masseter and temporal). She sought an emergency service on March 4th, 2018. After cranial tomography for the differential diagnosis in relation to a possible transitory stroke, the neurologist diagnostic was Bell's palsy. In our first evaluation (Figures 1 and 2), we classified the case as grade V (severe), according to the House-Brackmann Scale (Table 1). This classification will be detailed later in the discussion topic. Laser-photobiomodulation was proposed and initiated on March 5th.

2.1. Materials and Methods. A low-level laser (brand: DMC™) was previously measured to have a 100 mW output power density with a fiber diameter of 600 μm. The protocol was punctual application of 3.3 J per point (120 J/cm^2), 10 seconds each, in contact with the skin, infrared of 808 nm, and applied to ten points (Figure 3):

(i) Point 1: frontal muscle

(ii) Point 2: temporal muscle

(iii) Points 3, 4, and 5: zygomatic muscle

(iv) Point 6: buccinator muscle

(v) Points 7: lip elevator

(vi) Point 8: orbicularis of the lips

(vii) Point 9: lip depressor

(viii) Point 10: masseter

3. Results and Discussion

After the fifth session, the patient's recovery was remarkable, and she was both cooperative and satisfied. It should be pointed out that no other form of therapy was performed.

A total of 10 sessions were held, initially one session every 48 hours; after the fifth session, two weekly sessions were held until the remission of the condition. The treatment was ended on April 21st, 2018. Follow-up was performed every two weeks in May and June, followed by monthly evaluations to the present date, with no sequelae or recurrence (Figure 4). According to the HB Scale, the results indicate grade I (Table 1).

The results were evaluated according to the House-Brackmann Scale (1985).

Table 1: House-Brackmann Scale evaluates the level of facial nerve paralysis.

Grade	Function level	Symmetry at rest	Eyes	Mouth	Forehead
I	Normal	Normal	Normal	Normal	Normal
II	Mild	Normal	Easy and complete closure	Slightly asymmetrical	Reasonable function
III	Moderate	Normal	With effort complete closure	Slightly affected with effort	Slight to moderate
IV	Moderately severe	Normal	Incomplete closure	Asymmetrical with maximum effort	None
V	Severe	Asymmetry	Incomplete closure	Minimal movement	None
VI	Total paralysis	Total paralysis	Total paralysis	Total paralysis	Total paralysis

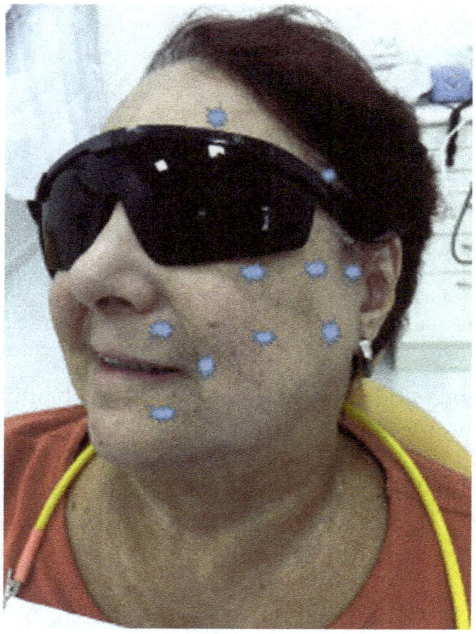

Figure 3: Laser application points.

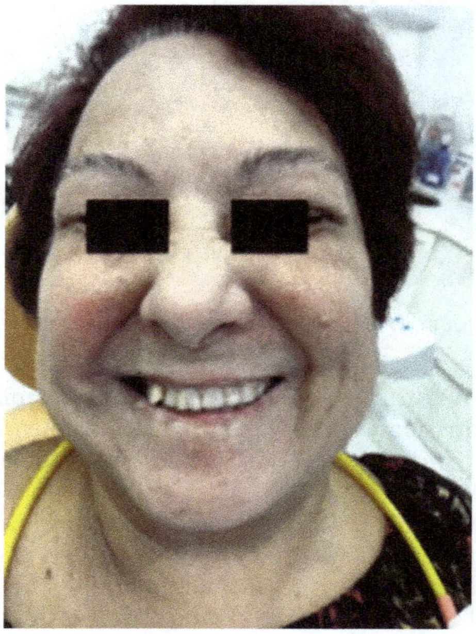

Figure 4: Results after ten sessions of L-PBM.

Bell's palsy is generally a self-limiting condition, with the return of functions within a six-month period and with no substantial sequelae in most cases. However, a significant portion of patients have more severe conditions. It is estimated that 71% of affected individuals recover completely, about 13% only achieve partial recovery, and approximately 4% experience severe paralysis [3].

The conventional therapies include drug therapy (corticosteroids and antiviral drugs), facial exercises, massage, thermotherapy, electrical stimulation, acupuncture, and laser-photobiomodulation [1–4, 15].

Regarding the recovery time, the literature shows that, with conventional therapies, 69.5% of patients have good recovery after 3 months, while 30.5% have poor results [20].

Recovery results are often evaluated by the House-Brackmann Scale, assessing the levels of facial nerve injury and proposing the following order: normal, soft, moderate, moderate/severe, severe dysfunction, and complete paralysis [20, 21].

Some studies have demonstrated that L-PBM enhances the regeneration of neurons, with local and systemic effects, directly restoring nerve structure and their communication with the central nervous system. Some researchers have demonstrated that laser increases microcirculation, activating angiogenesis and stimulating nerve regeneration [2]. Laser-photobiomodulation stimulates photoreceptors present on the mitochondrial membrane, converting light energy into chemical energy, increasing ATP that enhances cellular functions and regeneration [2]. One of the possible explanations of the low-level laser effects is that it increases the activity of the enzymes involved in the mitochondrial respiratory chain, leading to an increase in ATP production, directly acting on the oxidative stress, that is increased in Bell's palsy [1, 5, 22]. Low-level lasers also have an anti-inflammatory effect, explained by the reduction of proinflammatory cytokines and increasing anti-inflammatory growth factors [22]. Once inflammation is one of the factors involved in the pathophysiology of facial palsy, the L-PBM can improve the restoration of the homeostasis of the tissues [2].

A recent study reports that oxidative stress is high among individuals with Bell's palsy [5]. As one of the important mechanisms of action of L-PBM is the restoration of normal intratissue oxygen levels, this could be an important therapeutic modality for both minimizing the occurrence of sequelae and accelerating complete recovery. While some studies have demonstrated such effects [2, 4, 12, 16, 22], there remains a need for the establishment of standardized protocols. The present case report demonstrates that laser-photobiomodulation, when used in the early stages, can be an effective treatment for Bell's palsy.

4. Conclusion

Idiopathic facial paralysis (Bell's palsy) is an event that has a benign course in the majority of cases but can leave sequelae and have negative social, professional, and psychological impacts. Apparently, the early institution of therapeutic measures improves the chances of a complete recovery. Laser-photobiomodulation is a promising treatment option in such cases. However, controlled clinical trials are needed to enable the establishment of safe, adequate, and individualized protocols.

Authors' Contributions

Tanganeli JPC was assigned on the bibliographic survey, orientation of protocols, and drafting of the manuscript. Oliveira SSI was assigned on the execution of protocols. Silva T assisted in article writing. Fernandes KPS assisted in article writing. Motta LJ assisted in article writing. Bussadori SK was assigned on the orientation of protocols.

References

[1] A. Falavigna, A. R. Teles, A. D. Giustina, and F. D. Kleber, "Bell's palsy: pathophysiology and treatment," *Scientia Medica*, vol. 18, no. 4, pp. 177–183, 2008.

[2] B. Ordahan and A. Y. Karahan, "Role of low-level laser therapy added to facial expression exercises in patients with idiopathic facial (Bell's) palsy," *Lasers in Medical Science*, vol. 32, no. 4, pp. 931–936, 2017.

[3] D. Somasundara and F. Sullivan, "Management of Bell's palsy," *Australian Prescriber*, vol. 40, no. 3, pp. 94–96, 2016.

[4] T. F. Montero, M. S. H. Zayas, L. R. C. Andino, and V. C. Correoso, "Evaluación clínica y funcional de pacientes con parálisis de Bell tratados con láser," *Medisan*, vol. 19, no. 12, 2015.

[5] S. Terzi, E. Dursun, A. Yılmaz et al., "Oxidative stress and antioxidant status in patients with Bell's palsy," *Journal of Medical Biochemistry*, vol. 36, no. 1, pp. 18–22, 2017.

[6] S. Ş. Eliçora and D. Erdem, "Does Type 2 Diabetes Mellitus Affect the Healing of Bell's Palsy in Adults?," *Canadian Journal of Diabetes*, vol. 42, no. 4, pp. 433–436, 2018.

[7] T. J. Eviston, L. S. H. Chong, N. C. G. Kwai, J. R. Clark, and A. V. Krishnan, "Altered axonal excitability properties in facial palsy," *Muscle & Nerve*, vol. 57, no. 2, pp. 268–272, 2018.

[8] J. Kuya, K. Kuya, Y. Shinohara et al., "Usefulness of high-resolution 3D multi-sequences for peripheral facial palsy," *Otology & Neurotology*, vol. 38, no. 10, pp. 1523–1527, 2017.

[9] G. P. Wormser, D. McKenna, C. Scavarda, and C. Karmen, "Outcome of facial palsy from Lyme disease in prospectively followed patients who had received corticosteroids," *Diagnostic Microbiology and Infectious Disease*, vol. 91, no. 4, pp. 336–338, 2018.

[10] K. Shikino, S. Suzuki, T. Uehara, and M. Ikusaka, "Central nervous system lymphoma mimicking Bell palsys," *Cleveland Clinic Journal of Medicine*, vol. 85, no. 6, pp. 442-443, 2018.

[11] M. Calik and O. Ethemoglu, "Childhood peripheral facial palsy," *Child's Nervous System*, vol. 34, no. 8, pp. 1441-1442, 2018.

[12] C. R. Fontana and V. S. Bagnato, "Low-level laser therapy in pediatric Bell's palsy: case report in a Three-Year-Old child," *Journal of Alternative and Complementary Medicine*, vol. 19, no. 4, pp. 376–382, 2013.

[13] A. L. Lutley and S. M. Standridge, "A Case of An Unusual Bell's Palsy Mimic," *Seminars in Pediatric Neurology*, vol. 26, pp. 77–79, 2018.

[14] P. N. Patel, S. R. Owen, C. P. Norton et al., "Outcomes of buccinator treatment with botulinum toxin in facial synkinesis," *JAMA Facial Plastic Surgery*, vol. 20, no. 3, pp. 196–201, 2018.

[15] D. O. Alptekin, "Acupuncture and Kinesio Taping for the acute management of Bell's palsy: A case report," *Complementary Therapies in Medicine*, vol. 35, pp. 1–5, 2017.

[16] T. A. Alfaya, P. N. Tannure, E. C. Dip, L. Uemoto, R. Barcelos, and C. V. D. Gouvêa, "Association of Bell's palsy and temporomandibular dysfunction: clinical management," *Revista da Faculdade de Odontologia-UPF*, vol. 17, no. 2, pp. 222–227, 2012.

[17] Z. Ferraz, J. Parra, A. Areia, E. Vasco, and P. Moura, "Acute onset neurological disorders during pregnancy: a literature review," *Revista Brasileira de Ginecologia e Obstetrícia*, vol. 39, no. 10, pp. 560–568, 2017.

[18] T. Maller, S. Goldenstein, and O. Ronen, "Prevalence and characteristics of hearing loss in patients diagnosed with Bell's palsy," *European Archives of Oto-Rhino-Laryngology*, vol. 275, no. 1, pp. 99–102, 2018.

[19] J. H. Kim, L. M. Fisher, L. Reder, E. R. Hapner, and J. P. Pepper, "Speech and communicative participation in patients with facial paralysis," *JAMA Otolaryngology-Head & Neck Surgery*, vol. 144, no. 8, pp. 686–693, 2018.

[20] E. M. Khedr, N. Abo el-fetoh, D. H. el-Hammady et al., "Prognostic role of neurophysiological testing 3-7 days after onset of acute unilateral Bell's palsy," *Neurophysiologie Clinique*, vol. 48, no. 2, pp. 111–117, 2018.

[21] K. M. O. Fonseca, A. M. Mourão, A. R. Motta, and L. C. C. Vicente, "Escalas de grau da paralisia facial: analise de concordancia," *Brazilian Journal of Otorhinolaryngology*, vol. 81, no. 3, pp. 288–293, 2015.

[22] M. S. M. Alayat, A. M. Elsodany, and A. A. R. El Fiky, "Efficacy of high and low level laser therapy in the treatment of Bell's palsy: a randomized double blind placebo-controlled trial," *Lasers in Medical Science*, vol. 29, no. 1, pp. 335–342, 2014.

40

Acanthomatous Ameloblastoma: An Early Stage Case Report with Difficult Management

Roberto Pippi,[1] **Marcello Santoro,**[1] **Alessandra Pietrantoni**,[1] **and Angelina Pernazza**[2]

[1]*Department of Odontostomatological and Maxillo Facial Sciences, Sapienza University of Rome, Via Caserta 6, 00161 Rome, Italy*
[2]*Department of Molecular Medicine, Sapienza University of Rome, Italy*

Correspondence should be addressed to Alessandra Pietrantoni; alessandra.pietrantoni@uniroma1.it

Academic Editor: Giuseppe Colella

A case of a mandibular acanthomatous ameloblastoma, with an admixed little component of follicular type, is reported. The epidemiological features of the present case agree with those reported in the international literature. Clinico-radiographic differential diagnostic difficulties existed with several other noncystic osteolytic lesions of the mandible. Recurrence was diagnosed early 1 year after the initial excisional biopsy, and a definitive rim resection was therefore performed. No further recurrence occurred in the following 4-year follow-up.

1. Introduction

Ameloblastoma belongs to the benign epithelial odontogenic tumor subgroup, and it is probably one of the most controversial and enigmatic tumors of the facial skeleton, due to both clinical behavior and histological features [1–10].

The World Health Organization in 2005 [8] defined four variants: solid/multicystic (11-90%), unicystic (5-22%), desmoplastic (0.9-13%), and extraosseous/peripheral (0.5-9.3%) [5, 8, 9]; although in 2017 [11], the desmoplastic variant was included in the solid/multicystic forms, under the common term of ameloblastoma (9310/0 ICD-O code).

Unlike unicystic, peripheral, and desmoplastic types, which show a good response to the lowly invasive local excision, the solid/multicystic variant are more infiltrative with a high rate of local recurrence, especially following nonaggressive procedures, such as enucleation and curettage [1, 4, 6, 7].

The term acanthomatous is used in the presence of extensive squamous metaplasia and variable keratinization of stellate reticulum-like cells; in addition, the formation of squamous edges, in the center of the neoplastic nests, and calcification may be present. Acanthomatous ameloblastoma (AA) also presents histological features very similar to those of the squamous odontogenic tumor from which it differs since the peripheral cells are columnar instead of flat [9]. In an extensive review of 3,677 cases performed by Reichart et al. in 1995 [1], the AA was the third most frequent histological variant (12.1%) after the follicular (32.5%) and plexiform (28.2%) ones, although various histological aspects may be present in each ameloblastoma [11]. Very similar data were found in a multicenter study performed by Dhanuthai et al. [5] with a sample of 1,289 North American and Asian cases, on the basis of the 2005 WHO classification [8], with an incidence rate of 7.06% for the AA and 27.7% and 21.1% for the follicular and plexiform forms, respectively.

2. Case Presentation

A 78-year-old patient was first observed in December 2008 at the Complex Operative Unit of Oral Surgery at the Department of Odontostomatological and Maxillofacial Sciences of the "Sapienza" University of Rome due to a small, symptomless, localized swelling at the right inferior alveolar process, between the canine and the first premolar which appeared spaced several millimeters each other (Figure 1). The swelling was reported to appear a few months earlier and was hard fibrous and painless on palpation. The contiguous teeth were firm and vital to the cold test, and neither the involvement of the lingual aspect of the mandible nor of the regional lymph nodes was detected on clinical examination.

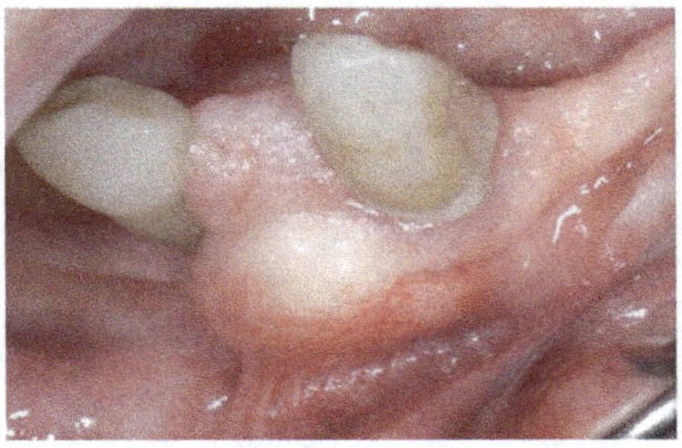

Figure 1: First visit clinical view shows a localized swelling at the right inferior alveolar process.

The patient was suffering from hemiparesis caused by cerebral ischemia in 2007, from noninsulin-dependent diabetes and from polio disability of the lower legs since he was 12 years old. The orthopantomography showed a homogeneous, radiolucent, oval-shaped, unilocular area, well-delimited by a peripheral radiopaque and slightly scalloped border, involving the roots of the canine and the first premolar and vertically oriented, from the top of the alveolar process up to about 1 cm below the apices of the neighboring teeth (Figure 2).

The en bloc excision of the lesion was directly performed under local anesthesia and after antibiotic prophylactic regimen (amoxicillin+clavulanic acid, 2 gr p. os, 1 hour before surgery) involving the overlying keratinized tissue and the 2 contiguous teeth, with a few millimeters of lateral and apical clinically healthy tissue and about 2 mm of residual bone cavity curettage. A surgical dressing was finally placed to support a secondary intention healing. No medical treatment was prescribed after surgery but only the use of a 0,20% chlorexidine mouthwash and analgesics as needed.

An acanthomatous ameloblastoma (AA), with a little component of follicular histo-type, was histologically diagnosed, and a microscopic amount of pathological tissue was identified at the deep edge of the surgical piece corresponding to the center of the residual bone cavity, while the lesion appeared completely removed from the contiguous soft and bone tissues.

A close clinical radiographic follow-up was therefore performed until, after approximately 1 year, a 5 mm radiolucent area was detected in the middle of the mineralized bone tissue (Figure 3).

A computed tomography (CT) with the Dentascan program was then performed (Figure 4) to better evaluate the morphology and the limits of the possible recurrence, and an incisional biopsy was performed to obtain microscopic confirmation.

Complete excision of the lesion was then performed by a rim resection involving a safety margin of about 7-8 mm of laterally and inferiorly radiographically healthy bone tissue, while preserving the integrity of the lingual cortical bone (Figure 5).

Histological examination of the surgically excised tissue confirmed the tumor recurrence (Figures 6–9).

No recurrence was observed at the radiographic 4-year follow-up (Figure 10), and no further diagnostic exams were performed due to the difficult clinical conditions of the patient who subsequently died due to other causes at the age of 83.

3. Discussion

The epidemiological features of the present case support those reported by the international literature regarding AA, despite the association of two different histo-types. Actually, the advanced age of the patient (78 years) is typical of the AA whose mean age at presentation (51 years) is more advanced than that of both the follicular (41 years) and the plexiform (39.1 years) subtypes [1]. Moreover, the mandibular canine-premolar localization of the present case corresponds to the generic ameloblastoma's predilection for the mandible (81%) and in particular to that of the AA for the mandibular incisor-canine area (42.8%), while the plexiform and follicular subtypes prefer both the molar area and the ascending branch (31.5%). No difference, on the other hand, was found in the literature with reference to gender and race [1, 10].

Although ameloblastomas with more than one epithelial hysto-type are not infrequent, mixed cases with acanthomatous hysto-type are rarely reported in the literature [12–14], and, to the best of the authors' knowledge, no cases of mixed ameloblastomas in which the acanthomatous component is so much represented, except for the present case, are reported in the international literature.

Pathogenesis of the coexistence of different hysto-types in the same tumor has not been explained yet. It is possible that it represents the different expression of the same neoformation process due to epithelial ameloblastic cells in different stages of maturation and morpho-differentiation—in relation to genetic mutations of their pathway of differentiation [15–17] or to different epigenetic or nongenetic time- and site-related stimuli [18]—or due to cells derived from different portions of the dental lamina, rather than the early or late association of different neoplasms or the conversion of one hysto-type into another, as already suggested in the past [19]. The genetic study of the various histological subtypes present in the mixed forms of ameloblastoma could provide useful information on their pathogenesis as well as allowing a targeted therapeutic strategy.

The clinical radiographic features of this case also support those described in the literature.

Actually, bone swelling seems to be the most common clinical sign of all types of ameloblastoma.

Other frequent events are pain, soft tissue ulceration, tooth eruption disorders, tooth mobility, and dislocation [1, 6, 8]. Dislocation was particularly evident in the present case, given the remarkable diastema between the involved teeth. Reichart et al. [1] already identified that AA caused cortical bone involvement more (50%) than all other types in the case of expansion of the involved bone segment, as in the present case.

All these clinical features, however, as well as the radiographic appearance, were not pathognomonic of ameloblastoma. Actually, differential diagnostic difficulties exist with several other noncystic osteolytic lesions of the mandible, since unilocular and multilocular aspects of the solid/multicystic forms seem to occur with approximately the same frequency [1, 5, 8].

The decision to first perform an excisional rather than an incisional biopsy of the lesion was made based on the

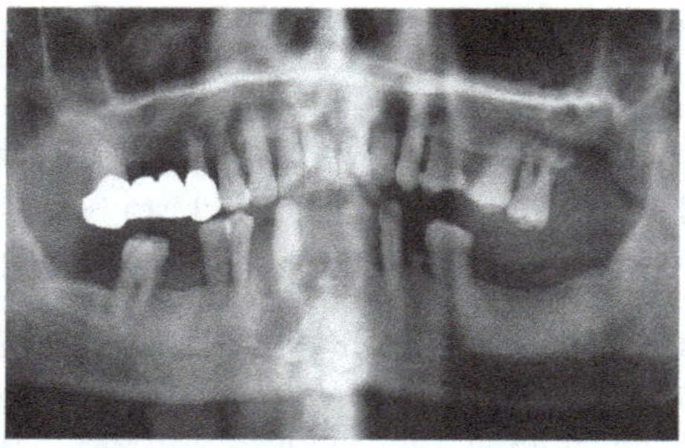

Figure 2: Orthopantomography at first visit showed a homogeneous, radiolucent, oval-shaped, unilocular area, which appeared quite well-delimited by a peripheral radiopaque and slightly scalloped border.

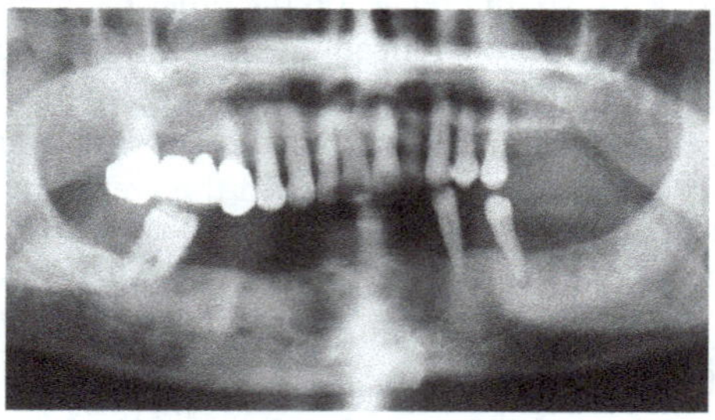

Figure 3: Orthopantomography 1 year after initial treatment: a radiolucent area was detected in the middle of the mineralizing bone tissue.

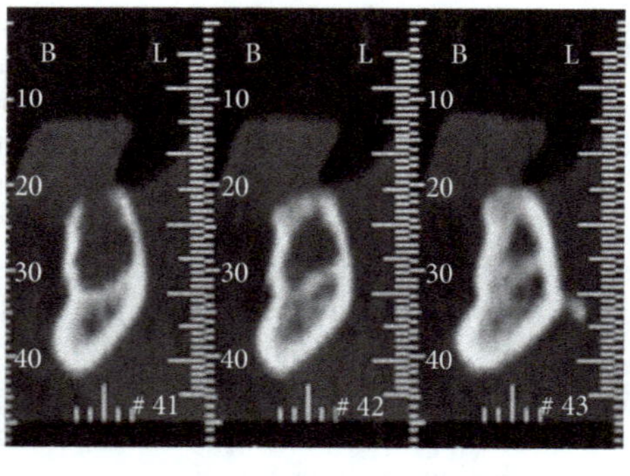

Figure 4: Dentascan CT: cross sections detail showed the limited involvement of the lingual cortical bone the limits of the recurrence.

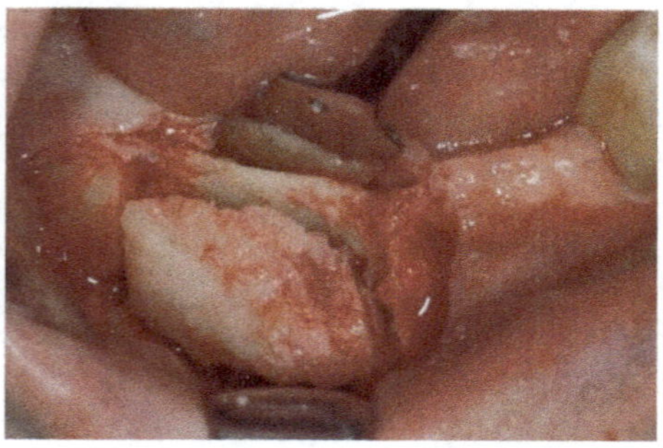

Figure 5: Rim resection intraoperative view.

following aspects: the diagnostic assumption of a benign neoformation due to the limited extension to the canine region in a subedentulous mandible; the lack of involvement of the nervous and vascular surrounding structures (mental bundle); the good radiographic peripheral demarcation, the radiographic appearance not pathognomonic of ameloblastoma; the hypothesis to resolve the pathological picture in a single surgical session, in view of the disability, with lack of mobility; the advanced age of the patient; and the notable distance of his home from the hospital. Actually, to the best of the authors' knowledge, there are no guidelines in the international literature on when to perform an excisional or incisional biopsy of jaw bone lesions. It therefore seems appropriate to obtain a precise histological diagnosis preoperatively using a preliminary incisional biopsy in the presence of an apparently benign osteolytic lesion of an

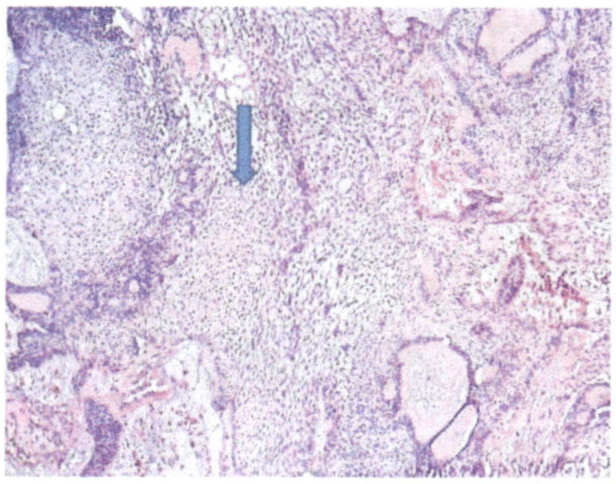

Figure 6: Histological preparation from the definitive surgically excised tissue, evidence of squamoid area (arrow), H&E ×4.

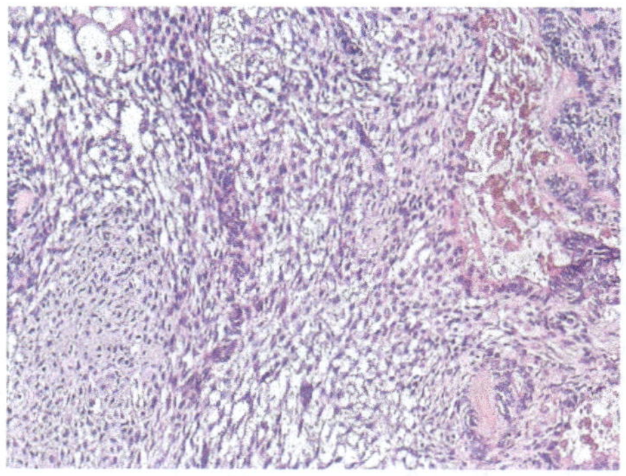

Figure 7: The tumor cells appear clear with eosinophilic cytoplasm, according to the differentiation H&E ×10.

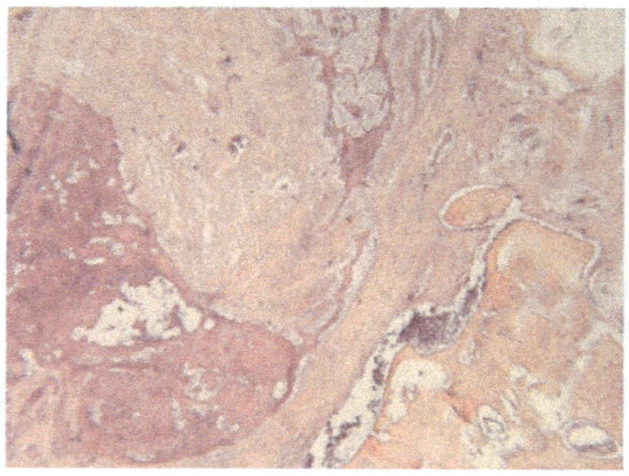

Figure 8: H&E ×25: mixed type of follicular and acanthomatous solid ameloblastoma.

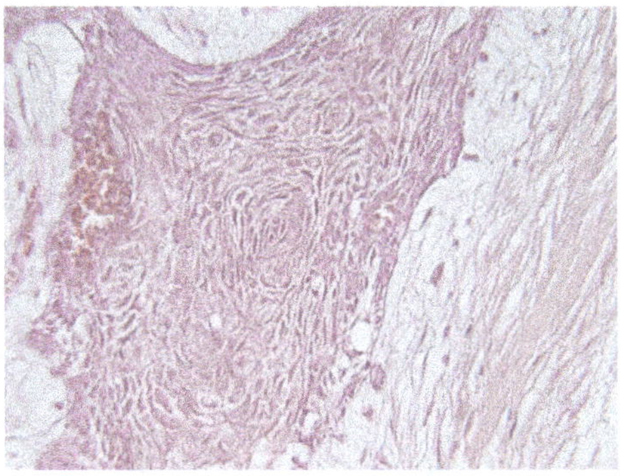

FIGURE 9: Detail from the previous histological preparation. H&E ×250: magnification of the acanthomatous component; Malpighian differentiation is highlighted by the presence of desmosomes.

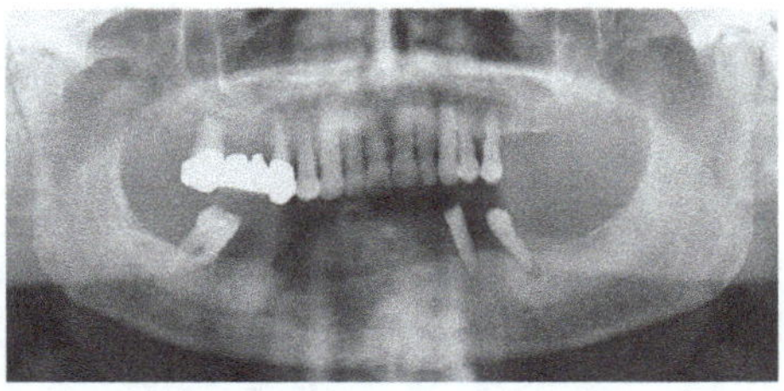

FIGURE 10: Four-year radiographic follow-up. No recurrence was detected.

uncertain nature, wide enough and/or involving important adjacent anatomical structures such as nerves, blood vessels, mucous membranes, and roots of many teeth, in order to perform a proper surgical planning, reducing the risk of recurrence caused by an incomplete intervention. Actually, the frequency of ameloblastoma recurrence, which may occur even many years after surgery, seems to depend on both the histological features of the tumor and the type of therapeutic approach used [1, 4, 6–8].

The extensive 1995 literature review by Reichart et al. [1] (3,677 cases) showed that tumors of follicular and plexiform subtypes resulted having a high frequency of recurrence (16.7% and 29.5%, respectively) compared to the acanthomatous, unicystic, and peripheral subtypes which, instead, appeared associated with a relatively lower recurrence rate (4.5%, 13.7%, and 9.1%, respectively).

However, the most recent study by Hong et al. [4] with 305 cases reported a 26.47% recurrence rate for AA, comprised between that of the follicular/granular cell subtypes and that of the plexiform/unicystic subtypes [5–7, 9]. The current WHO classification of odontogenic tumors [11] finally reports that the hystological type does not condition the prognosis, and it is therefore possible to argue, in the same way, that the presence of different histological types in the same tumor does not determine an evident improvement or worsening of the average tumor prognosis, and, probably, the different therapeutic approach is the most important factor in recurrence frequency which seems related to an uncompleted tumor removal [11], as happened in the present case, as well as to the tumor genetic profile, which were both found to be independent, statistically significant predictor factors of recurrence [17].

Since the simple enucleation or curettage of solid/multicystic ameloblastoma has 60-80% recurrence rate, especially in the presence of high-risk histologic variants such as the follicular one, lesion excision with an adequate safety margin is necessary [4, 7].

Histological sections showed tumor cells at a distance of 8 mm from the clinical and radiographic limit of the lesion, so the elimination of at least 1 cm of peripheral bone margin and the removal of at least 1 tissue plane surrounding the tumor when the soft tissues are involved seem to ensure the complete elimination of all possible peripheral tumor nuclei and may therefore significantly reduce the recurrence rates [4, 7].

The close clinical radiographic follow-up of the patient was therefore essential for early detection of recurrence and for its rapid treatment. Its small size compared to that of the initial mass also allowed to perform a much less aggressive or radical surgery, compared to what could have been in the first instance. Such a procedure allowed the removal of about 7-8 mm of clinically and radiographically healthy bone tissue, laterally and inferiorly to the lesion, and the simultaneous preservation of the lingual cortical bone integrity, in order to reduce surgical invasiveness and promote better tissue healing. The decision to conservatively treat the recurrence with a rim resection took into account its small size, histological type, and the advanced age and the clinical conditions of the patient. Actually, although neoplastic projections are able to spread easily through the marrow spaces of the spongy bone, it is unusual that the tumor tissue infiltrates the compact bone as well as the neural structures such as the inferior alveolar nerve [1, 4].

Finally, since the slow growth of these tumors can take many years (even 20 years) before a recurrence may be seen, although it most commonly appears 2-5 years later, the surgical site clinical radiographic follow-up is highly recommended for at least 10 years [4, 7, 9]. In the present case, follow-up was not possible because of the patient's death which occurred 5 years after surgery due to other causes.

4. Conclusions

Clinical and radiographic features of an early stage ameloblastoma can be not pathognomonic, so a preliminary histological diagnosis, through an incisional biopsy, seems highly indicated. During surgery, the preservation of the lingual cortical is advisable unless it is not clearly compromised by the tumor, in order to preserve bone continuity. Acanthomatous ameloblastoma is not frequent, but its complete excision, with adequate peripheral safety margin, is of paramount importance in reducing the risk of recurrence.

References

[1] P. A. Reichart, H. P. Philipsen, and S. Sonner, "Ameloblastoma: biological profile of 3677 cases," *European Journal of Cancer. Part B, Oral Oncology*, vol. 31, no. 2, pp. 86–99, 1995.

[2] S. G. Kim and H. S. Jang, "Ameloblastoma: a clinical, radiographic, and histopathologic analysis of 71 cases," *Oral Surgery, Oral Medicine, Oral Pathology, Oral Radiology, and Endodontics*, vol. 91, no. 6, pp. 649–653, 2001.

[3] J. George and M. Kamboj, "Ameloblastoma-an enigma," *Journal of Oral Biology and Craniofacial Research*, vol. 2, no. 3, pp. 203–205, 2012.

[4] J. Hong, P. Y. Yun, I. H. Chung et al., "Long-term follow up on recurrence of 305 ameloblastoma cases," *International Journal of Oral and Maxillofacial Surgery*, vol. 36, no. 4, pp. 283–288, 2007.

[5] K. Dhanuthai, S. Chantarangsu, S. Rojanawatsirivej et al., "Ameloblastoma: a multicentric study," *Oral Surgery, Oral Medicine, Oral Pathology, Oral Radiology*, vol. 113, no. 6, pp. 782–788, 2012.

[6] C. H. Siar, S. H. Lau, and K. H. Ng, "Ameloblastoma of the jaws: a retrospective analysis of 340 cases in a Malaysian population," *Journal of Oral and Maxillofacial Surgery*, vol. 70, no. 3, pp. 608–615, 2012.

[7] M. A. Pogrel and D. M. Montes, "Is there a role for enucleation in the management of ameloblastoma?," *International Journal of Oral and Maxillofacial Surgery*, vol. 38, no. 8, pp. 807–812, 2009.

[8] L. Barnes, J. W. Eveson, P. Reichart, and D. Sidransky, *World Health Organization Classification of Tumours. Pathology and genetics. Head and neck tumours*, International Agency for Research on Cancer, Lyon, 2005.

[9] P. Reichard and H. P. Philipsen, *Odontogenic Tumours and Allied Lesions*, Quintessence Publishing Co Ltd, London, 2004.

[10] M. Bansal, T. P. Chaturvedi, R. Bansal, and M. Kumar, "Acanthomatous ameloblastoma of anterior maxilla," *Journal of the Indian Society of Pedodontics and Preventive Dentistry*, vol. 28, no. 3, pp. 209–211, 2010.

[11] M. Vened, S. Muller, and K. Heikinheimo, *Benign Epithelial Odontogenic Tumours*, A. K. El-Naggar, C. JKC, T. T. Grandis, T. Takata, and P. J. Slootweg, Eds., WHO classification of head and neck tumours. International Agency for Research on Cancer, Lyon, 2017.

[12] J. K. Brooks, H. al-Mubarak, M. J. Ribera, P. D. Cohen, D. S. Ross, and M. A. Scheper, "Diminutive, interradicular "hybrid" desmoplastic/acanthomatous ameloblastoma," *Quintessence International*, vol. 41, no. 3, pp. 209–212, 2010.

[13] K. Jain, G. Sharma, P. Kardam, and M. Mehendiratta, "Unicystic ameloblastoma of mandible with an unusual diverse histopathology: a rare case report," *Journal of Clinical and Diagnostic Research*, vol. 11, no. 4, pp. ZD04–ZD05, 2017.

[14] C. R. Lakshmi, S. M. Bhavana, S. M. Nallamilli, M. P. Prabhat, G. Sarat, and C. Anuradha, "Hybrid ameloblastoma of the maxilla: a puzzling pathology," *Iranian Journal of Medical Sciences*, vol. 41, no. 4, pp. 340–344, 2016.

[15] R. T. Sweeney, A. C. McClary, B. R. Myers et al., "Identification of recurrent _SMO_ and _BRAF_ mutations in ameloblastomas," *Nature Genetics*, vol. 46, no. 7, pp. 722–725, 2014.

[16] A. P. Dodds, R. E. Cannon, C. A. Suggs, and J. T. Wright, "mRNA expression and phenotype of odontogenic tumours in the v-Ha-ras transgenic mouse," *Archives of Oral Biology*, vol. 48, no. 12, pp. 843–850, 2003.

[17] N. A. Brown, D. Rolland, J. B. McHugh et al., "Activating FGFR2-RAS-BRAF mutations in ameloblastoma," *Clinical Cancer Research*, vol. 20, no. 21, pp. 5517–5526, 2014.

[18] R. Pippi, "Odontomas and supernumerary teeth: is there a common origin?," *International Journal of Medical Sciences*, vol. 11, no. 12, pp. 1282–1297, 2014.

[19] H. P. Philipsen, P. A. Reichart, and T. Takata, "Desmoplastic ameloblastoma (including "hybrid" lesion of ameloblastoma). Biological profile based on 100 cases from the literature and own files," *Oral Oncology*, vol. 37, no. 5, pp. 455–460, 2001.

41

Reconstruction of Natural Smile and Splinting with Natural Tooth Pontic Fiber-Reinforced Composite Bridge

Maryam S. Tavangar[1] **Fatemeh Aghaei**[2] **and Massoumeh Nowrouzi**[3]

[1]*Oral and Dental Disease Research Center, Department of Operative Dentistry, Dental Faculty, Shiraz University of Medical Sciences, Shiraz, Iran*
[2]*Department of Operative Dentistry, School of Dentistry, Isfahan University of Medical Sciences, Isfahan, Iran*
[3]*Department of Periodontics, School of Dentistry, Hormozgan University of Medical Sciences, Bandar Abbas, Iran*

Correspondence should be addressed to Maryam S. Tavangar; tavangarm@yahoo.com
and Fatemeh Aghaei; m_aghaei878@yahoo.com

Academic Editor: Andrea Scribante

Teeth replacement is challenging in old patients with severe periodontal disease, limiting prosthetics treatment options. Here, we report a fiber-reinforced composite (FRC) resin bridge using natural tooth pontic in a patient with severe periodontitis. A 60-year-old lady complaining of teeth mobility was diagnosed with severe periodontitis, recession, bone loss, and crowding in the anterior maxillary teeth. Due to a hopeless periodontal prognosis, lateral incisors were extracted and sectioned using a cylindrical diamond bur. The pulp chamber was debrided and filled with self-adhesive flowable composite resin. After three weeks, the pontics were fixed in proximal contact areas, and the FRC bridge was fabricated directly using the resin fiber strip followed by occlusion adjustment, finishing, and polishing. Esthetic, occlusion, and periodontal status were re-evaluated after six months. Here, FRC using natural pontic could successfully reconstruct a natural smile, splint the adjacent teeth, eliminate crowding, and provide stable occlusion. Therefore, this method may be considered for similar cases.

1. Introduction

With an increase in the elderly population in recent years and advances in oral health, the number of natural teeth in the elderly population has increased, leading to more demands for conservative and esthetic dental treatments [1, 2]. There are some considerations for dental treatments in this population due to age-related changes in the oral soft and hard tissues, such as increased prevalence and severity of periodontal disease [3], gingival recession, and changes in the texture and composition of the enamel, dentin, and cementum [4]. Extraction of sound anterior teeth due to poor periodontal prognosis is common among the elderly and may compromise the patient's self-confidence and affect the quality of life due to loss of esthetic and difficulties in speaking [5, 6]. Replacement of these teeth for the re-establishment of esthetic and function is challenging, since a previous bone loss would limit prosthetics treatment options, such as implant-supported restorations, removable partial denture (RPD), and fixed partial denture (FPD) [7].

Resin-bonded bridge (RBB) is a conservative fixed partial prosthesis that provides esthetic and some functional demands, such as speaking, space maintenance, and lip support in anterior regions [8]. RBBs are used to replace a single missed tooth, whereas the adjacent abutment teeth are sound and have enough enamel available for adhesion [9]. In comparison to conventional FPD, RRBs need minimally invasive preparations and consequently cause less tooth sensitivity and less caries susceptibility. They also need fewer visits and have lower costs. In addition, RBBs can splint the mobile teeth where indicated, to improve patient comfort and spread occlusal forces across multiple abutment teeth [9].

With recent advances in adhesive materials as well as composite resins, an RBB may be fabricated with fiber-reinforced composite (FRC) resin instead of older metal

Table 1: Peridontal indices at different stages of treatment.

		18	17	16	15	14	13	12	11	21	22	23	24	25	26	27	28
Indices before periodontal treatments																	
Tooth number		18	17	16	15	14	13	12	11	21	22	23	24	25	26	27	28
Recession* (mm)	B		221		332	120	020	020	011	110	—	122	020	030	020	240	232
	P		112		342	—	—	—	—	—	—	—	—	010	010	252	233
Pocket depth** (mm)	B		332		223	534	437	633	733	322	225	824	435	525	523	326	624
	P		533		324	435	637	744	733	434	424	835	535	525	534	435	323
Mobility***		I		I	I	II	+	II	+	+	III	—	I	+	I	+	
Indices 4 weeks after periodontal treatments																	
Tooth number		18	17	16	15	14	13	12	11	21	22	23	24	25	26	27	28
Recession (mm)	B		222		443	221	231	131	211	210	—	223	231	121	121	343	232
	P		322		352	111	020	—	111	—	—	110	010	010	010	263	233
Pocket depth (mm)	B		322		222	222	216	612	522	322	224	522	224	313	422	225	523
	P		422		323	223	426	643	322	324	424	733	323	225	423	323	323
Mobility		I		I	I	I	+	II	+	+	III	—	I	+	I	I	
Indices six-month after restorative treatments																	
Tooth number		18	17	16	15	14	13	12	11	21	22	23	24	25	26	27	28
Recession (mm)	B		322		333	222	343	343	221	221	101	221	343	121	121	444	333
	P		322		352	121	132	—	111	—	110	—	011	010	010	243	233
Pocket depth (mm)	B		322		222	212	223	411	—	212	212	—	312	212	212	223	222
	P		222		323	213	323	411	—	212	212	—	312	213	212	213	211
Mobility		I		I	—	+	—	—	—	—	—	—	+	+	I	I	

Recession: exposure of the tooth via the apical migration of the gingiva is called gingival recession or atrophy. Pocket depth is the distance between the base of the pocket and the crest of the gingival margin. Miller's classification of mobility: grade I (−0.2 < horizontal movement ≥ 1 mm), grade II (−1 < horizontal movement ≥2 mm), and grade III (2 < vertical or/and horizontal movement). Abbreviations: B = buccal; P = palatal.

frameworks and can provide better adhesion of the luting agent to the framework, less total expenses, and more esthetic [10]. FRCs are composite materials with three different components: the matrix (continuous phase), the fibers (dispersed phase), and the zone in between (interphase). FRC materials present high stiffness and strength per weight when compared with other structural materials along with adequate toughness [11]. The pontic of the FRC bridge may be fabricated using acrylic resin, porcelain, processed laboratory composite materials, or even natural tooth pontic [12]. Natural tooth pontic leads to the highest esthetic results for those patients who are already satisfied with the size, shade, and morphology of their natural teeth. It provides the highest biocompatibility to the oral environment, which can be achieved in the least amount of time and lowest cost [13].

Here, we report an FRC bridge treatment with natural tooth pontic in a patient with severe chronic periodontitis to replace and splint her anterior teeth.

2. Case Report

A 60-year-old female patient was referred to the Department of Periodontology with the chief complaint of mobility of the maxillary anterior teeth. The patient was diagnosed with generalized severe chronic periodontitis and gingival recession due to bone loss in the central and lateral incisors, as well as canines. In addition, lateral incisors were rotated in place and were in an overlapped position on the central incisors, which caused crowding in the anterior maxillary segment. The same problem was previously addressed in her mandibular incisor with implant-supported FPD, but the periodontal prognosis was not acceptable, and the patient was unsatisfied with the esthetic and functional results.

Supra-gingival scaling and sub-gingival scaling were performed using Ultrasonic Piezo Scaler (DTE, Wuhan, China) and Gracey curette (Hu-Friedy Mfg. Co., LLC, Chicago, IL, USA), respectively. The periodontal indices were measured using a color-coded Michigan Williams probe (Premium Instruments, Ronkonkoma, NY, USA) after 4 weeks. They include gingival recession, pocket depth, and tooth mobility, as are shown and defined in Table 1 [14]. As the maxillary right and lateral incisors had grade II and III mobility with probing depths of 7 and 8 mm and more than 50% bone loss, respectively, with a hopeless periodontal prognosis, their extraction was recommended (Figures 1(a) and 1(b)). All the possible treatment modalities for the replacement of the lateral incisors and their costs, benefits, and prognosis were explained to the patient. After obtaining informed written consent, we chose and initiated the treatment plan with FRC bridge using natural tooth pontics.

The maxillary right and left lateral incisors were extracted under local anesthesia (1 cartridge of xylopen 2%; lidocaine 12 mg/epinephrine 12.5 μg/ml, Exir, Borujerd, Iran), and the extraction was performed atraumatically with no need of suture. The extracted teeth were scaled and polished thoroughly to remove all the deposits on them and kept in distilled water at the temperature of 4°C until the restorative procedure (Figure 2(a)).

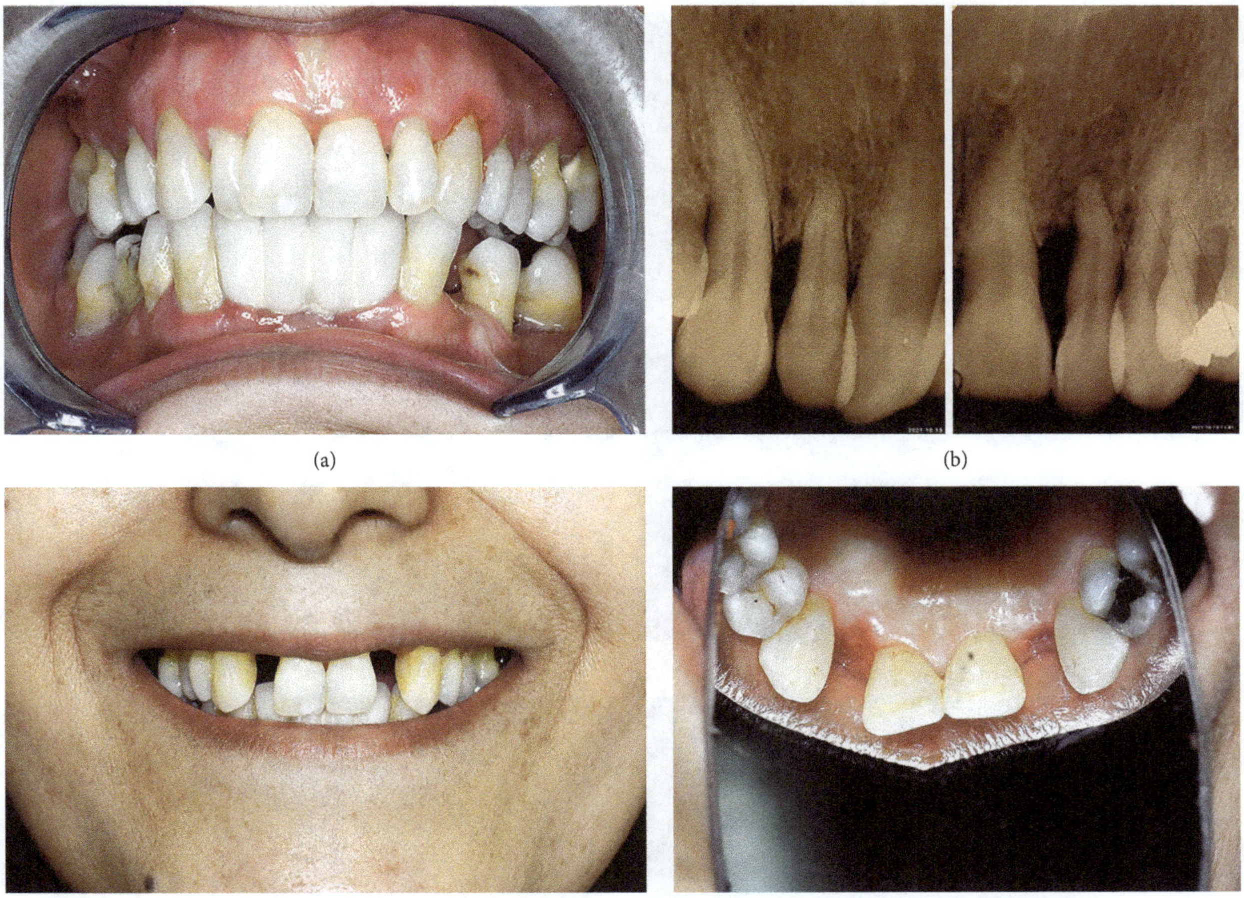

(a) (b) (c) (d)

FIGURE 1: (a) Frontal view and (b) peripapical radiogarphy showing crowding, gingivitis, severe periodontitis, and severe bone loss at lateral incisors periodontal tissue. (c) Frontal and (d) occlusal views three weeks after extraction of lateral incisors.

After three weeks, the healing of the extraction socket was re-evaluated, and the stable periodontal status was affirmed (Figures 1(c) and 1(d)). An impression of the maxillary arch with c-silicon material (Speedex, Coltene, Langenau, Germany) and the study model was made in order to adjust the length and proximal contours of pontics and correct the crowding in the anterior maxillary segment. The approximate cutting location on the root of the lateral incisors was marked while holding the teeth near their previous location on the study model. The root section was initiated using a cylindrical diamond bur in a way that the remained tooth portion consisted of an anatomical crown, in addition to a part of the root due to mimicking the gingival recession (Figure 2(b)). The pontics seem shorter than the natural teeth due to the root section. However, the remained tooth structure represents the clinical crown of pontics in harmony with the appearance of adjacent teeth.

The opening of the root canal was enlarged in the tissue side of the pontics with round diamond bur (Jota, Rüthi, Switzerland; Figure 2(c)). The root canal space was instrumented (K-file, Dentsply-Maillefer, Tulsa, OK, USA) and then debrided with sodium hypochlorite (NaOCl) 2.5% (Sigma-Aldrich, St. Louis, MO, USA) and remained in place for 10 minutes followed by irrigation with normal saline (Figure 2(d)). The pontics were kept in distilled water at 4°C for one week in order to prevent the detrimental effect of NaOCl on the bond strength.

Then, the root canal space was washed with distilled water, dried using paper points, and filled with Vertise™ Flow as a Self-Adhering Flowable Composite (Kerr Dental, Kloten, Switzerland); it was cured (BlueLEX, GT 1200, New Taipei City, Taiwan) at the light intensity of $1200\,mW/cm^2$ and wavelength of 470 nm for 40 seconds from each aspect of the pontics [15] (Figure 2(e)). Then, the proximal contours of the pontics were stripped using cylindrical diamond bur (Jota) in order to achieve the appropriate intra-arch position and correct the crowding in the anterior maxillary segment. There was no need for occlusal plan correction before the placement of RBB due to the corrected alignment of pontics in the arch. The tissue side of the pontics was formed in a sanitary ovate shape in a way that it could be cleansable by dental floss. Proximal contacts and soft tissue contact of the pontics were assessed intraorally, and the final adjustment was done to ensure there would be cleansable embrasures and optimized soft tissue contact of the pontics to establish the physiological massage of the edentulous ridge soft tissue. The tissue edentulous as the adjusted proximal contour of the pontics was then finished and polished using the OptiDisk Finishing and Polishing system (Kerr Dental, Brea, CA, USA) in 4 sequences.

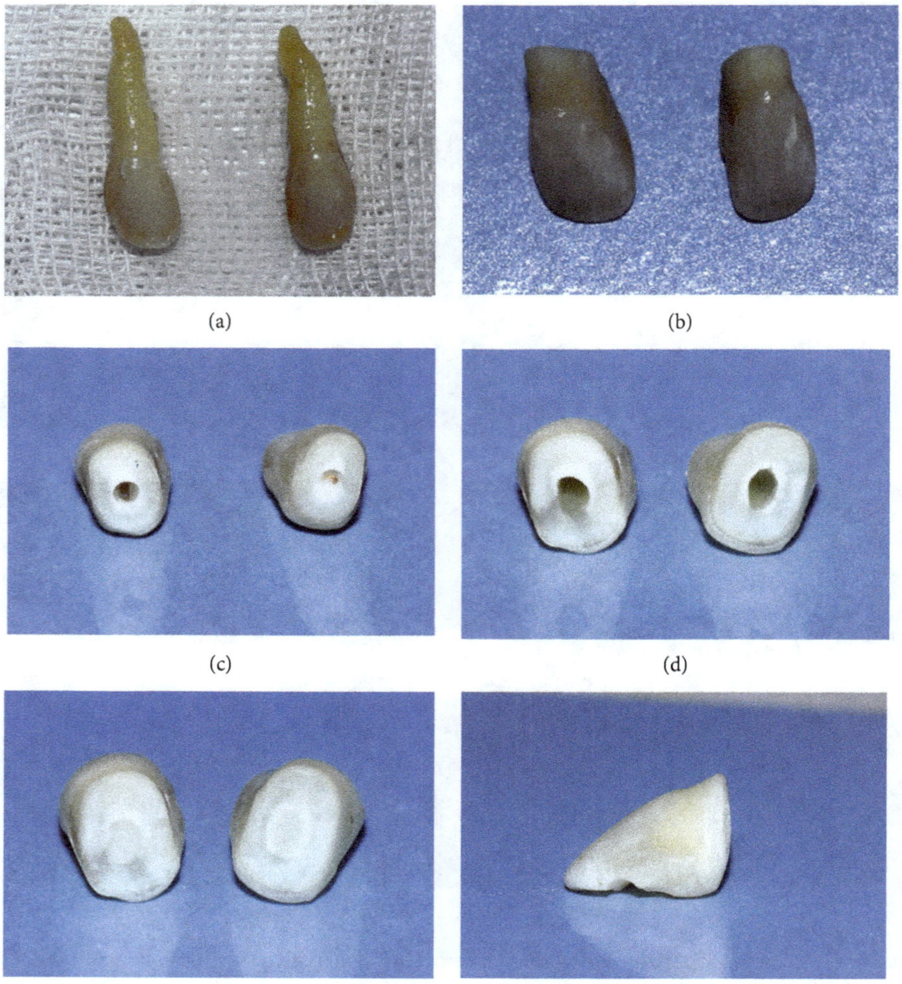

(a) (b) (c) (d) (e) (f)

Figure 2: (a) Extracted lateral incisors. (b) Initial root section. (c) Access opening for debridement of the pulp chamber. (d) The lateral incisors after cleaning and shaping the pulp chamber. (e) Tissue surface of natural tooth pontics after root canal filling. (f) Palatal surface preparation in lateral incisors.

On the middle third of the palatal surfaces of pontics and abutments (from the middle of the right canine to the middle part of the left one), preparation of 2 mm incisogingival width and 1.5 mm depth to preserve the enamel substrate was performed using a round diamond bur number 1 (Figure 2(f)). The prepared palatal surfaces were etched (Scotchbond™ Etchant, 3M ESPE, Washington, DC, USA) for 20 seconds, then rinsed, and dried (Figure 3(a)). Total etch adhesive (Adper Single Bond 2, 3M ESPE) was applied and light cured according to the manufacturer's instructions. The pre-impregnated resin fiber strip (Interlig, Angelus, Londrina, Brazil) was adopted in prepared surfaces, covered by flowable composite resin (Universal flow, Tokuyama, Encinitas, CA, USA), and then light cured for 20 seconds on each tooth. The pontics were fixed in place with Universal flow (Tokuyama) in proximal contact areas of pontics and light cured for 20 seconds. Universal composite resin (Estelite®Sigma Quick, Tokuyama) was applied and cured in some areas as needed for providing smooth contour (Figure 3(b)).

The occlusion was evaluated in centric position, protrusive, and lateral movements, and adjusted to remove heavy occlusion force in the pontics in the middle third portion where fiber was placed (Figures 3(c) and 3(d)). Then, the palatal surfaces were finished with football shape medium grit diamond bur and polished with impregnated silicon rubber points. The chronological order of all the clinical procedures is shown in Table 2.

The RBB was re-evaluated after 6 months in the point of esthetic, occlusion, soft tissue contact of the pontics, and periodontal status of abutments and restored part of retainers and pontics (Figures 3(e), 3(f), 3(g) and 3(h)). There was no sign of microleakage in the palatal surface of the retainers and pontics. Pontics showed no color change and were completely in accordance with adjacent retainers in appearance, color, and optical properties. The patient was satisfied with her smile and appreciated. Periodontal examination showed a stable condition without any mobility in abutments, and no edema, recession, or proliferation was detected in the soft tissue (Table 1). Follow-up evaluation

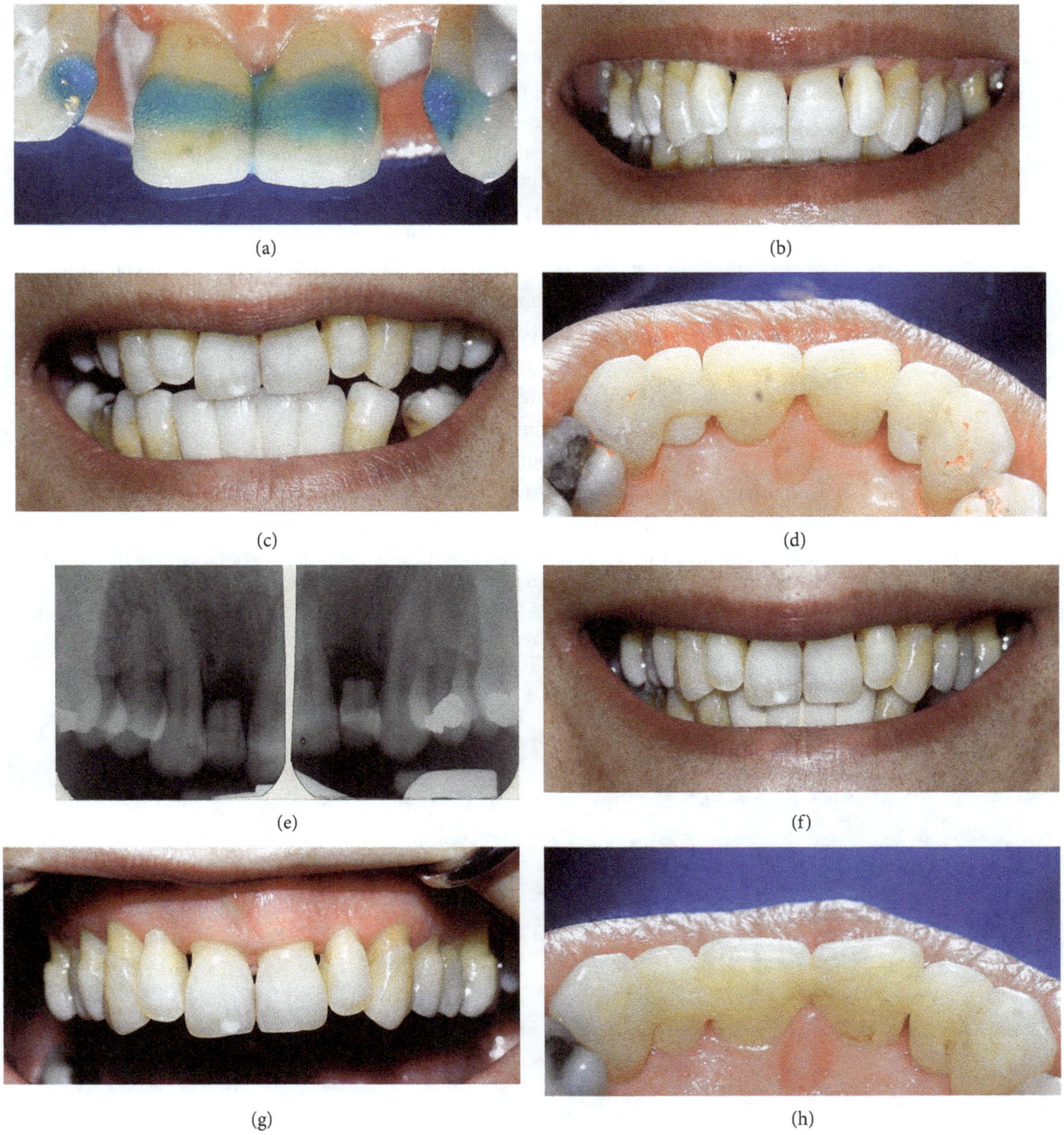

FIGURE 3: (a) Etching the prepared surface. (b) Close-up frontal view immediately after resin-bonded bridge (RBB) fabrication: reconstruction of natural smile and correction of crowding (c) occlusal contact in protrusive movement. (d) Palatal view before finishing and polishing. (e) Six-month follow-up: X-ray radiography. (f) Six-month follow-up: smile view. (g) Well adoption of pontics to the ridge six-month follow-up, there is no evidence of inflammation or recession in the soft tissue. (h) Palatal view of RBB after six months.

after 1 year was still satisfactory without apparent complication (Figures 4(a), 4(b), 4(c) and 4(d)).

3. Discussion

Here, we reported a successful reconstruction of a natural smile and accompanying splinting with a natural tooth pontic FRC bridge in a case of anterior maxillary tooth loss due to severe bone resorption and periodontitis.

Various treatment options are available for the replacement of a single tooth, such as an implant, FPD, and RPD. However, the lack of enough supporting tissue may limit the treatment options or decrease their success rate significantly. Implant-supported crown has been proven to be a successful treatment to replace a single tooth [16]. However, there may be some limitations, especially in cases where severe bone loss has led to tooth extraction. In these situations, there would be a need for regenerative surgery to provide sufficient bone for fixture placement and an ideal or acceptable appearance of the supported crown. [17] It should be considered that localized bone augmentation in the vertical defect is one of the most challenging procedures with a significant complication rate, and its outcome is questionable [18]. In addition, the risk of biomechanical problems in prosthetic components may be enhanced due to the increased crown-to-implant ratio [19]. In patients with

Table 2: Procedures checklist and their chronological order.

1	First session	Examination, and supra- and sub-gingival scaling.
2	After 4 weeks	Measuring periodontal indices.
		Extraction of the maxillary right and lateral incisors.
		The healing of the extraction socket was re-evaluated and restorative procedure was initiated by impression-taking the study model was made.
		Roots were sectioned and the proximal contours of the pontic were stripped to achieve the appropriate intra-arch position and correct the crowding.
		Root canal space was debrided, cleaned, and filled with a self-adhering flowable composite.
		The tissue side of the pontics was formed in a sanitary ovate shape.
3	After 3 weeks	Proximal contacts and soft tissue contact of the pontics were assessed intraorally and the final adjustment was done.
		Pontics were finished and polished.
		On the middle third of the palatal surfaces of pontics a preparation was performed
		Acid etchant and adhesive were applied.
		The pontics were fixed in place.
		Pre-impregnated resin fiber strip was applied and covered by a resin composite.
		Occlusion adjustment, finishing, and polishing.
4	After 6 months	Follow-up: Evaluated in the point of esthetic, occlusion, soft tissue contact of the pontics, and periodontal status of abutments and restored part of retainers and pontics. X-ray radiography was taken.
5	After 12 months	Follow-up: Evaluated in the point of esthetic, occlusion, soft tissue contact of the pontics, and periodontal status of abutments and restored part of retainers and pontics. X-ray radiography was taken.

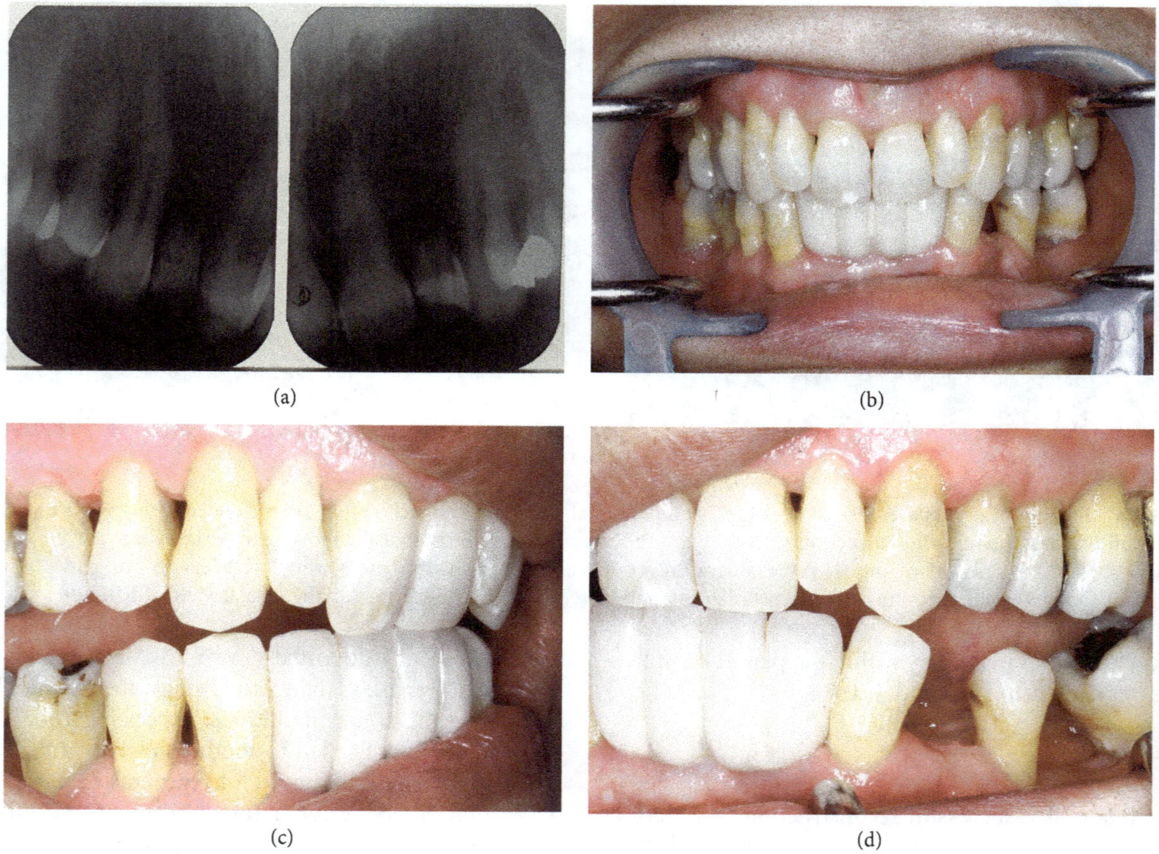

Figure 4: One-year follow-up. (a) X-ray radiography. (b) Retracted view. (c) Lateral movement in right side. (d) lateral movement in left side.

a history of periodontal disease and bone loss, RPDs make retainers prone to tooth mobility as well as plaque accumulation and tooth caries [20]. An FPD was a viable treatment option as well. However, when the adjacent teeth are sound, it would be an aggressive treatment as it needs full crown preparation [21]. In addition, the bone loss and variable degrees of mobility in abutment teeth lead to a crown–root ratio that is less than ideal. In addition, for patients avoiding removable dentures is satisfactory, as removable dental prostheses usually lead to lower satisfaction than FDPs. In an investigation by Malmstrom et al., high levels of patient satisfaction were reported when assessed by a Visual Analogue Scale at a 2-year follow-up visit [22].

Since the lack of enough supporting tissue limited the treatment options due to a probable failure and lack of satisfaction of patients with these treatments for mandibular incisors, we decided to use a natural tooth pontic FRC bridge. Fabrication of a pontic that mimics the natural color, optical properties, surface texture, and characterization of the adjacent natural teeth is one of the most important esthetic challenges in the replacement of a single missing tooth, especially in old patients with gingival recession, visible root surfaces, and altered appearance characteristics of the remained teeth [4]. There would also be some limitations to mimicking the natural appearance root portion in the crown or reconstruction of the gingiva with pink porcelain [23]. None of the artificial tooth pontic materials, such as direct and indirect composites, acrylic resins, or even porcelain, can be well-matched to the adjacent teeth in terms of color and optical properties, size, and morphology. As this patient was highly concerned with her 'natural teeth' appearance, the possibility of using the clinical crowns of the extracted teeth as natural tooth pontics being incorporated into FRC RBBs was proposed.

In the presented case, the Vertise™ Flow was used to fill the pulp chamber due to its ease of use and handling as a flowable composite resin. In addition, this composite has the advantage of being self-adhesive and requires no further steps for etching or applying adhesives [24]. These characteristics were highly beneficial in this case, since there was limited access to the restoration area. No internal discoloration was seen in the pontics after 6 months of follow-up, which demonstrates complete debridement and irrigations of the pulp chamber.

The loss of anterior teeth can be functionally and socially damaging. FRC bridges are a cost-effective, esthetically favorable, and minimally invasive method for the replacement of missing teeth. Minimal invasiveness is the main advantage of an FRC bridge, and it can maintain the maximum possible amount of tooth substance, which helps to conserve dental hard tissues for any further possible treatments [25]. Furthermore, using the extracted natural tooth as a pontic offers the benefits of it being the right shape, color, and size providing a good appearance and functional results. It is also noteworthy that FRC bridges showed a promising survival rate. A systematic review investigating the longevity of FRC bridges involving the placement of 592 FRC bridges with follow-up periods of up to 8 years showed an overall survival rate of 94.4% at 4.8 years [26]. Most of the failures are usually due to the debonding and delamination of veneering composites [27]. In most cases, these failures could be repaired, and the repairability of FRC bridges could lengthen the longevity of the restoration. Consequently, FRC bridges can be a good alternative method for rehabilitating teeth that need extraction.

Using FRC bridges for the replacement of a lost tooth may face some limitations. Some risk factors may decrease the longevity of an FRC bridge. Occlusion seems to represent a major risk factor for damage to FRC bridges [28]. Therefore, in this case, the load of occlusion on the pontics was adjusted to inhibit heavy occlusion forces in protrusive and lateral movements. Based on previous studies, ensuring macro-mechanical retention of a natural tooth pontic to the FRC framework is very important to diminish the tensile stresses at the bonding interface [29]. In this case, this retention is provided by preparing a groove into the pontic to resist dislodgement forces. Generally, the FRCs are recommended as a short-to-medium-term restorative option in previous studies [10]. Therefore, the patient was informed about the limitations of this treatment option, such as the risk of deboning of natural tooth pontics and fracture of supporting framework in the long term. Future investigations are needed to assess the durability of this treatment compared to other treatment options for a missing tooth.

It can be concluded that an FRC bridge using a natural pontic can be considered as a treatment option for replacing the extracted anterior tooth due to periodontal disease. In the presented case, this method could successfully reconstruct a natural smile, splint the abutments to decrease the adjacent teeth's mobility, eliminate crowding in the anterior teeth, and provide stable occlusion.

Acknowledgments

The authors would like to thank Shiraz University of Medical Sciences, Shiraz, Iran, and also the Center for Development of Clinical Research of Nemazee Hospital, Shiraz, Iran, and Dr. Nasrin Shokrpour for editorial assistance.

References

[1] H. Maeda, "Aging and senescence of dental pulp and hard tissues of the tooth," *Frontiers in Cell and Developmental Biology*, vol. 8, p. 605996, 2020.

[2] R. Guiglia, A. Musciotto, D. Compilato et al., "Aging and oral health: effects in hard and soft tissues," *Current Pharmaceutical Design*, vol. 16, no. 6, pp. 619–630, 2010.

[3] P. A. Razak, K. J. Richard, R. P. Thankachan, K. A. Hafiz, K. N. Kumar, and K. Sameer, "Geriatric oral health: a review article," *Journal of International Oral Health*, vol. 6, no. 6, pp. 110–116, 2014.

[4] G. Mckenna and F. M. Burke, "Age-related oral changes," *Dental Update*, vol. 37, no. 8, pp. 519–523, 2010.

[5] P. H. M. P. Tolentino, L. G. Rodrigues, É. M. de Torres, A. Franco, and R. F. Silva, "Tooth extractions in patients with periodontal diseases and clinical decision-making process," *Acta Stomatologica Croatica*, vol. 53, no. 2, pp. 141–149, 2019.

[6] M. S. Patil and S. B. Patil, "Geriatric patient–psychological and emotional considerations during dental treatment," *Gerodontology*, vol. 26, no. 1, pp. 72–77, 2009.

[7] R. R. Nadig, G. Usha, V. Kumar, R. Rao, and A. Bugalia, "Geriatric restorative care - the need, the demand and the challenges," *Journal of Conservative Dentistry*, vol. 14, no. 3, pp. 208–214, 2011.

[8] K. Durey, P. Nixon, S. Robinson, and M.-Y. Chan, "Resin bonded bridges: techniques for success," *British Dental Journal*, vol. 211, no. 3, pp. 113–118, 2011.

[9] J. S. Gulati, S. Tabiat-Pour, S. Watkins, and A. Banerjee, "Resin-bonded bridges–the problem or the solution? Part 1: assessment and design," *Dental Update*, vol. 43, no. 6, pp. 506–521, 2016.

[10] M. Miettinen and B. Millar, "A review of the success and failure characteristics of resin-bonded bridges," *British Dental Journal*, vol. 215, no. 2, p. E3, 2013.

[11] A. Scribante, P. K. Vallittu, and M. Özcan, "Fiber-reinforced composites for dental applications," *BioMed Research International*, vol. 2018, 2018.

[12] A. Gupta, R. K. Yelluri, and A. Munshi, "Fiber-reinforced composite resin bridge: a treatment option in children," *International Journal of Clinical Pediatric Dentistry*, vol. 8, no. 1, pp. 62–65, 2015.

[13] A. Khetarpal, S. Talwar, and M. Verma, "Creating a single-visit, fibre-reinforced, composite resin bridge by using a natural tooth pontic: a viable alternative to a PFM bridge," *Journal of Clinical and Diagnostic Research*, vol. 7, no. 4, pp. 772–775, 2013.

[14] M. Newman, I. Dragan, S. Elangovan, and A. Karan, *Newman and Carranza's Essentials of Clinical Periodontology*, Elsevier, 1st edition, 2022.

[15] A. R. Alpöz, F. Ertugrul, D. Cogulu, A. T. Ak, M. Tanoglu, and E. Kaya, "Effects of light curing method and exposure time on mechanical properties of resin based dental materials," *European Journal of Dentistry*, vol. 2, no. 1, pp. 37–42, 2008.

[16] R. E. Jung, B. E. Pjetursson, R. Glauser, A. Zembic, M. Zwahlen, and N. P. Lang, "A systematic review of the 5-year survival and complication rates of implant—supported single crowns," *Clinical Oral implants Research*, vol. 19, no. 2, pp. 119–130, 2008.

[17] Z. Sheikh, C. Sima, and M. Glogauer, "Bone replacement materials and techniques used for achieving vertical alveolar bone augmentation," *Materials*, vol. 8, no. 6, pp. 2953–2993, 2015.

[18] S. S. Jensen and H. Terheyden, "Bone augmentation procedures in localized defects in the alveolar ridge: clinical results with different bone grafts and bone-substitute materials," *The International Journal of Oral & Maxillofacial Implants*, vol. 24, Suppl, pp. 218–236, 2009.

[19] K. X. Michalakis, P. Calvani, and H. Hirayama, "Biomechanical considerations on tooth-implant supported fixed partial dentures," *Journal of Dental Biomechanics*, vol. 3, p. 1758736012462025, 2012.

[20] M. Saito, K. Notani, Y. Miura, and T. Kawasaki, "Complications and failures in removable partial dentures: a clinical evaluation," *Journal of Oral Rehabilitation*, vol. 29, no. 7, pp. 627–633, 2002.

[21] B. E. Pjetursson, K. Tan, N. P. Lang, U. Brägger, M. Egger, and M. Zwahlen, "A systematic review of the survival and complication rates of fixed partial dentures (FPDs) after an observation period of at least 5 years implant-supported FPDs," *Clinical Oral Implants Research*, vol. 15, no. 6, pp. 625–642, 2004.

[22] H. Malmstrom, A. Dellanzo-Savu, J. Xiao et al., "Success, clinical performance and patient satisfaction of direct fibre-reinforced composite fixed partial dentures - a two-year clinical study," *Journal of Oral Rehabilitation*, vol. 42, no. 12, pp. 906–913, 2015.

[23] M. S. Gowd, T. Shankar, R. Ranjan, and A. Singh, "Prosthetic consideration in implant-supported prosthesis: a review of literature," *Journal of International Society of Preventive & Community Dentistry*, vol. 7, Suppl 1, pp. S1–S7, 2017.

[24] N. Tuloglu, E. Sen Tunc, S. Ozer, and S. Bayrak, "Shear bond strength of self-adhering flowable composite on dentin with and without application of an adhesive system," *Journal of Applied Biomaterials & Functional Materials*, vol. 12, no. 2, pp. 97–101, 2014.

[25] G. Heo, E. H. Lee, J. W. Kim, K. M. Cho, and S. H. Park, "Fiber-reinforced composite resin bridges: an alternative method to treat root-fractured teeth," *Restorative Dentistry and Endodontics*, vol. 45, no. 1, p. e8, 2020.

[26] K. E. Ahmed, K. Y. Li, and C. A. Murray, "Longevity of fiber-reinforced composite fixed partial dentures (FRC FPD)–systematic review," *Journal of Dentistry*, vol. 61, pp. 1–11, 2017.

[27] O. Kumbuloglu and M. Özcan, "Clinical survival of indirect, anterior 3-unit surface-retained fibre-reinforced composite fixed dental prosthesis: up to 7.5-years follow-up," *Journal of Dentistry*, vol. 43, no. 6, pp. 656–663, 2015.

[28] P. K. Vallittu, A. Shinya, A. Baraba et al., "Fiber-reinforced composites in fixed prosthodontics—quo vadis?," *Dental Materials*, vol. 33, no. 8, pp. 877–879, 2017.

[29] L. Perea-Lowery and P. K. Vallittu, "Framework design and pontics of fiber-reinforced composite fixed dental prostheses—an overview," *Journal of Prosthodontic Research*, vol. 62, no. 3, pp. 281–286, 2018, PubMed PMID: 29759826.

Permissions

All chapters in this book were first published by Hindawi Publishing Corporation; hereby published with permission under the Creative Commons Attribution License or equivalent. Every chapter published in this book has been scrutinized by our experts. Their significance has been extensively debated. The topics covered herein carry significant findings which will fuel the growth of the discipline. They may even be implemented as practical applications or may be referred to as a beginning point for another development.

The contributors of this book come from diverse backgrounds, making this book a truly international effort. This book will bring forth new frontiers with its revolutionizing research information and detailed analysis of the nascent developments around the world.

We would like to thank all the contributing authors for lending their expertise to make the book truly unique. They have played a crucial role in the development of this book. Without their invaluable contributions this book wouldn't have been possible. They have made vital efforts to compile up to date information on the varied aspects of this subject to make this book a valuable addition to the collection of many professionals and students.

This book was conceptualized with the vision of imparting up-to-date information and advanced data in this field. To ensure the same, a matchless editorial board was set up. Every individual on the board went through rigorous rounds of assessment to prove their worth. After which they invested a large part of their time researching and compiling the most relevant data for our readers.

The editorial board has been involved in producing this book since its inception. They have spent rigorous hours researching and exploring the diverse topics which have resulted in the successful publishing of this book. They have passed on their knowledge of decades through this book. To expedite this challenging task, the publisher supported the team at every step. A small team of assistant editors was also appointed to further simplify the editing procedure and attain best results for the readers.

Apart from the editorial board, the designing team has also invested a significant amount of their time in understanding the subject and creating the most relevant covers. They scrutinized every image to scout for the most suitable representation of the subject and create an appropriate cover for the book.

The publishing team has been an ardent support to the editorial, designing and production team. Their endless efforts to recruit the best for this project, has resulted in the accomplishment of this book. They are a veteran in the field of academics and their pool of knowledge is as vast as their experience in printing. Their expertise and guidance has proved useful at every step. Their uncompromising quality standards have made this book an exceptional effort. Their encouragement from time to time has been an inspiration for everyone.

The publisher and the editorial board hope that this book will prove to be a valuable piece of knowledge for researchers, students, practitioners and scholars across the globe.

List of Contributors

Masahiko Okubo
Department of Oral and Maxillofacial Surgery, Faculty of Medicine, Saitama Medical University, 38 Morohongo, Moroyama-machi, Iruma-gun, Saitama 350-0495, Japan

Yoshie Sano, Yosuke Fukushima and Taketo Tomoda
Kamimura Dental and Orthodontic Clinic, 3-246-1, Sagami-chou, Koshigaya-shi, Saitama 343-0823, Japan

Tsuyoshi Sato
Department of Oral and Maxillofacial Surgery, Faculty of Medicine, Saitama Medical University, 38 Morohongo, Moroyamamachi, Iruma-gun, Saitama, Japan
Kamimura Dental and Orthodontic Clinic, 3-246-1, Sagami-chou, Koshigaya-shi, Saitama 343-0823, Japan

Shoichiro Kokabu
Division of Molecular Signaling and Biochemistry, Department of Health Improvement, Kyushu Dental University, 2-6-1 Manazuru, Kokurakita-ku, Kitakyusyu-shi, 803-8580, Japan

Ibrahim Tulunoglu and Samuel Cohen
Case Western Reserve University School of Dental Medicine, Department of Comprehensive Care, 2124 Cornell Rd, Cleveland, 44106 OH, USA

Eger V. Korolevsky and Denise Foran
Department of Veterans Affairs, New York Harbor Healthcare System, New York City, NY, USA

Takashi Komabayashi
Department of Veterans Affairs, New York Harbor Healthcare System, New York City, NY, USA
University of New England College of Dental Medicine, Portland, ME, USA

Eve Malthiery, Marie-Alix Fauroux and Jacques-Henri Torres
Service d'Odontologie, Centre Hospitalier Universitaire, 34295 Montpellier Cedex 5, France

Valérie Costes-Martineau
Laboratoire d'Anatomie et de Cytologie Pathologiques, Centre Hospitalier Universitaire, 34295 Montpellier Cedex 5, France

Dulyapong Rungraungrayabkul, Naruemon Panpradit and Nis Okuma
Department of Oral Medicine and Periodontology, Faculty of Dentistry, Mahidol University, 6 Yothi Rd. Rajthewee, Bangkok, Thailand 10400

Puangwan Lapthanasupkul
Department of Oral and Maxillofacial Pathology, Faculty of Dentistry, Mahidol University, 6 Yothi Rd. Rajthewee, Bangkok, Thailand 10400

Isao Hoshi, Kei Onodera, Yu Ohashi, Tadashi Kawai, Ikuya Miyamoto and Hiroyuki Yamada
Division of Oral and Maxillofacial Surgery, Department of Reconstructive Oral and Maxillofacial Surgery, School of Dentistry, Iwate Medical University, Morioka 020-8505, Japan

Ryosuke Abe
Department of Oral and Maxillofacial Surgery, Iwate Prefectural Central Hospital, Morioka 020-0066, Japan

Toshimi Chiba
Division of Internal Medicine, Department of Oral Medicine, Iwate Medical University, Morioka 020-8505, Japan

Yasunori Takeda
Division of Clinical Pathology, Department of Oral and Maxillofacial Reconstructive Surgery, School of Dentistry, Iwate Medical University, Morioka 020-8505, Japan

Federica Pulicari, Massimo Porrini and Francesco Spadari
Maxillo-Facial and Odontostomatology Unit, Fondazione IRCCS Cà Granda Ospedale Maggiore Policlinico, Milan 20122, Italy
Department of Biomedical, Surgical and Dental Sciences, University of Milan, Via della Commenda 10, Milan 20122, Italy

Matteo Pellegrini
Section of Dentistry, Department of Clinical, Surgical, Diagnostic and Pediatric Sciences, University of Pavia, Pavia 27100, Italy

Maurizio Pascadopoli and Andrea Scribante
Unit of Orthodontics and Pediatric Dentistry, Section of Dentistry, Department of Clinical, Surgical, Diagnostic and Pediatric Sciences, University of Pavia, Pavia 27100, Italy

Elisabetta Kuhn
Department of Biomedical, Surgical and Dental Sciences, University of Milan, Via della Commenda 10, Milan 20122, Italy
Division of Pathology, Fondazione IRCCS Ca' Granda Ospedale Maggiore Policlinico, 20122 Milan, Italy

Yumiko Nagao
Department of Public Health, Graduate School of Medicine, Juntendo University, Bunkyo-ku, Tokyo 113-8421, Japan

Hitomi Nakagaki and Masahide Tsuji
Tsuji Dental & Oral Surgery Clinic, Shiragane Machi, Omuta, Fukuoka 836-0052, Japan

Bassel Tarakji
Department of Oral and Maxillofacial Surgery and Diagnostic Sciences, College of Dentistry Prince Sattam Bin Abdulaziz University, Al-Kharj, Saudi Arabia

Yuki Kojima
Department of Anesthesiology, Asahi General Hospital, Chiba, Japan

Ryozo Sendo
Department of Anesthesiology, Imakiire General Hospital, Kagoshima, Japan

Jaahnavi Lanka and Santhosh Kumar
Department of Periodontology, Manipal College of Dental Sciences, Manipal, Manipal Academy of Higher Education, Manipal, 576104, Udupi, Karnataka, India

Wakako Nawata
The Center for Visiting Dental Service, Fukuoka Dental College Medical and Dental General Hospital, Fukuoka, Japan
Division of Dental Hygiene, Fukuoka Dental College Medical and Dental General Hospital, Fukuoka, Japan

Yojiro Umezaki and Masahiro Yamaguchi
The Center for Visiting Dental Service, Fukuoka Dental College Medical and Dental General Hospital, Fukuoka, Japan
Section of Geriatric Dentistry, Department of General Dentistry, Fukuoka Dental College, Fukuoka, Japan

Masato Nakajima
The Center for Visiting Dental Service, Fukuoka Dental College Medical and Dental General Hospital, Fukuoka, Japan
Section of General Dentistry, Department of General Dentistry, Fukuoka Dental College, Fukuoka, Japan

Michiko Makino and Hiromitsu Morita
The Center for Visiting Dental Service, Fukuoka Dental College Medical and Dental General Hospital, Fukuoka, Japan

Masahiro Yoneda and Takao Hirofuji
Section of General Dentistry, Department of General Dentistry, Fukuoka Dental College, Fukuoka, Japan

Takafumi Yamano
Section of Otorhinolaryngology, Department of General Medicine, Fukuoka Dental College, Fukuoka, Japan

Hiroaki Ooboshi
Section of Internal Medicine, Department of General Medicine, Fukuoka Dental College, Fukuoka, Japan

Fahd A. Aljarbou
Department of Restorative Dental Sciences, Division of Endodontics, College of Dentistry, King Saud University, Riyadh, Saudi Arabia

Luka Morelato
Department of Oral Surgery, Faculty of Dental Medicine, University of Rijeka, Croatia

Igor Smojver
Special Hospital, St. Catherine, Zagreb, Croatia

Sven Seiwerth
Department of Pathology, School of Medicine, University of Zagreb, Croatia

Dragana Gabrić
Department of Oral Surgery, School of Dental Medicine, University of Zagreb, Croatia

Mattia Manfredini, Susanna Ferrario, Luca Creminelli and Pier Paolo Poli
Implant Center for Edentulism and Jawbone Atrophies, Maxillofacial Surgery and Odontostomatology Unit, Fondazione IRCCS Cà Granda Ospedale Maggiore Policlinico, Milan, Italy
Department of Biomedical, Surgical and Dental Sciences, University of Milan, Milan, Italy

Akari Noda, Takahiro Abe and Kazuto Hoshi
Department of Oral & Maxillofacial Surgery, University of Tokyo Hospital, Tokyo, Japan

Masanobu Abe
Department of Oral & Maxillofacial Surgery, University of Tokyo Hospital, Tokyo, Japan
Division for Health Service Promotion, University of Tokyo, Tokyo, Japan

Aya Shinozaki-Ushiku
Department of Pathology, Graduate School of Medicine, University of Tokyo, Tokyo, Japan

Yae Ohata
Department of Oral Pathology, Graduate School of Medical and Dental Sciences, Tokyo Medical and Dental University, Tokyo, Japan

Liang Zong
Graduate School of Medicine, The University of Tokyo, Tokyo, Japan
Department of Gastrointestinal Surgery, Peking University Cancer Hospital & Institute, Beijing, China

Masahiko Okubo
Department of Oral and Maxillofacial Surgery, Faculty of Medicine, Saitama Medical University, 38 Morohongo, Moroyamamachi, Iruma-gun, Saitama, Japan
Kamimura Dental and Orthodontics Clinic, 3-246-1, Sagami-chou, Koshigaya-shi, Saitama, Japan

Hideyuki Kamimura
Kamimura Dental and Orthodontics Clinic, 3-246-1, Sagami-chou, Koshigaya-shi, Saitama, Japan

Shoichiro Kokabu
Division of Molecular Signaling and Biochemistry, Department of Health Improvement, Kyushu Dental University, 2-6-1 Manazuru, Kokurakita-ku, Kitakyusyu-shi, Japan

Shinichi Sato
Oral and Maxillofacial Surgery, Japan Community Health Care Organization Sendai Hospital, 3-16-1 Tsutsumimachi, Aoba-ku, Sendai 981-8501, Japan
Division of Oral and Maxillofacial Surgery, Tohoku University Graduate School of Dentistry, 4-1, Seiryo-machi, Aoba-ku, Sendai 980-8575, Japan

Masato Takahashi
Oral and Maxillofacial Surgery, Japan Community Health Care Organization Sendai Hospital, 3-16-1 Tsutsumimachi, Aoba-ku, Sendai 981-8501, Japan

Tetsu Takahashi
Division of Oral and Maxillofacial Surgery, Tohoku University Graduate School of Dentistry, 4-1, Seiryo-machi, Aoba-ku, Sendai 980-8575, Japan

Layla Louise de Amorim Rocha and Matheus Francisco Barros Rodrigues
Dentistry Course, Faculdade Cathedral, Boa Vista 69307-053, Brazil

Rodrigo da Franca Acioly and Daniel do Carmo Carvalho
Department of Oral and Maxillofacial Surgery and Traumatology, Hospital Geral, Boa Vista 69305-455, Brazil

Cristofe Coelho Lopes da Rocha
Department of Infrastructure, Federal Institute, Boa Vista 69303-340, Brazil

Takahiro Kaneko, Shunsuke Hino, Yosuke Iijima, Miki Yamada and Norio Horie
Department of Oral and Maxillofacial Surgery, Saitama Medical Center, Saitama Medical University, Saitama, Japan

Shohei Takaoka, Makiko Okubo-Sato and Satoshi Fukuzawa
Department of Oral and Maxillofacial Surgery, University of Tsukuba Hospital, Tsukuba, Ibaraki 305-8576, Japan

Kenji Yamagata, Fumihiko Uchida, Naomi Ishibashi-Kanno and Hiroki Bukawa
Department of Oral and Maxillofacial Surgery, Institute of Clinical Medicine, Faculty of Medicine, University of Tsukuba, Tsukuba, Ibaraki 305-8575, Japan

Camillo D'Arcangelo, Mirco Vadini, Matteo Buonvivere and Francesco De Angelis

Unit of Restorative Dentistry and Endodontics, Department of Medical, Oral and Biotechnological Science, School of Dentistry, "G. D'Annunzio" University of Chieti, Chieti, Italy

Lara Schorn, Christoph Sproll, Rita Depprich, Norbert R. Kübler, Majeed Rana, Daman D. Singh and Julian Lommen
Department of Oral, Maxillofacial and Facial Plastic Surgery, University Hospital Düsseldorf, Düsseldorf, Germany

Kazuhiro Murakami, Kazuhiko Yamamoto, Tsutomu Sugiura and Tadaaki Kirita
Department of Oral and Maxillofacial Surgery, Nara Medical, University, Kashihara City, Nara, Japan

Rafael Martins Afonso Pereira, Patrícia Cristine de Oliveira Afonso Pereira, Vitor Carvalho Rodrigues, Luiz Fernando Braga de Andrade, Elisa Morais de Carvalho and Helvécio Marangon Júnior
School of Dentistry, University Center of Patos de Minas (UNIPAM), Patos de Minas, Minas Gerais, Brazil

Andrea E. Borgonovo, Simone L. M. Galbiati and Dino Re
Department of Aesthetic Dentistry, University of Milan, Istituto Stomatologico Italiano, Milan, Italy

Kamichika Hayashi, Takeshi Onda, Takahiro Iwasaki, Takahiko Shibahara and Masayuki Takano
Department of Oral and Maxillofacial Surgery, Tokyo Dental College, Tokyo, Japan

Mitsuru Takata, Kiyotaka Mori, Hiroyuki Matsuda, Shinya Watanabe and Hidetoshi Tamura
Oral and Maxillofacial Surgery, Kameda General Hospital, Chiba, Japan

Kenichi Sato, Mami Chikuda, Yoshihisa Miyamae and Miwako Kan
Division of Dental Anesthesiology, Department of Reconstructive Oral and Maxillofacial Surgery, School of Dentistry, Iwate Medical University, 19-1 Uchimaru, Morioka, Iwate 020-8505, Japan

Archana P. Kanteti and Ernesto Martinez Duarte
Department of Pathology and Microbiology, University of Nebraska Medical Center, USA

W. Patrick Kelsey
Creighton University School of Dentistry, USA

Shinsuke Yamamoto and Toshihiko Takenobu
Department of Oral and Maxillofacial Surgery, Kobe City Medical Center General Hospital, Kobe, Hyogo 650-0047, Japan

Shigeo Hara
Department of Pathology, Kobe City Medical Center General Hospital, Kobe, Hyogo 650-0047, Japan

Philippe Bousquet
Department of Periodontology and Implantology, Faculty of Dentistry, University of Montpellier, Montpellier, France
Laboratoire Bioingenierie et Nanosciences UR-UM104, University of Montpellier, Montpellier, France

Delphine Carayon
Department of Prosthetic Dentistry, Faculty of Dentistry, University of Montpellier, Montpellier, France

Jean-Cedric Durand
Laboratoire Bioingenierie et Nanosciences UR-UM104, University of Montpellier, Montpellier, France
Department of Prosthetic Dentistry, Faculty of Dentistry, University of Montpellier, Montpellier, France

Motohiko Sano
Division of Applied Pharmaceutical Education and Research Hoshi University, Tokyo, Japan

Riccardo Aiuto and Christian Barbieri
Department of Biomedical, Surgical, and Dental Science, University of Milan, Italy

Daniele Garcovich
Universidad Europea de Valencia, Spain

Mario Dioguardi
Department of Clinical and Experimental Medicine, University of Foggia, Italy

Mattia Redaelli
Private Practice, Albavilla, Como, Italy

Luca De Micheli
Department of Periodontology, Italian Stomatological Institute, Milan, Italy

Brenton J. Wilson and Phoebe E. O'hare
James Cook University, Cairns, Australia

John Zacariah
Oral Health Services Northern Territory, Australia

Julian Leow and Robin Amanullah
Eastman Dental Hospital, 256 Grays Inn Rd, London WC1X 8LD, UK

Korehide Arai, Yuto Tanaka, Tomohiko Okamura, Kazufumi Iwayama and Yoshiaki Ono
Department of Special Care Dentistry, Osaka Dental University Hospital, Osaka, Japan

Shinsuke Matsuda
Matsuda Oral Appliance, Osaka, Japan

Abdulrahman Aseri
Department of Preventive Dental Sciences, Faculty of Dentistry, Najran University, Saudi Arabia

João Paulo Colesanti Tanganeli
Post-Doctoral Student Program in Biophotonics Applied to Health Sciences, University Nove de Julho, SP, Brazil

Simone Saldanha Ignácio de Oliveira
PhD University of São Paulo, SP, Brazil

Tamiris da Silva
Post-Graduate Program in Biophotonics Applied to Health Sciences, University Nove de Julho, SP, Brazil

Kristianne Porta Santos Fernandes, Lara Jansiski Motta and Sandra Kalil Bussadori
PhD Biophotonics Applied to Health Sciences, University Nove de Julho, SP, Brazil

Roberto Pippi, Marcello Santoro and Alessandra Pietrantoni
Department of Odontostomatological and Maxillo Facial Sciences, Sapienza University of Rome, Via Caserta 6, 00161 Rome, Italy

Angelina Pernazza
Department of Molecular Medicine, Sapienza University of Rome, Italy

Maryam S. Tavangar
Oral and Dental Disease Research Center, Department of Operative Dentistry, Dental Faculty, Shiraz University of Medical Sciences, Shiraz, Iran

Fatemeh Aghaei
Department of Operative Dentistry, School of Dentistry, Isfahan University of Medical Sciences, Isfahan, Iran

Massoumeh Nowrouzi
Department of Periodontics, School of Dentistry, Hormozgan University of Medical Sciences, Bandar Abbas, Iran

Index

www.ingramcontent.com/pod-product-compliance
Lightning Source LLC
LaVergne TN
LVHW082224200926
848484LV00008B/2299
9798887406398